Evaluation, Pathophysiology and Treatment of Kidney Diseases

Evaluation, Pathophysiology and Treatment of Kidney Diseases

Editor: Donald Moore

AMERICAN
MEDICAL PUBLISHERS
www.americanmedicalpublishers.com

AMERICAN
MEDICAL PUBLISHERS
www.americanmedicalpublishers.com

Cataloging-in-Publication Data

Evaluation, pathophysiology and treatment of kidney diseases / edited by Donald Moore.
p. cm.
Includes bibliographical references and index.
ISBN 979-8-88740-224-6
1. Kidneys--Diseases. 2. Kidneys--Diseases--Diagnosis. 3. Kidneys--Disease--Pathophysiology.
4. Kidneys--Diseases--Treatment. 5. Nephrology. I. Moore, Donald.
RC902 .E93 2023
616.61--dc23

American Medical Publishers,
41 Flatbush Avenue,
1st Floor, New York,
NY 11217, USA

ISBN 979-8-88740-224-6 (Hardback)

Contents

Preface

The purpose of the book is to provide a glimpse into the dynamics and to present opinions and studies of some of the scientists engaged in the development of new ideas in the field from very different standpoints. This book will prove useful to students and researchers owing to its high content quality.

The kidneys are two bean-shaped organs that are roughly the size of a fist. They are located on each side of the spine and just below the rib cage. Kidney diseases refer to those conditions in which kidneys get damaged and are unable to filter blood normally. There are various types of kidney diseases, such as chronic kidney disease, cystinosis, IgA nephropathy, polycystic kidney disease, lupus nephritis, glomerulonephritis, Fabry disease, etc. The diagnosis of kidney diseases is done through urine and blood tests. The key markers utilized for assessing kidney function include estimated glomerular filtration rate (eGFR) and abnormal urine albumin levels. Treatment often comprises of measures to control signs and symptoms, slow disease progression and decrease complications. Kidney transplantation and dialysis are two treatments that are utilized for end-stage kidney disease. This book elucidates the innovative researches around prospective developments with respect to kidney diseases. It addresses the causes, diagnoses and therapies for these diseases. The extensive content of this book provides the readers with a thorough understanding of this medical condition.

At the end, I would like to appreciate all the efforts made by the authors in completing their chapters professionally. I express my deepest gratitude to all of them for contributing to this book by sharing their valuable works. A special thanks to my family and friends for their constant support in this journey.

Editor

1

Primary synovial sarcoma of the kidney: A case report of complete pathological response at a Lebanese tertiary care center

Alissar El Chediak[1], Deborah Mukherji[1], Sally Temraz[1], Samer Nassif[2], Sara Sinno[2], Rami Mahfouz[2] and Ali Shamseddine[1*]

Abstract

Background: Primary synovial sarcoma of the kidney is a rare type of soft tissue sarcoma. Its presenting features can resemble those of other renal tumors; rendering its early diagnosis, a dilemma. Several cases of renal synovial sarcoma have been reported in the literature with varying treatment options and outcomes. This article describes a rare case of primary renal synovial sarcoma and reviews all cases in the literature.

Case presentation: A 26-year-old male presented with flank pain and hematuria. Initially diagnosed with Wilm's tumor, revision of pathology and histology, along with the immunohistochemical profile, confirmed, nevertheless, the diagnosis of primary monophasic synovial sarcoma of the kidney with the SYT-SSX2 fusion transcript. Follow-up, post nephrectomy, revealed recurrence within the lungs and at the surgical bed. Surgical resection followed by adjuvant chemotherapy regimen constituting of Doxorubicin and Ifosfamide, achieved complete pathological response.

Conclusion: In this case report, we emphasize the need for accurate diagnosis and prompt treatment. We propose multimodality treatment approach including surgery along with anthracycline-based chemotherapy to induce complete remission.

Keywords: Synovial sarcoma, SYT-SSX, Doxorubicin, Ifosfamide, Pathological response, Survival

Background

Soft tissue sarcoma (STS) is a rare malignant tumor of mesenchymal origin having an incidence of 2–3 cases per 100,000, thus contributing to less than 1% of all adult malignancies [1, 2]. Synovial sarcoma (SS), or sarcoma of tissues adjacent to joints, is a rare type of STS, and represent 5 to10% of all STSs [1]. SS is commonly found in the proximal limb of young adults and has a male predominance [3]. Other unusual sites of occurrence include the head and neck, heart, lungs, and kidneys [4]. Very few reports have tackled this tumor due to its rarity and difficulty to distinguish from other renal pathologies. The first case of primary SS of the kidney has been reported by Faria et al. in 1999 [5]. We present a case of primary synovial sarcoma of the kidney, initially thought to be a Wilm's tumor, along with patient follow-up, showing complete pathological response to treatment, followed by a literature review of this disease entity.

Case presentation

A 26-year-old male experienced recurrent flank pain and gross hematuria over several months duration. Kidney ultrasound showed a lower pole mass concerning for renal cell carcinoma. After confirmation of a right kidney tumor, measuring 6 cm, by an enhanced CT scan, he underwent right radical nephrectomy with para-caval lymph node dissection, at another institute, with pathology there, read initially as adult type Wilm's tumor. After referral to our institute for rereading of the pathological slides, the morphological and immunostaining profiles were analyzed, and results came out to be consistent with synovial sarcoma of the right kidney. The tumor was monophasic and showed a cellular spindle cell proliferation with a prominent perivascular growth

* Correspondence: as04@aub.edu.lb
[1]Department of Internal Medicine, Division of Hematology/Oncology, American University of Beirut - Medical Center, P.o.Box: 11-0236, Riad El Solh, Beirut 110 72020, Lebanon
Full list of author information is available at the end of the article

pattern and partial necrosis. It was positive for vimentin, BCL-2, CD56, MCK (partial), and negative for CD10, 31, 34, 99, 117, CK7, Desmin, SMA, MyoD1, EMA, WT-1, S100, RCC, PAX8, GATA-3, and Synaptophysin (Fig. 1).

Molecular studies on the paraffin-embedded blocks were performed to test for the t(X; 18) SYT/SSX fusion transcript, using RT-PCR, at the University of Michigan Health System. RT-PCR amplification was performed using fluorescent dye-labeled primers, specific for the SYT-SS18 and SYT-SSX genes. The PCR products were then detected and sized by capillary electrophoresis to identify the presence of chimeric transcripts. A concurrent internal control was run to ensure the integrity of the mRNA. FISH analysis was also performed using a break-apart style probe. The results were unfortunately negative due to the low quality samples.

According to these findings, a diagnosis of primary monophasic SS of the kidney was made. It was elected for serial follow up and no adjuvant treatment, thereafter. Six months later, a follow up CT scan detected a 1. 5cmx1.7 cm left lower lobe lung nodule suggestive of metastasis. Consequently, he underwent a smooth left lower lobe wedge resection. Fusion gene product analysis on the resected lung tissue, via FISH, revealed SYT-SSX 2 gene rearrangement confirming the SS diagnosis. Three months afterwards, CT scan of the chest, abdomen, and pelvis revealed another disease recurrence in the nephrectomy surgical bed, with tumor invasion of the inferior vena cava and the presence of conglomerate suspicious aorto-iliac lymph nodes. A multidisciplinary team approach decided to start the patient on Doxorubicin 50 g/m^2 and Ifosfamide 5 g/m^2 chemotherapeutic regimen. Following the third cycle, CT scan and MRI showed a 30 to 50% interval decrease in size of tumor masses in the right nephrectomy bed and adjacent retroperitoneum, IVC tumor, and distal aortocaval lymph nodes, indicating partial treatment response. The patient were received a total of 5 cycles, with no adjunct side effects.

A follow-up MRI, several months later, showed continued decrease in the size of 3 masses at the previous surgical site, IVC tumor invasion, and aortocaval lymph nodes, indicating continued response to treatment. One of the small masses in the nephrectomy bed almost completely resolved, on imaging, with no new progression. It was then decided to have the patient undergo surgical resection of the residual masses at the previous surgical bed with removal of the aorto-caval lymph nodes, thrombectomy with vena caval repair. All surgical margins were negative. Final pathology came out to be necrosis, with no viable tumor identified. Thus, a complete pathological response was achieved using the Adriamycin/Ifosfamide regimen, a year after the initial nephrectomy. A sample of the kidney lysate was again tested for the (X; 18) SYT/SSX fusion transcript via RT-PCR and FISH, and results were negative, suggestive of complete treatment response.

Discussion

Synovial sarcoma is a mesenchymal spindle cell tumor which displays variable epithelial differentiation and has a specific chromosomal translocation t(X; 18) (p11; q11), which results from the fusion of the SYT gene on chromosome 18 to exon 5 of either SSX1 or SSX2 genes

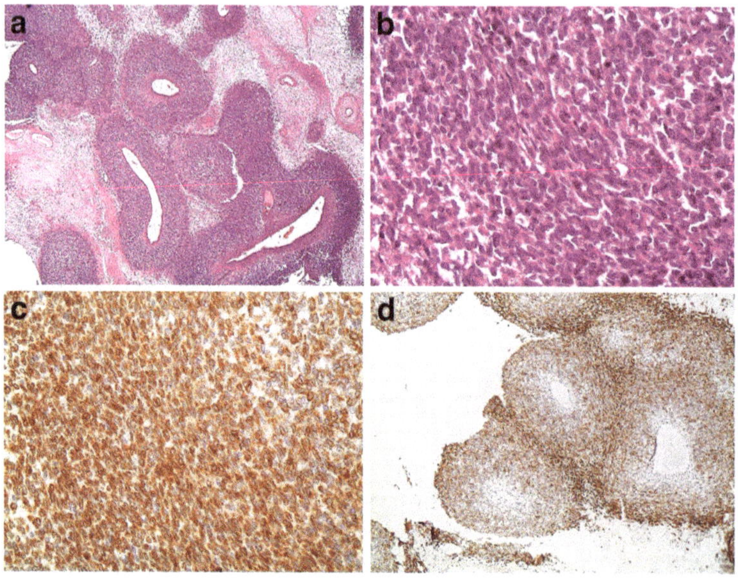

Fig. 1 Partially necrotic, densely cellular proliferation with a prominent perivascular growth pattern (**a**, H&E stain, 40×). Tumor cells are essentially spindle in appearance (**b**, H&E stain, 400×), and express vimentin (not shown), focal keratin (not shown), BCL-2 (**c**, 400×), and CD56 (**d**, 100×)

on chromosome X [6]. It was recently reported that the SSX4 gene is also involved in such a translocation [6, 7]. Nonetheless, SS of the kidney can be first misdiagnosed as a renal cell carcinoma due to similar clinical presentation [3]. The identification of the monophasic type of renal SS is also controversial as it has similar microscopic features to other spindle cell tumors, such as fibrosarcoma, leiomyosarcoma, malignant peripheral nerve sheath tumors, adult Wilm's tumor, spindle cell carcinoma and spindle cell melanoma [3]. While monophasic SS of the kidney is made up exclusively of monomorphic spindle cells, the biphasic type is a mixture of both spindle-shaped cells and epithelial cells. SS of the kidney is a rare disease such as 64 cases have been reported since the Faria et al. cases up to 2012 [6]. We conducted a literature review using Embase and PubMed databases and included all cases (even those published in languages other than English) till the year 2016. This yielded a total of 114 cases (Table 1) constituting the largest series of renal SS cases to be reported. Noteworthy, our case is the first to be reported from the Middle East.

The median age of patients with renal SS was 40.5 (15–78) years, which is half the median age for diagnosis of renal cell carcinoma [7]. The female to male ratio was 1:1. Regarding the predominant presentation symptoms, data was only available for 82 cases. The most frequently reported symptom on presentation was isolated flank/lumbar pain which was found in 20 patients (24.4%).This is in concordance with a review conducted on older data where this same predominant symptom occurred in 55. 5% of cases [8]. Hematuria was present in 37 patients (44%) upon presentation. Kohle et al. reported similar data, albeit smaller sample size, where 98% of their patients were symptomatic at the time of presentation, with 67% having pain and 38% having hematuria [6]. These figures are in concordance with our analysis of the world literature.

According to our analysis, the leading fusion variant was the SYT-SSX 2, detected in 42 (36.8%) patients, as opposed to the SYT-SSX 1 variant, detected in 23 (20.2%) patients, in total (Table 1).

Data on metastasis and disease recurrence was available for 70 and 57 patients, respectively. 19 (27.1%) patients had metastasis, whereas 14 (24.6%) patients had tumor recurrence on follow-up. These numbers are similar to what was published in previous series [9].

A 30 to 50% of the patients who underwent surgical resection of their primary tumor were reported to witness metastasis to the lungs or liver [10]. Our patient is of no exception. In terms of median survival for patients with localized disease, size represents an important prognostic factor [10]. A retrospective analysis was done on 135 consecutive patients with extremity and truncal variant of synovial sarcomas, seen at three institutions in Boston, between years 1961 and 1996. Patients with localized synovial sarcomas, less than 5 cm in longest diameter, had a survival at 10 years equivalent to 88%, compared with a 10-year survival of 38 and 8% for 5 to 10 cm and greater than 10 cm sarcomas, respectively [10]. Similar results were reported by Singer et al. on 48 consecutive patients with extremity and truncal synovial sarcomas, seen between years 1966 and 1994 [11].

SS of the kidneys presents a diagnostic dilemma, as it resembles renal cell carcinoma amongst other tumors. Diagnosis can be based on morphological (spindle cell) and immunological tumor profile. It can also be established by genetic analysis via FISH and RT-PCR, demonstrating the SYT18-SSX gene translocation. Demonstrating which translocation, the tumor possesses, has been a delicate matter. For instance, a SS case that was previously shown to be negative for SYT/SSX1 and SYT/SSX2 gene expression by conventional RT-PCR, was instead found to be SYT/SSX4 positive, as the sole fusion transcript expressed in this tumor sample, when the RT-PCR was redesigned [6]. This might have explained our negative results, when trying to identify the translocations, since our RT-PCR was only designed to detect SYT/SSX1 and SYT/SSX2 fusion gene variants.

Moreover, the value of TLE1 antibody in the diagnosis of SS has also been examined. TLE1 was found to be an excellent discriminator of SS from other sarcomas, in a study by Terry et al. [12]. They reported that TLE1 monoclonal and polyclonal antibodies gave intense and/or diffuse nuclear staining in 91 out of 94 molecularly confirmed synovial sarcoma patients. In contrast, TLE1 staining has been detected much less frequently and at lower levels, if et al.l, in 40 other mesenchymal tumors; thereby making this a robust immunohistochemical marker for SS. Jagdis et al. also supported this view as their findings confirmed that TLE1 was more sensitive and specific for synovial sarcoma, than any other currently available immunohistochemical kits [13]. Kosemehmetoglu et al. confirmed the sensitivity, but not the specificity, of TLE1 antibodies in diagnosing synovial sarcomas [14].

The prognostic implication of SYT-SSX fusion type in synovial sarcomas is still under debate. The SYT-SSX fusion type and the presence of metastasis, at diagnosis, were both proven to be important prognostic indicators [15]. Kawai et al. analyzed SYT–SSX fusion transcripts in 45 synovial sarcomas by reverse-transcriptase polymerase chain reaction, and compared the results with relevant clinical and pathological data [16]. SYT- SSX2 fusion type carried a significant positive prognosis for overall survival [16]. This was thought to be due to an association with a lower prevalence of metastatic disease at diagnosis, in patients having this rearrangement [16]. In another study by Ladanyi et al., the SYT–SSX2 fusion

Table 1 List of 114 cases of renal SS published in the literature

Case Report/ Series	Author/ Year of publication	No of cases	Age(Y)/Gender (M/F)	Presenting symptoms	Fusion gene Variant	Treatment	Outcome
1	Argani P et al.; 2000 [5]	17	10 M 7 F Median age: 35	Abdominal pain; hematuria; incidental finding for hypertension workup; other data not available	1: SYT-SSX1; 4: SYT-SSX2	Radical nephrectomy	N/A
2	Kim DH et al.; 2000 [17]	2	53/M 47/M	Rt flank pain Rt flank pain, gross hematuria	SYT-SSX2;	Rt radical nephrectomy; Rt radical nephrectomy with IVC thrombectomy	No recurrence 6 mons later; lung mets 5 mons later, death 10mons post-op
3	Chen S et al.; 2001 [18]	1	48/M	Hematuria	SYT-SSX 2	Lt radical nephroureterectomy; Radiation to surgical bed; 4 cycles of ifosfamide and Doxorubicin	N/A
4	Koyama S et al.; 2001 [8]	1	47/F	Right back pain	SYT-SSX 2	Rt radical nephrectomy	No recurrence 17 mons later
5	Bella AJ et al.; 2002 [25]	1	24/M	Gross hematuria	SYT-SSX t(X;18)	Rt radical nephrectomy, adjuvant Actinomycin + Vincristine	No clinical evidence of disease 18 mons after nephrectomy
6	Dai YC et al.; 2002 [26]	1	19/F	Abdominal Pain, 3 mons of amenorrhea	SYT-SSX t(X;18)	Rt nephrectomy	Recurrence of tumor in retroperitoneum and abdominal wall 9 mons after surgery
7	Vesoulis Z et al.; 2003 [27]	1	38/M	Acute abdominal pain	SST-SSX1	Lt radical nephrectomy	N/A
8	Moch H et al.; 2003 [28]	2	47/M 56/F	Renal mass	SST-SSX1/ SYT-SSX2	Nephrectomy/ Rt nephrectomy	Local recurrence 11 years later/ N/A
9	Chen PC et al.; 2003 [29]	1	19/M	left flank pain and intermittent hematuria	N/A	Lt radical nephrectomy + IVC thrombectomy; adjuvant Ifosfamide + Etoposide	died of sepsis 1 month after surgery
10	Park SJ et al.; 2004 [9]	1	32/F	Intermittent abdominal pain	N/A	Lt radical nephrectomy + thormbectomy; 6 cycles Ifosfamide + Doxorubicin	Metastasis to lung 4 mons post-op, complete remission after chemotherapy
11	Jun SY t al; 2004 [30]	3	27, 35/F 26/M	Rt flank pain	SYT-SSX2	Rt radical nephrectomies	1F: disease free 5 mons post-op; 2F: lumbar vertebral mets 5 mons post-op, 6 mons disease free post-resection; 3 M: bilateral hemothorax; death 34 days post-op
12	Tornkvist M et al.; 2004 [24]	1	34/F	N/A	SYT-SSX 2	Rt nephrectomy, chemotherapy	Visceral recurrence; lung metastases
13	Schaal CH et al.; 2004 [14]	1	27/M	Hematuria and large abdominal mass	N/A	Ifosfamide and Adriamycin, followed by Rt Radical nephrectomy	No recurrence after one year
14	Shao L et al.; 2004 [31]	4	N/A	N/A	N/A	N/A	N/A

Table 1 List of 114 cases of renal SS published in the literature *(Continued)*

Case Report/ Series	Author/ Year of publication	No of cases	Age(Y)/Gender (M/F)	Presenting symptoms	Fusion gene Variant	Treatment	Outcome
15	Shannon BA et al.; 2005 [32]	1	60/M	Hematuria	SYT-SSX 2	Rt radical nephrectomy, Imatinib, 5 cycles of adjuvant chemotherapy	Pulmonary metastasis 6 mons after surgery; death 12 mons later
16	Perlmutter AE et al.; 2005 [33]	1	61/F	Right flank pain and gross hematuria	SYT-SSX 2	Rt nephrectomy, refused adjuvant chemotherapy	No recurrence 5 mons post-surgery
17	Stage et al.; 2005 [34]	1	51/F	Renal masses incidentally found	N/A	N/A	N/A
18	Paláu L MA et al.; 2007 [35]	1	71/F	Flank pain and gross hematuria	SYT-SSX 2	Lt nephrectomy	Recovery in 22 mons after surgery
19	Drozenova et al.; 2008 [36]	2	33/M 57/F	Rt flank pain Lt flank pain	SYT-SSX1/ SYT-SSX1	Rt Radical nephrectomy/ Lt Radical nephrectomy	Local recurrence and lung mets; death 6 mons later/ N/A
20	Mirza M et al.; 2008 [37]	1	17/M	Flank pain and gross hematuria	SYT-SSX 2	Lt radical nephrectomy	No recurrence 1 year later
21	Gabilondo F et al.; 2008 [38]	1	32/F	Mild abdominal pain; gross hematuria	SYT-SSX t(X;18)	Rt radical nephrectomy	N/A
22	Zakhary MM et al.; 2008 [39]	1	52/F	Right flank pain	N/A	Rt nephrectomy	N/A
23	Chung SD et al.; 2008 [40]	2	30/F 49/F	Rt flank pain Lt loin pain	SYT-SSX1	Rt radical nephrectomy/ Lt radical nephrectomy	No recurrence 15 mons post-op/ No recurrence 27 mons post-op
24	Erturhan S et al.; 2008 [41]	1	59/M	Right lumbar pain and palpable mass	N/A	N/A	N/A
25	Divetia M et al.; 2008 [42]	7	2-M 5-F (15–46 years)	Abdominal lump, hematuria	3 SYT-SSX1/ 1 SYT-SSX2	Radical nephrectomy	Lung mets in 2 patients; death at 6 and 12 mons, respectively
26	Dassi V et al.; 2009 [43]	1	20/F	Flank pain	SYT-SSX t(X;18)	Lt radical nephrectomy	N/A
28	Kawahara et al.; 2009 [44]	1	40/F	Abdominal pain	SYT-SSX 1	Radical nephrectomy	N/A
29	Long JA et al.; 2009 [45]	3	(Age range: 27–33 years)	Back pain and spontaneous rupture	SYT-SSX t(X;18)	2 Rt radical nephrectomy; 1 Lt radical nephrectomy	2 patients: total remission 25 mons post-op; 1 patient: death 24 mons post-op
30	Wezel F et al.; 2010 [46]	1	47/M	Hematuria, abdominal pain, weight loss	SYT-SSX t(X;18)	Nephrectomy	No recurrence 18 weeks after surgery
31	Wang Z-H et al.; 2009 [47]	4	2/F 2/M 32 to 48 years	Low back pain, hematuria	SYT-SSX1	Radical nephrectomy; 3 Lt side, 1 Rt side	Liver + lung metastasis; death at 5, 8, 18, and 21 mons post-op, respectively
32	Kageyama S et al.; 2010 [48]	1	67/M	Gross hematuria and right flank pain	SYT-SSX 2	Rt nephroureterectomy, Ifosfamide and Etoposide regimen	Tumor recurrence 33 mons post nephrectomy; Liver mets; death 4 years later
33	Tan YS et al.; 2010 [49]	4	N/A	N/A	N/A	N/A	N/A
34	Romero-Rojas AE et al.; 2013 [50]	1	15/M	Lt abdominal pain; weight loss	N/A	Neoadjuvant chemotherapy followed by Lt radical nephrectomy	Death 1.8 years later
35	Lakshmaiah KC et al.; 2010 [51]	2	50/F 45/M	Rt flank pain/ Lt flank pain, hematuria	SYT-SSX2/ NOT DONE	Radical nephrectomy	No recurrence 2 years post-op/ lost to follow-up

Table 1 List of 114 cases of renal SS published in the literature *(Continued)*

Case Report/ Series	Author/ Year of publication	No of cases	Age(Y)/Gender (M/F)	Presenting symptoms	Fusion gene Variant	Treatment	Outcome
36	Kataria et al.; 2010 [52]	1	52/F	Renal mass	SYT-SSX 2	Radical nephrectomy IVC thrombectomy; adjuvant chemo-radiation	Mets to lung
37	Grampurohit VU et al.; 2011 [53]	1	21/F	Fever, hematuria; right flank pain	SYT-SSX t(X;18)	Rt nephrectomy	No recurrence 6 mons post-surgery
38	Ozkan EE et al.; 2011 [20]	1	68/F	Right flank pain and abdominal distention	N/A	Rt nephroureterectomy, 4 cycles Ifosfamide and Doxorubicin	No recurrence one year later
39	Karafin M et al.; 2011 [54]	3	39/F 41/M 53/M	N/A	SYT-SSX2 SYT-SSX2 N/A	N/A	N/A
40	Nishida T et al.; 2011 [55]	1	63/F	Dysuria, hematuria	SYT-SSX 1 & 2	Rt Radical nephrectomy	No recurrence one year postop
41	Pitino A et al.; 2011 [8]	1	67/M	Lumbar pain, gross hematuria	SYT-SSX 2	Lt Nephroureterectomy; adjuvant Epirubicin post-op	Local recurrence of disease 24 mons post- surgery
42	Bakhshi et al.; 2012 [56]	1	33/F	Abdominal pain and gross hematuria	SYT-SSX 2	Lt radical nephrectomy; external radiotherapy	No recurrence at 2 years
43	Lopes et al.; 2013 [3]	1	19/M	Lumbar pain, gross hematuria	Negative translocation	Lt nephrectomy, thrombectomy; 5 cycles of doxorubicin	Lung mets several mons post-op
44	Pereira E Silva R et al.; 2013 [57]	1	17/M	Incidental large renal mass after workup for secondary hypertension	Negative translocation	Radical nephrectomy followed by ifosfamide	No recurrence 29 mons later
45	Marković-Lipkovski J et al.; 2013 [12]	1	38/M	Rt flank pain; fever; hematuria	SYT-SSX2	Rt radical nephrectomy	Died three mons later
46	Moorthy et al.; 2014 [58]	1	46/M	Flank pain	SYT-SSX 2	Lt radical nephrectomy	N/A
47	Majumber et al.; 2014 [59]	1	46/F	Flank pain, hematuria	N/A	Rt radical nephrectomy	No evidence of disease after 2 mons follow up
48	Schoolmeester JK et al.; 2014 [60]	16	9M/7F 17-78 yrs.; Median: 46 yrs	N/A; Rt: 10; Lt: 6;	SYT-SSX2: 10; SYT-SSX1: 5; 1: failed	14: Radical nephrectomy; 1: partial nephrectomy; 1: needle biopsy	6: death within 1–58 mons (mean 31mons); 5: no recurrence 12–77 mons (39 mons); 1: alive with spine mets 11mons later
49	Kim MS et al.; 2014 [61]	1	38/F	Lt flank pain	SYT-SSX2	Lap Lt radical nephrectomy followed by radiation to surgical bed	Recurrence at the distal ureter and uretero-vesical junction 6 mons post- surgery
50	Ozkanli SS et al.; 2014 [62]	1	45/M	Flank pain; macroscopic hematuria	SYT-SSX t(X;18)	Lt radical nephrectomy	N/A
51	Mishra S et al.; 2015 [13]	1	60/M	Flank pain, hematuria	SYT-SSX t(X;18)	Radical nephrectomy	N/A
52	Wang Z et al.; 2015 [61]	1	54/F	Flank pain, hematuria	SYT-SSX 1	Radical nephrectomy	No recurrence 12 mons post-surgery
53	Vedana M et al.; 2015 [63]	1	76/F	Flank pain; hematuria	SYT-SSX t(X;18)	Rt radical nephro-ureterectomy	No recurrence 20 mons post-surgery

Table 1 List of 114 cases of renal SS published in the literature *(Continued)*

Case Report/ Series	Author/ Year of publication	No of cases	Age(Y)/Gender (M/F)	Presenting symptoms	Fusion gene Variant	Treatment	Outcome
54	Lv X-F et al.; 2015 [64]	5	2F/3M (15–43 yrs.; Median: 27.4 yrs)	N/A	N/A	N/A	N/A
55	Present case El Chediak A. et al.; 2016	1	26/M	Rt flank pain; hematuria	SYT-SSX2	Rt radical nephrectomy, Doxorubicin Ifosfamide	Lung metastasis 6 mons post nephrectomy; no recurrence one year post chemotherapy

M Males, *F* Females, *Yrs* Years, *Rt* Right, *Lt* Left, *Mets* Metastasis, *Mons* Months, *IVC* Inferior vena cava, *N/A* Not Applicable

transcript had a significantly longer metastasis-free survival [15]. On the contrary, Japanese patients, with synovial sarcoma, having positive SYT-SSX fusion transcript, were retrospectively analyzed [17]. They concluded that *SYT-SSX* fusion type was not found to be a significant prognostic factor, unlike tumor size and histological grading, for patients with localized synovial sarcoma [17]. Another study by Guillou et al. also confirmed that histologic grading, and not SYT-SSX fusion type, was a stronger predictor of survival, by collecting retrospective data on 165 SS patients [18].

In our sample, staging information was available for 46 patients, based on the 7th edition TNM staging for soft tissue sarcomas. Among the patients having the SYT-SSX2 fusion protein. 53.8% were stage II and 34.6% were of stage III. 33 and 25% of patients with SYT-SSX1 transcript were stage II and III, respectively. 25% of patients with SYT-SSX1 were of stage IV, versus only 7.7% for SYT-SSX2 patients.

Lungs were the most common metastatic site, regardless of the fusion type. However, 50% of patients with SYT-SSX2 fusion type had metastasis to the liver. Although lungs and liver are common sites for metastasis for renal SS [19, 20], it was not reported before whether there is a relation between the site of metastasis and the type of fusion transcript. From the above, it appears that SYT-SSX 1 behaves more aggressively. However, studies with a larger number of patients and longer follow-up periods are needed to verify these observations, especially in the light of the contradicting data, presenting on the prognostic value of the SYT-SSX fusion protein.

Although SS is considered an aggressive form of STS where metastasis can occur in 50% of the cases, it was found to be sensitive to Anthracycline based chemotherapy [21]. However, due to the rarity of the tumor, a standard therapy has not been established. Treatment modalities include surgical resection and chemotherapy. A combination of chemotherapy (Ifosfamide and Doxorubicin) and surgery has yielded positive results [6, 9, 12, 13]. Based on our review of the literature, 10 patients took Ifosfamide and Doxorubicin, either together or in combination with other chemotherapeutic agents. 5 out of 10 cases were reported to have complete remission. This further corroborates the effectiveness of giving Ifosfamide and Doxorubicin as a regimen to treat primary renal SS. The basis for chemotherapy was tumor volume reduction, mainly attributed to Ifosfamide. In one case report, the combination of Ifosfamide and Doxorubicin lead to a 50% reduction of the tumor before consequent resection [14]. The controversy of the impact of adjuvant chemotherapy on overall survival, in SS patients, is limited by randomized clinical trials'(RCTs) sample size and varied chemotherapy regimens with discrepant results [22]. The Sarcoma Meta-analysis Collaboration (SMAC) group performed a meta-analysis of all known randomized clinical trials in 1997. Their results indicated that doxorubicin-based chemotherapy served to significantly improve time to local and distant recurrence, as well as overall recurrence-free survival in comparison to patients who were just observed [23]. An increase in overall survival was not statistically significant [23]. Another meta-Analysis of RCTs of adjuvant chemotherapy for localized resectable STS was conducted by Pervais et al. where they built on the results of the SMAC study and narrowed the confidence intervals [24]. This meta-analysis demonstrated marginal efficacy of doxorubicin based chemotherapy with respect to local recurrence, distant recurrence, overall recurrence, and overall survival, in comparison to those who did not receive adjuvant chemotherapy [22].

Conclusion

In conclusion, primary SS of the kidney is an aggressive rare disease that can be mistaken for other types of renal cell carcinomas. Its diagnosis is based on morphological and molecular studies demonstrating spindle cells and the SYT-SSX translocation. However, establishing a correct diagnosis may be difficult. Prognosis can be enhanced by use of anthracycline based chemotherapy. Moreover, the combination of surgery and chemotherapy has shown positive results. Particularly, we propose the use of Ifosfamide and Doxorubicin as a standard chemotherapy to induce complete remission. Since the disease may have rapid course with unfavorable outcomes, clinicians need to be aware of the existence of this rare entity, so that timely and appropriate therapy can be initiated.

Abbreviations

CT: Computer tomography; FISH: fluorescence in situ hybridization; IVC: Inferior vena cava; MRI: Magnetic resonance imaging; N/A: Not available; RCT: Randomized clinical trials; RT-PCR: reverse transcriptase-polymerase chain reaction; SS: Synovial sarcoma; STS: Soft tissue sarcoma

Authors' contributions

EA was involved in acquisition, analysis, and interpretation of data (literature), and manuscript writing. SN and SS performed histological examination of the resected tumor and provided the pathological images in our manuscript. MR performed molecular analysis of the tumor sample. Both MD and TS were involved in manuscript writing and editing. SA was involved in data analysis, interpretation of data (literature), and revising the manuscript. He also gave final approval of the version prior to submission. All authors read and approved the final manuscript.

Author details

[1]Department of Internal Medicine, Division of Hematology/Oncology, American University of Beirut - Medical Center, P.o.Box: 11-0236, Riad El Solh, Beirut 110 72020, Lebanon. [2]Department of Pathology and Laboratory Medicine, American University of Beirut - Medical Center, Beirut, Lebanon.

References

1. Fletcher CD. The evolving classification of soft tissue tumours - an update based on the new 2013 WHO classification. Histopathology. 2014;64(1):2–11.
2. Goldblum JR, Weiss SW, Andrew L. Folpe Enzinger and Weiss's soft tissue tumors. sixth ed. St Louis, Missouri: Saunders; 2001. 1176.
3. Lopes H, et al. Primary monophasic synovial sarcoma of the kidney: a case report and review of literature. Clin Med Insights Oncol. 2013;7:257–62.
4. Spillane AJ, et al. Synovial sarcoma: a clinicopathologic, staging, and prognostic assessment. J Clin Oncol. 2000;18(22):3794–803.
5. Argani P, et al. Primary renal synovial sarcoma: molecular and morphologic delineation of an entity previously included among embryonal sarcomas of the kidney. Am J Surg Pathol. 2000;24(8):1087–96.
6. Kohle O, et al. Soft tissue sarcomas of the kidney. Rare Tumors. 2015;7(1):5635.
7. Namita Chittoria, B.I.R. Renal Cell Carcinoma. 2013 [cited 2016; Available from: http://www.clevelandclinicmeded.com/medicalpubs/diseasemanagement/nephrology/renal-cell-carcinoma/#top. Accessed 25 May 2017.
8. Pitino A, et al. Primary synovial sarcoma of the kidney. A case report with pathologic appraisal investigation and literature review. Pathologica. 2011; 103(5):271–8.
9. Park SJ, et al. A case of renal synovial sarcoma: complete remission was induced by chemotherapy with doxorubicin and ifosfamide. Korean J Intern Med. 2004;19(1):62–5.
10. Deshmukh R, Mankin HJ, Singer S. Synovial sarcoma: the importance of size and location for survival. Clin Orthop Relat Res. 2004;419:155–61.
11. Singer S, et al. Synovial sarcoma: prognostic significance of tumor size, margin of resection, and mitotic activity for survival. J Clin Oncol. 1996;14(4): 1201–8.
12. Markovic-Lipkovski J, et al. Rapidly progressive course of primary renal synovial sarcoma–case report. Srp Arh Celok Lek. 2013;141(11–12):814–8.
13. Mishra S, et al. Primary synovial sarcoma of the kidney. Saudi J Kidney Dis Transpl. 2015;26(5):996–9.
14. Schaal CH, Navarro FC, Moraes Neto FA. Primary renal sarcoma with morphologic and immunohistochemical aspects compatible with synovial sarcoma. Int Braz J Urol. 2004;30(3):210–3.
15. Ladanyi M. Fusions of the SYT and SSX genes in synovial sarcoma. Oncogene. 2001;20(40):5755–62.
16. Kawai A, et al. SYT-SSX gene fusion as a determinant of morphology and prognosis in synovial sarcoma. N Engl J Med. 1998;338(3):153–60.
17. Kim DH, et al. Primary synovial sarcoma of the kidney. Am J Surg Pathol. 2000;24(8):1097–104.
18. Chen S, et al. Primary synovial sarcoma of the kidney: a case report with literature review. Int J Surg Pathol. 2001;9(4):335–9.
19. Iacovelli R, et al. Clinical and pathological features of primary renal synovial sarcoma: analysis of 64 cases from 11 years of medical literature. BJU Int. 2012;110(10):1449–54.
20. Ozkan EE, Mertsoylu H, Ozardali HI. A case of renal synovial sarcoma treated with adjuvant ifosfamide and doxorubicin. Intern Med. 2011;50(15):1575–80.
21. Karavasilis V, Seddon BM, Ashley S, Al-Muderis O, Fisher C, Judson I. Significant clinical benefit of first-line palliative chemotherapy in advanced soft-tissue sarcoma: retrospective analysis and identification of prognostic factors in 488 patients. Cancer. 2008;112(7):1585–91. https://www.ncbi.nlm.nih.gov/pubmed/18278813.
22. Pervaiz N, et al. A systematic meta-analysis of randomized controlled trials of adjuvant chemotherapy for localized resectable soft-tissue sarcoma. Cancer. 2008;113(3):573–81.
23. Adjuvant chemotherapy for localised resectable soft tissue sarcoma in adults. Cochrane Database Syst Rev, 2000(4): p. Cd001419.
24. Tornkvist M, et al. A novel case of synovial sarcoma of the kidney: impact of SS18/SSX analysis of renal hemangiopericytoma-like tumors. Diagn Mol Pathol. 2004;13(1):47–51.
25. Bella AJ, Winquist EW, Perlman EJ. Primary synovial sarcoma of the kidney diagnosed by molecular detection of SYT-SSX fusion transcripts. J Urol. 2002;168(3):1092–3.
26. Dai YC, et al. A rare synovial sarcoma of the kidney exhibiting translocation (X;18) and SYT-SSX2 fusion gene. Zhonghua Yi Xue Za Zhi (Taipei). 2002; 65(6):293–7.
27. Vesoulis Z, et al. Fine needle aspiration biopsy of primary renal synovial sarcoma. A case report. Acta Cytol. 2003;47(4):668–72.
28. Moch H, et al. Primary renal synovial sarcoma. A new entity in the morphological spectrum of spindle cell renal tumors. Pathologe. 2003;24(6): 466–72.
29. Chen PC, et al. Primary renal synovial sarcoma with inferior vena cava and right atrium invasion. Int J Urol. 2003;10(12):657–60.
30. Jun SY, et al. Synovial sarcoma of the kidney with rhabdoid features: report of three cases. Am J Surg Pathol. 2004;28(5):634–7.
31. Shao L, Hill DA, Perlman EJ. Expression of WT-1, Bcl-2, and CD34 by primary renal spindle cell tumors in children. Pediatr Dev Pathol. 2004;7(6):577–82.
32. Shannon BA, Murch A, Cohen RJ. Primary renal synovial sarcoma confirmed by cytogenetic analysis: a lesion distinct from sarcomatoid renal cell carcinoma. Arch Pathol Lab Med. 2005;129(2):238–40.
33. Perlmutter AE, et al. Primary synovial sarcoma of the kidney. Int J Urol. 2005; 12(8):760–2.
34. Stage AC, Pollock RE, Matin SF. Bilateral metastatic renal synovial sarcoma. Urology. 2005;65(2):389.
35. Palau LM, et al. Primary synovial sarcoma of the kidney with rhabdoid features. Int J Surg Pathol. 2007;15(4):421–8.
36. Drozenova J, et al. Primary synovial sarcoma of the kidney. Cesk Patol. 2008; 44(1):20–2.
37. Mirza M, Zamilpa I, Bunning J. Primary renal synovial sarcoma. Urology. 2008;72(3):716. e11-2
38. Gabilondo F, et al. Primary synovial sarcoma of the kidney: corroboration with in situ polymerase chain reaction. Ann Diagn Pathol. 2008;12(2):134–7.
39. Zakhary MM, et al. Magnetic resonance imaging features of renal synovial sarcoma: a case report. Cancer Imaging. 2008;8:45–7.
40. Chung, S.D., et al., Primary synovial sarcoma of the kidney. J Formos Med Assoc, 2008. 107(4): 344–347.
41. Erturhan S, et al. Primary synovial sarcoma of the kidney: use of PET/CT in diagnosis and follow-up. Ann Nucl Med. 2008;22(3):225–9.
42. Divetia M, et al. Synovial sarcoma of the kidney. Ann Diagn Pathol. 2008; 12(5):333–9.
43. Dassi V, et al. Primary synovial sarcoma of kidney: a rare tumor with an atypical presentation. Indian J Urol. 2009;25(2):269–71.
44. Kawahara T, et al. Primary synovial sarcoma of the kidney. Case Rep Oncol. 2009;2(3):189–93.
45. Long JA, et al. Primitive renal synovial sarcoma: a cystic tumor in young patients. Prog Urol. 2009;19(7):474–8.
46. Wezel F, et al. Primary biphasic synovial sarcoma of the kidney. Urologe A. 2010;49(3):411–4.
47. Wang ZH, Wang XC, Xue M. Clinicopathologic analysis of 4 cases of primary renal synovial sarcoma. Chin J Cancer. 2010;29(2):212–6.
48. Kageyama S, et al. Primary synovial sarcoma arising from a crossed ectopic kidney with fusion. Int J Urol. 2010;17(1):96–8.
49. Tan YS, et al. Synovial sarcoma of the kidney: a report of 4 cases with pathologic appraisal and differential diagnostic review. Anal Quant Cytol Histol. 2010;32(4):239–45.
50. Romero-Rojas AE, et al. Early age renal synovial sarcoma. Arch Esp Urol. 2010;63(6):464–71.

51. Lakshmaiah KC, et al. Primary synovial sarcoma of kidney-a report of 2 cases and review of literature. J Egypt Natl Canc Inst. 2010;22(3):149–53.
52. Kataria T, et al. Pulmonary metastasis from renal synovial sarcoma treated by stereotactic body radiotherapy: a case report and review of the literature. J Cancer Res Ther. 2010;6(1):75–9.
53. Grampurohit VU, Myageri A, Rao RV. Primary renal synovial sarcoma. Urol Ann. 2011;3(2):110–3.
54. Karafin M, et al. Diffuse expression of PAX2 and PAX8 in the cystic epithelium of mixed epithelial stromal tumor, angiomyolipoma with epithelial cysts, and primary renal synovial sarcoma: evidence supporting renal tubular differentiation. Am J Surg Pathol. 2011;35(9):1264–73.
55. Nishida T, et al. Monophasic primary renal synovial sarcoma accompanied with a hemorrhagic cyst. Urol J. 2011;8(3):244–7.
56. Bakhshi GD, et al. Primary renal synovial sarcoma. Clin Pract. 2012;2(2):e44.
57. Pereira ESR, et al. Primary synovial sarcoma of the kidney with unusual follow up findings. Can J Urol. 2013;20(2):6734–6.
58. Moorthy HK, Pillai BS, Varghese J. Primary renal synovial sarcoma: an oncologic surprise. Urol Case Rep. 2014;2(5):152–3.
59. Majumder A, et al. Primary renal synovial sarcoma: a rare tumor with an atypical presentation. Arch Iran Med. 2014;17(10):726–8.
60. Schoolmeester JK, Cheville JC, Folpe AL. Synovial sarcoma of the kidney: a clinicopathologic, immunohistochemical, and molecular genetic study of 16 cases. Am J Surg Pathol. 2014;38(1):60–5.
61. Wang Z, et al. Primary synovial sarcoma of the kidney: a case report. Oncol Lett. 2015;10(6):3542–4.
62. Ozkanli SS, et al. Primary synovial sarcoma of the kidney. Urol Int. 2014;92(3): 369–72.
63. Vedana M, et al. Primary synovial cell sarcoma of the kidney: case report and review of the literature. Case Reports in Oncology. 2015;8(1):128–32.
64. Lv XF, et al. Primary renal synovial sarcoma: computed tomography imaging findings. Acta Radiol. 2015;56(4):493–9.

2

Kidney stone formers have more renal parenchymal crystals than non-stone formers, particularly in the papilla region

Atsushi Okada*, Shuzo Hamamoto, Kazumi Taguchi, Rei Unno, Teruaki Sugino, Ryosuke Ando, Kentaro Mizuno, Keiichi Tozawa, Kenjiro Kohri and Takahiro Yasui

Abstract

Background: We investigated the renoprotective ability of healthy people against kidney stone formation. To clarify intratubular crystal kinetics and processing in human kidneys, we performed a quantitative and morphological observation of nephrectomized renal parenchyma tissues.

Methods: Clinical data and pathological samples from 60 patients who underwent radical nephrectomy for renal cancer were collected from June 2004 to June 2010. The patients were retrospectively classified as stone formers (SFs; $n = 30$, kidney stones detected by preoperative computed tomography) and non-stone formers (NSFs; $n = 30$, no kidney stone history). The morphology of parenchymal intratubular crystals and kidney stone-related gene and protein expression levels were examined in noncancerous renal sections from both groups.

Results: SFs had a higher smoking rate ($P = 0.0097$); lower red blood cell, hemoglobin, and hematocrit values; and higher urinary red blood cell, white blood cell, and bacterial counts than NSFs. Scanning electron microscopy revealed calcium-containing crystal deposits and crystal attachment to the renal tubular lumen in both groups. Both groups demonstrated crystal transmigration from the tubular lumen to the interstitium. The crystal diffusion analysis indicated a significantly higher crystal existing ratio in the medulla and papilla of SFs and a significantly higher number of papillary crystal deposits in SFs than NSFs. The expression analysis indicated relatively high osteopontin and CD68, low superoxide dismutase, and significantly lower Tamm–Horsfall protein expression levels in SFs. Multivariate logistic regression analysis involving the above factors found the presence of renal papillary crystals as a significant independent factor related to SFs (odds ratio 5.55, 95% confidence interval 1.08–37.18, $P = 0.0395$).

Conclusions: Regardless of stone formation, intratubular crystals in the renal parenchyma seem to transmigrate to the interstitium. SFs may have reduced ability to eliminate renal parenchymal crystals, particularly those in the papilla region, than NSFs with associated gene expression profiles.

Keywords: Kidney stones, Macrophages, Osteopontin, Oxidative stress, Tamm-Horsfall protein

Background

Since the introduction of extracorporeal shock-wave lithotripsy in 1980, [1] fewer opportunities for open surgery have led to fewer chances for pathological investigations of kidney stone formation (KSF) using human kidney parenchymal tissue. Therefore, studies of human KSF tend to focus on urinary inorganic concentrations [2, 3] and epidemiological data, such as those investigating the relationship with diabetes [4] and metabolic syndrome [5]. Recent progress in endoscopic technology has directed attention to Randall's plaque [6]; interstitial apatite crystal deposits beginning at the basement membranes of the thin loops of Henle seem to be sites of calcium oxalate (CaOx) stone formation [7–9]. However, intraparenchymal events involving the kinetics of intratubular crystals have not been elucidated.

Previous basic studies using hyperoxaluric-animal and cell-culture models led to the detection of morphological

* Correspondence: a-okada@med.nagoya-cu.ac.jp
Department of Nephro-urology, Nagoya City University Graduate School of Medical Sciences, 1 Kawasumi, Mizuho-cho, Mizuho-ku, Nagoya, Aichi 467-8601, Japan

and genetic events in the renal parenchyma via the detection of stone matrix protein, [10] completion of the human genome project, and technological progress related to recombinant gene analysis [11–13]. In particular, the factors currently considered to affect calcium kidney stone formation are stone matrix proteins, cell injury caused by oxidative stress, monocyte/macrophage induction, and urinary stone inhibitors.

Osteopontin (OPN), the main component of stone matrix protein, is a glycoprotein present in human calcium-containing kidney stones [10] that may play an important role in crystal conversion to stones. OPN antisense-expressing cultured renal tubular cells demonstrate reduced aggregation of CaOx crystals and crystal-cell interactions [14] and OPN-knockout mice show reduced growth of renal crystals [12]. OPN is also involved in the formation of the organic layer of apatite plaque particles in the renal inner medulla of CaOx stone formers (SFs) [15]. Furthermore, renal tubular-cell injury caused by oxidative stress is essential for kidney stone formation [16]. Some studies have indicated that tubular-cell apoptosis caused by deviated free radicals and diminished superoxide dismutase (SOD) expression, [17] and collapsed organelles, including mitochondria and fragmented microvilli in the renal tubular lumen, lead to stone nidus formation [18]. We reported renal intratubular crystal elimination in a mouse model, increased expression of macrophage-related inflammatory genes in a DNA microarray analysis of stone-forming kidneys, [13] and phagocytosis of interstitial crystals by macrophages under transmission electron microscopy, [19] suggesting the kidney stone-preventive ability of macrophages by crystal processing. Moreover, Umekawa et al. [20] demonstrated that exposure to CaOx crystals promotes the expression of monocyte chemotactic protein-1 (MCP-1) and induces macrophage migration. Finally, Tamm–Horsfall protein (THP), a urinary inhibitor of stone formation, has been studied because THP-deficient mice demonstrate spontaneous calcium crystal formation [21].

The above experimental findings suggest that intratubular crystal formation involves several steps and that animal models may have the ability to eliminate the crystals. However, among the possible mechanisms of stone formation, these processes are thought to model Randall's plug due to hyperoxaluria or cystinuria rather than Randall's plaque. However, there is no definitive evidence to confirm this assumption. With the above in mind, we aimed to elucidate the intratubular crystal kinetics and processing in human kidneys using nephrectomized parenchymal tissues.

Methods

Patients

We obtained clinical data and pathological samples from 60 patients who underwent radical nephrectomy for stage I renal cell carcinoma (RCC) from June 2004 to June 2010. The Institutional Review Board of Nagoya City University Hospital approved the study design (Approval No. 551). The patients were retrospectively classified as SFs (30 patients with renal stones detected by preoperative computed tomography [CT]) and non-stone formers (NSFs; 30 age [± 1 year] - and sex-adjusted patients without renal stone and kidney disease history). In SFs, all stones were also detectable by abdominal X-ray and were presumed to be non-uric acid stones.

Clinical data analysis

We evaluated basic clinical and pathological data, comorbidities, and lifestyle factors. The preoperative laboratory data analyses included complete blood count, coagulability tests, and biochemical analyses. Using spot urine sampling, qualitative analysis of specific gravity, pH, protein, and glucose and flow cytometry-based quantitative analysis of urinary red blood cells (RBCs), white blood cells (WBCs), epithelial cells, and bacteria were conducted.

Aortic calcification index

Because of the similarity between atherosclerosis formation and kidney stone formation, [22] we calculated the aortic calcification index of both groups as the degree of calcification at the aortic arterial wall as follows: grade 0, none; grade 1, < 120 degrees of calcification; grade 2, ≥ 120 degrees but < 240 degrees of calcification; and grade 3, ≥ 240 degrees of calcification.

Detection and quantification of renal crystal deposits

Paraffin-embedded tissue blocks prepared from formalin-fixed excised kidneys were sliced to a 4-μm thickness and stained with hematoxylin and eosin (H&E). Crystal deposits in the normal renal parenchyma were detected by polarized light optical microphotography of the H&E-stained samples. The number of crystal deposits was quantified by counting the crystals per 100 visual fields (magnification, × 100) in noncancerous sections of the renal cortex, medulla, and papilla and as the existing ratio (number of kidneys with crystal deposits/whole kidneys). CaOx crystals were detected by Pizzolato staining [23].

Scanning electron microscopy (SEM) analysis

Dewaxed paraffin-embedded sections (4-μm thickness) were washed with a phosphoric acid buffer, re-fixed with 2.5% glutaraldehyde and subsequently with 2% osmium liquid, dehydrated in a 50–100% ethanol series, and embedded in epoxy resin. After sputtering a platinum filter on a stage, SEM specimens were prepared using electrical conduction. The crystal ultrastructure was then examined by SEM. The elemental spectra of the crystal deposits were determined by energy-dispersive X-ray spectroscopy (EDX).

Immunohistochemistry (IHC)

IHC for OPN, SOD, CD68 (a macrophage surface marker), and THP was performed using 4-μm-thick cross-sections. The tissues were autoclaved for antigen activation at 121 °C for 5 min, blocked with 0.5% hydrogen peroxide in methanol for 30 min, washed with 0.01 M phosphate-buffered saline (PBS), and treated with skimmed milk in PBS for 1 h at room temperature. They were then incubated overnight at 4 °C with the following polyclonal antibodies: rabbit anti-human OPN (Immuno-Biological Laboratories Co., Ltd., Gunma, Japan), rabbit anti-human CD68 (Santa Cruz Biotechnology, Santa Cruz, CA, USA), rabbit anti-human THP (Santa Cruz Biotechnology), and goat anti-human SOD (Santa Cruz Biotechnology). The reacted antibodies were detected using a Histofine simple stain kit for goat or rabbit immunoglobulin G (Nichirei Biosciences, Inc., Tokyo, Japan) according to the manufacturer's instructions.

Quantitative reverse transcription-polymerase chain reaction (qRT-PCR) analysis

Total RNA from noncancerous kidney sections was extracted using NucleoSpin FFPE RNA (Macherey-Nagel GmbH & Co., Düren, Germany) according to the manufacturer's instructions. All RNA samples were reverse-transcribed to complementary DNA with a High Capacity cDNA reverse transcription kit (Applied Biosystems, Life Technologies, Carlsbad, CA, USA). According to the annotation information of each gene, the TaqMan gene expression assay product, a 20× assay mix of forward and reverse primer sets, and TaqMan MGB probe (FAM dye labeled) with complementary sequences to each messenger RNA sequence were obtained. The qPCR was performed with the TaqMan Universal PCR master mix (404,437, Applied Biosystems) using the 7500 FAST real-time PCR system (Applied Biosystems). After denaturation at 95 °C for 10 min, PCR was initiated at 95 °C for 15 s and completed at 60 °C for 1 min. The reaction was repeated 45 times. The expression of each sample was determined as a ratio to the expression of the glyceraldehyde 3-phosphate dehydrogenase gene (*GAPDH*; internal control). TaqMan gene expression assay probe kits were used for the secreted phosphoprotein-1 gene (*SPP1*, encoding OPN; Hs00959010_m1), *SOD1* (Hs00533490_m1), *CD68* (Hs00154355_m1), uromodulin gene (*UMOD*, encoding THP; Hs00358451_m1), and *GAPDH* (Hs03929097_g1).

Statistical analysis

We used the chi-square test using a 2 × 2 table to compare the comorbidities and lifestyle factors. The clinical and basic laboratory data were compared using Student's *t*-test. Furthermore, the pathological data, aortic calcification grades, urinalysis results, number of crystal deposits, and messenger RNA expression levels were analyzed using the Mann–Whitney *U*-test. The categorical pathological patient data, comorbidity data, and lifestyle factor data were assessed using the chi-square test. Repeated-measures analysis of variance (ANOVA) was used to compare the renal crystal distribution between the groups. Based on each analysis, the extracted factors were evaluated for their relationship with kidney stone formation using multivariate logistic regression analysis. In these analyses, a *P*-value < 0.05 was considered to indicate a statistically significant difference.

Results

Clinical findings

The groups were not significantly different in terms of clinical data. No significant sex difference was detected between the groups (Table 1). Both groups were predominantly composed of patients with clear-cell RCC. There were no significant differences in pathological diagnoses, grades, stages, and affected sides between the groups (Table 2). Comorbidities did not differ between the groups (Table 3). However, SFs had a significantly higher smoking rate than NSFs ($P = 0.0097$).

Although the RBC, hemoglobin, and hematocrit (Ht) values of SFs were within the normal limits, they were significantly lower than those of NSFs ($P = 0.0290$, 0.0360, and 0.0268, respectively; Table 4). The coagulation-related and blood biochemical data were not significantly different between the groups. Furthermore, no significant differences in urinalysis results were noted. However, SFs had significantly higher urinary RBC, WBC, and bacterial count values ($P = 0.0343$,

Table 1 Clinical patient data

Parameter	Total, mean (SD)		*P*-value*	Men, mean (SD)		*P*-value*	Women, mean (SD)		*P*-value*
	SFs	NSFs		SFs	NSFs		SFs	NSFs	
Age (years)	62.1 (10.6)	61.7 (10.9)	0.8856	62.7 (10.3)	63.0 (10.3)	0.9336	56.6 (13.3)	57.6 (12.2)	0.8856
Height (cm)	164.6 (7.4)	165.3 (6.7)	0.7016	166.1 (6.6)	166.7 (5.9)	0.7282	156.8 (6.6)	157.6 (5.2)	0.8366
Weight (kg)	62.2 (12.1)	66.0 (10.5)	0.1933	64.0 (11.7)	67.2 (9.6)	0.2902	53.2 (10.4)	59.8 (13.8)	0.4181
Body mass index (kg/m^2)	22.9 (3.4)	24.0 (3.7)	0.2149	23.2 (3.4)	24.0 (3.0)	0.3587	21.6 (2.9)	24.2 (6.6)	0.4455
Abdominal circumference (cm)	77.7 (8.1)	80.4 (8.3)	0.2027	78.2 (8.1)	80.5 (8.1)	0.3260	74.9 (8.0)	79.8 (10.2)	0.4243

SD standard deviation, *SFs* stone formers, *NSFs* non-stone formers
*$P < 0.05$ indicates statistically significant differences by Student's *t*-test

Table 2 Pathological patient data

Parameter	Number of SFs (%)	Number of NSFs (%)	*P*-value*
Diagnosis			0.7879
Clear cell RCC	27 (90.0)	28 (93.3)	
Papillary RCC	1 (3.3)	1 (3.3)	
Chromophobe RCC	1 (3.3)	0 (0)	
Collecting duct carcinoma	1 (3.3)	1 (3.3)	
Grade			0.3529
1	8 (26.7)	9 (30.0)	
2	20 (66.7)	21 (70.0)	
3	2 (6.7)	0 (0)	
INF			0.5194
a	18 (64.3)	20 (69.0)	
b	10 (35.7)	8 (27.6)	
c	0	1 (3.4)	
pT			0.7249
1a	12 (40.0)	13 (43.3)	
1b	9 (30.0)	11 (36.7)	
2	2 (6.7)	1 (3.3)	
3a	2 (6.7)	3 (10.0)	
3b	5 (16.7)	2 (6.7)	
Side			0.0705
Right	12 (40.0)	19 (63.3)	
Left	18 (60.0)	11 (36.7)	

SFs stone formers, *NSFs* non-stone formers, *RCC* renal cell carcinoma
$^*P < 0.05$ indicates statistically significant differences by the chi-square test

0.0117, and 0.0014, respectively); male patients had similar values for the above parameters ($P = 0.0108$, 0.0036, and 0.0010, respectively). Qualitative analysis of urinary protein and glucose levels did not yield significant differences between the groups (Table 5).

Table 3 Comparison of the comorbidities and lifestyle factors

Parameter	Number of SFs (%)	Number of NSFs (%)	*P*-value*
Comorbidity			
Hypertension	15 (50.0)	14 (46.7)	0.7961
Heart disease	4 (15.4)	3 (11.1)	0.6876
Cerebrovascular disease	0 (0.0)	2 (6.7)	0.1503
Diabetes	2 (6.7)	7 (23.3)	0.0706
Habituation			
Smoking	19 (63.3)	9 (30.0)	**0.0097**
Drinking	11 (36.7)	6 (20.0)	0.1520

SFs stone formers, *NSFs* non-stone formers
The bold number indicates a statistically significant difference ($^*P < 0.05$) by the chi-square test for a 2 × 2 table

Aortic calcification rates

The aortic calcification rates of SFs and NSFs were 80.0 and 63.3%, respectively (Table 6). SFs tended to have an insignificantly higher incidence of aortic calcification ($P = 0.3032$); a similar tendency was observed in both sexes.

Morphology and composition of renal crystals

Polarized light optical microphotography revealed renal crystal deposits with birefringence in both groups (Fig. 1a). SEM demonstrated no significant difference in crystal morphology and crystal attachment to the tubular walls between the groups (Fig. 1b). EDX showed that the main component of the deposits was calcium-containing crystals (Fig. 1c).

Crystal transmigration

Pizzolato staining revealed renal intratubular CaOx crystals (Fig. 2). The cortex crystals existed in the tubular lumen and adapted to the tubular walls (Fig. 2a). In the medullary regions, crystal-attached tubular epithelial cells were abraded and crystal transmigration into the interstitium was observed (Fig. 2b). In the papillary region, almost all crystals were detected in the interstitium (Fig. 2c). These findings were the same in both groups.

Crystal distribution

In the renal cortex, the incidence ratios of SFs and NSFs were 48.1 and 40.7%, respectively ($P = 0.3190$; Fig. 3a). SFs had significantly higher incidence ratios in the medulla (40.9% vs. 23.1%, $P = 0.0064$) and papilla (55.6% vs. 30.8%, $P = 0.0004$). There were no significant differences in the number of crystal deposits (Fig. 3b) in the cortex (2.41 [0.63] vs. 1.44 [0.43], $P = 0.3833$) and medulla (1.84 [0.53] vs. 1.56 [0.63], $P = 0.4079$) between SFs and NSFs. However, SFs had a significantly higher number of papillary crystal deposits than NSFs (7.58 [2.42] vs. 2.75 [1.14], $P = 0.0235$). Furthermore, SFs had a significantly greater number of crystal deposits overall ($P = 0.0187$).

Kidney stone-related gene and protein expression levels

OPN was expressed at the apical side of the distal tubular cells (Fig. 4a). SOD expression was diffusely detected among the proximal tubular cells. CD68-positive cells were detected mainly at the interstitial area of the renal papilla and tubular lumen. THP expression was diffusely detected among the distal tubular cells. As shown in Fig. 4b, SFs had a relatively high expression level of *SPP1* ($P = 0.4959$) and relatively low expression levels of *SOD1* ($P = 0.0790$) and *CD68* ($P = 0.2764$). Finally, SFs had a significantly lower expression level of *UMOD* ($P = 0.0392$) than NSFs.

Table 4 Preoperative laboratory patient data

Parameter	Total, mean (SD)		*P*-value*	Men, mean (SD)		*P*-value*	Women, mean (SD)		*P*-value*
	SFs	NSFs		SFs	NSFs		SFs	NSFs	
WBC (× 10^3/μL)	5.7 (1.4)	6.4 (1.8)	0.1172	5.9 (1.4)	6.7 (1.8)	0.0870	5.1 (0.9)	5.0 (1.2)	0.8366
Neutrophil (%)	62.1 (8.6)	62.4 (6.5)	0.8800	62.4 (8.9)	62.8 (6.0)	0.8742	59.3 (7.4)	61.1 (9.3)	0.8125
Eosinophil (%)	3.3 (3.3)	3.0 (2.3)	0.7481	3.6 (3.4)	3.1 (2.4)	0.5742	1.4 (0.80)	2.7 (1.9)	0.2588
Basophil (%)	0.4 (0.3)	0.5 (0.4)	0.3021	0.5 (0.3)	0.5 (0.4)	0.5532	0.2 (0.20)	0.5 (0.1)	0.0656
Monocyte (%)	5.2 (1.6)	5.5 (1.7)	0.5208	5.4 (1.4)	5.6 (1.2)	0.7515	3.6 (1.90)	4.9 (3.3)	0.5034
Lymphocyte (%)	27.6 (6.0)	28.7 (6.2)	0.5075	27.4 6.0)	28.3 (6.3)	0.6122	29.1 (6.9)	30.8 (5.1)	0.6899
RBC (×10^6/μL)	4.3 (0.6)	4.6 (0.6)	**0.0290**	4.3 (0.5)	4.7 (0.6)	0.0592	4.1 (0.40)	4.5 (0.3)	0.8366
Hemoglobin (g/dL)	13.0 (1.9)	14.0 (1.8)	**0.0360**	13.2 (1.8)	14.3 (1.7)	**0.0393**	11.8 (1.8)	12.4 (1.0)	0.4845
Hematocrit (%)	39.5 (4.7)	42.3 (4.8)	**0.0268**	40.1 (4.6)	43.2 (4.7)	**0.0248**	36.9 (4.4)	38.2 (2.7)	0.6088
Platelets (×10^3/μL)	216.0 (56.5)	211.7 (46.1)	0.7496	215.4 (61.9)	212.5 (46.4)	0.8554	218.9 (18.6)	207.4 (49.7)	0.6434
APTT (%)	97.1 (13.4)	96.3 (12.9)	0.8171	96.2 (12.1)	96.0 (13.7)	0.9551	101.4 (19.7)	97.9 (8.2)	0.7198
PT (%)	96.6 (13.2)	102.2 (14.5)	0.1611	86.1 (11.3)	102.7 (17.3)	0.1310	98.4 (21.8)	99.5 (12.8)	0.9303
PT/INR	1.04 (0.10)	1.01 (0.10)	0.2293	1.04 (0.09)	1.00 (0.11)	0.2641	1.04 (0.10)	1.01 (0.08)	0.6996
Fibrinogen (mg/dL)	327.8 (93.5)	319.6 (70.4)	0.7069	336.6 (98.2)	319.0 (74.1)	0.4818	285.4 (54.4)	322.8 (54.5)	0.3090
TP (g/dL)	7.3 (0.4)	7.33 (0.4)	0.6528	7.2 (0.4)	7.3 (0.5)	0.6805	7.5 (0.50)	7.6 (0.2)	0.8124
Albumin (g/dL)	4.3 (0.5)	4.33 (0.4)	0.9494	4.3 (0.60)	4.3 (0.4)	0.9010	4.6 (0.21)	4.4 (0.2)	0.3126
GOT (U/L)	20.8 (5.7)	23.3 (9.8)	0.2365	21.3 (5.9)	22.2 (8.0)	0.6390	18.4 (4.5)	28.6 (16.4)	0.2170
GPT (U/L)	20.9 (10.4)	26.2 (19.2)	0.1947	21.7 (10.3)	24.2 (11.6)	0.4303	16.8 (11.0)	36.0 (41.6)	0.3476
LDH (U/L)	198.1 (33.2)	185.8 (29.9)	0.1619	196.2 (34.9)	181.2 (24.6)	0.0975	212.3 (11.2)	213.5 (46.8)	0.9686
ALP (U/L)	233.6 (63.0)	241.3 (64.5)	0.6470	236.7 (57.9)	237.0 (62.2)	0.9828	219.0 (90.4)	262.4 (35.4)	0.4428
γ-GTP (U/L)	51.6 (63.2)	28.1 (10.2)	0.5916	60.5 (67.4)	29.0 (10.8)	0.1430	14.0 (0.1)	25.3 (0.1)	0.0771
Creatinine (mg/dL)	0.9 (0.2)	0.82 (0.2)	0.4937	0.9 (0.2)	0.9 (0.2)	0.4700	0.7 (0.2)	0.6 (0.0)	0.8480
Uric acid (mg/dL)	6.0 (1.7)	6.14 (1.6)	0.6891	6.1 (1.7)	6.5 (1.4)	0.4115	5.1 (1.3)	4.2 (1.2)	0.4009
BUN (mg/dL)	15.9 (4.9)	15.3 (3.3)	0.5500	15.9 (4.6)	15.5 (3.4)	0.7763	16.2 (6.6)	15.0 (2.6)	0.5092
Glucose (mg/dL)	122.5 (31.8)	129.2 (47.2)	0.5253	121.0 (33.4)	132.0 (49.6)	0.3690	130.0 (23.6)	115.4 (30.9)	0.4252
Calcium (mg/dL)	9.8 (0.3)	9.71 (0.4)	0.5741	9.8 (0.3)	9.7 (0.4)	0.3148	9.7 (0.3)	9.9 (0.1)	0.2483
e-GFR	71.4 (20.7)	74.9 (18.3)	0.4961	71.0 (20.8)	72.7 (14.0)	0.7287	73.4 (22.5)	85.2 (32.5)	0.5226
Urinary specific gravity	1.016 (0.006)	1.016 (0.006)	0.8782	1.016 (0.006)	1.016 (0.006)	0.9044	1.013 (0.006)	1.016 (0.009)	0.6434
Urinary pH	6.0 (0.7)	6.32 (0.8)	0.0899	5.9 (0.6)	6.3 (0.8)	0.0604	6.3 (1.2)	6.4 (0.8)	0.8783
Urinary RBC (/μL)	68.3 (37.8)	11.9 (5.5)	**0.0343**	80.1 (45.8)	5.7 (1.4)	**0.0108**	14.0 (9.1)	43.1 (30.9)	0.4647
Urinary WBC (/μL)	56.7 (38.7)	11.5 (7.4)	**0.0117**	54.5 (46.5)	3.6 (0.8)	**0.0036**	66.5 (40.5)	50.9 (43.4)	0.7540
Urinary epithelium (/μL)	4.0 (1.1)	2.66 (1.0)	0.1073	2.9 (1.0)	1.3 (0.2)	0.1428	9.4 (3.4)	9.7 (4.8)	0.6761
Urinary casts (/μL)	0.4 (0.1)	0.2 (0.1)	0.2339	0.5 (0.1)	0.1 (0.0)	0.1217	0.2 (0.2)	0.5 (0.4)	0.8345
Urinary bacteria (×10^3/μL)	5.4 (3.0)	1.12 (0.2)	**0.0014**	2.4 (0.6)	0.9 (0.1)	**0.0010**	19.2 (16.8)	2.3 (0.9)	0.4647
Urinary volume (L/day)	1.4 (0.5)	1.6 (0.6)	0.1511	1.4 (0.5)	1.6 (0.3)	0.3038	0.9 (0.4)	1.5 (0.7)	0.2225

SD standard deviation, *SFs* stone formers, *NSFs* non-stone formers, *WBC* white blood cell, *RBC* red blood cell, *APTT activated partial thromboplastin time*, *PT* prothrombin time, *PT/INR* prothrombin time international normalized ratio, *TP* total protein, *GOT* glutamic oxaloacetic transaminase, *GPT* glutamic pyruvic transaminase, *LDH lactate dehydrogenase*, *ALP* alkaline phosphatase, *γ-GTP* γ-glutamyl transpeptidase, *BUN blood urea nitrogen*, *e-GFR* estimated glomerular filtration rate
The bold numbers indicate statistically significant differences (*$P < 0.05$) by Student's *t*-test or the Mann–Whitney *U*-test

Multivariate analysis of the relationship between extracted factors and SFs

Multivariate logistic regression analysis was used to assess the relationship of the following factors with SFs: smoking habits, RBC, Ht, urinary RBC, urinary bacteria, existence of renal papillary crystals, and UMOD expression ratio. Continuous variables were adopted for analysis as two nominal scales with cut-off values set at the median values. The presence of renal papillary crystals was found to be a significant independent factor related to SFs (odds ratio 5.55, 95% confidence interval 1.08–37.18, $P = 0.0395$) (Table 7).

Table 5 Qualitative analysis of urinary protein and glucose

Parameter	Group	−, *n* (%)	±, *n* (%)	+, *n* (%)	++, *n* (%)	*P*-value*
Urinary protein	SFs	19 (63.3)	3 (19.0)	7 (23.3)	1 (3.33)	0.7007
	NSFs	20 (66.7)	5 (16.7)	4 (13.3)	1 (3.33)	
Urinary glucose	SFs	29 (96.7)	0 (0.0)	1 (3.3)	0 (0.0)	0.1785
	NSFs	23 (76.7)	1 (3.3)	3 (10.0)	3 (10.0)	

SFs stone formers, *NSFs* non-stone formers
*$P < 0.05$ indicates statistically significant differences by the Mann-Whitney *U*-test

Discussion

Kohri et al. [10] suggested that calcium kidney stone formation involves the expression of several stone matrix proteins, mainly OPN, in renal tubular cells, indicating that the phenomenon is inducible by both environmental and genetic factors [24]. However, their explanation has two major problems: (i) because kidney stone formation is asymptomatic, patients do not recognize its onset until colic pain occurs due to stone descent or chance detection by imaging studies; and (ii) due to the spread of extracorporeal shock wave lithotripsy, it has become difficult to extract tissues ethically from living kidneys, making it impossible to conduct detailed studies on kidney tissues, in contrast to the situation when open surgery was common. Due to the recent development of endoscopic instruments, morphological and pathological studies on Randall's plaque have become more common. We recently conducted a genome-wide study of plaque tissue, resulting in the confirmation of inflammatory cytokine expression, increased immune cell number, and cellular apoptosis in renal papilla stone tissue [25]. However, these findings were limited to the renal papilla tissue and represent only the change in expression levels after stone formation. To resolve these problems, we enrolled patients with asymptomatic stones detected contingently by preoperative CT for the diagnosis of renal tumors and investigated renal parenchyma integrally using pathological whole-kidney samples. Specifically, we analyzed the crystal morphology and transmigration in addition to kidney stone-related gene and protein expression.

Table 6 Analysis of aortic calcification grades

	Group	Grade 0, *n* (%)	Grade 1, *n* (%)	Grade 2, *n* (%)	Grade 3, *n* (%)	*P*-value*
Total	SFs	6 (20.0)	13 (43.3)	6 (20.0)	5 (16.7)	0.3032
	NSFs	11 (36.7)	10 (33.3)	4 (13.3)	5 (16.7)	
Men	SFs	5 (20.0)	11 (44.0)	5 (20.0)	4 (16.0)	0.4672
	NSFs	8 (32.0)	10 (40.0)	2 (8.0)	5 (20.0)	
Women	SFs	1 (20.0)	2 (40.0)	1 (20.0)	1 (20.0)	0.3808
	NSFs	3 (60.0)	0 (0.0)	2 (40.0)	0 (0.0)	

SFs stone formers, *NSFs* non-stone formers
*$P < 0.05$ indicates a statistically significant difference by the Mann–Whitney *U*-test

We found that SF group had a significantly higher smoking rate than NSFs. Słojewski et al. [26] did not detect significant correlations between smoking and kidney stone composition. Smoking is a significant, independent risk factor for atherosclerosis via the oxidative stress associated with mitochondrial damage [27]. Considering the similarity between kidney stone and atherosclerosis formation, [22] smoking might conceivably affect stone formation or crystal kinetics. The precise relationship between the risk of stone formation and smoking should be investigated in future studies.

SFs had significantly lower RBC, hemoglobin, and Ht values than NSFs. Renal ischemia via anemia could lead to renal tubular-cell injury, [28] implying that anemia might be involved in stone formation. However, patients with kidney stones have erythropoietin resistance caused by bone marrow oxalosis [29]. Furthermore, the increase in urine RBC, WBC, and bacterial counts may be the result of the erosion of the renal pelvic mucosa on Randall's plaque in patients with stones [30]. Unfortunately, we did not consider the existence of plaque in this study.

The notable findings of this study are as follows: (i) regardless of kidney stone history, intratubular crystal deposits were detectable in the renal parenchymal tissues; (ii) the crystals transmigrated from the tubular lumen to the papillary interstitium; and (iii) SFs had a significantly higher number of crystal deposits in the renal papilla. Bergsland et al. [31] noted that SFs, especially those with idiopathic hypercalciuria, have higher urinary calcium molarity than NSFs and that the difference becomes significant at night. CaOx supersaturation but not calcium phosphate supersaturation is higher in SFs than in NSFs, which could also explain CaOx stone formation on papillary Randal's plaques. CaOx crystal residues in the renal papilla could be another factor related to CaOx stone formation. Furthermore, Vervaet et al. [32] used hyperoxaluric rat model and human renal biopsy samples to indicate the gradual migration of intratubular crystals to the interstitium. In the hyperoxaluric mouse model we previously established, [11] intratubular crystal deposits were eliminated in about 6 days. The crystals were englobed and fragmented by macrophages and crystal deposits were undetectable in the renal papillary region at all time points. Boonla et al. [33] investigated MCP-1 and interleukin (IL)-6 messenger RNA expression in renal biopsy samples from SFs and extracted kidney samples from patients with renal cancer; they demonstrated relatively low MCP-1 and IL-6 expression levels in the cancerous samples compared to those in noncancerous tissues. In the present study, the significantly higher number of interstitial crystal deposits in

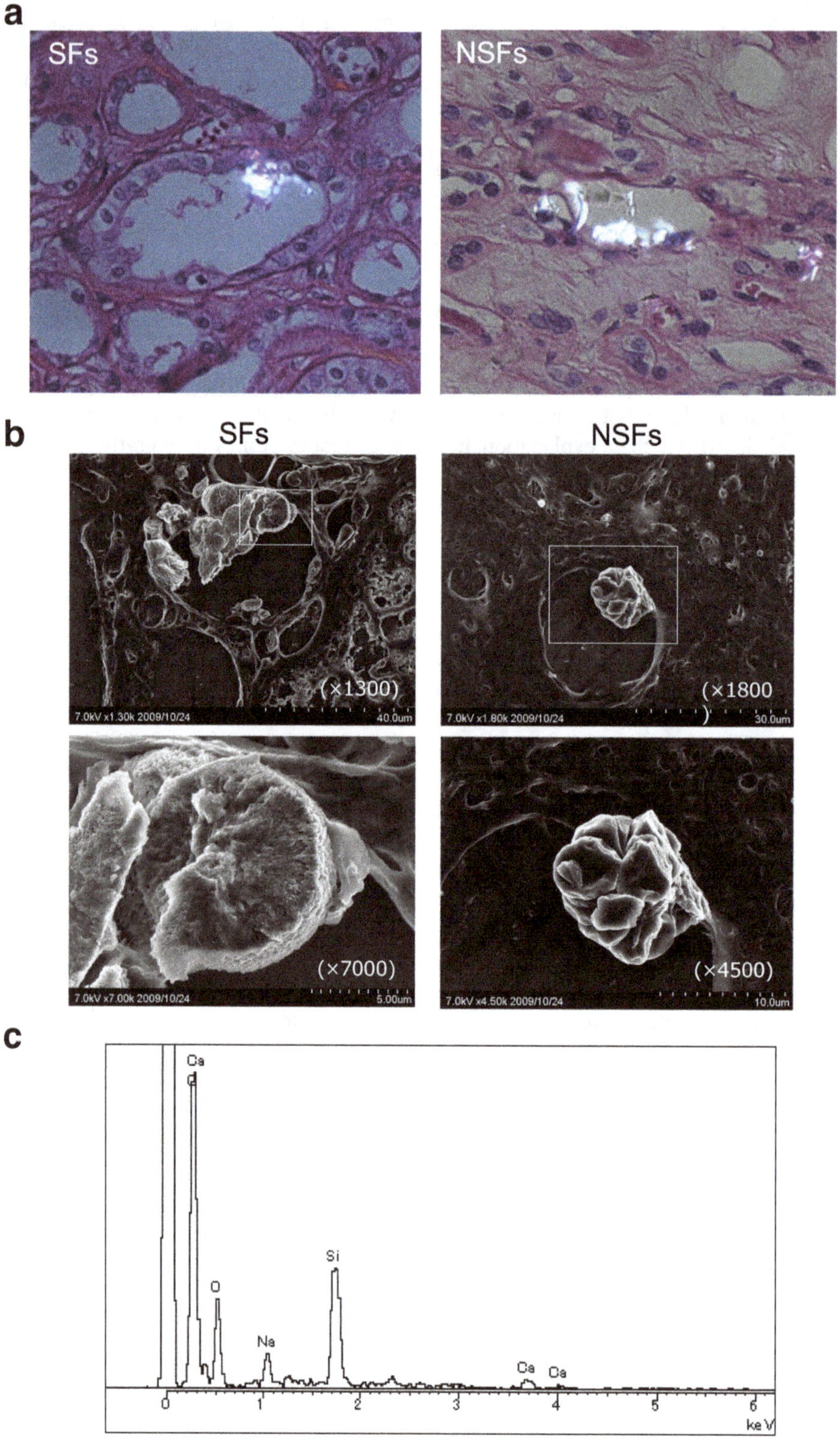

Fig. 1 Morphology and composition of renal tubular crystal deposits in stone formers (SFs) and non-stone formers (NSFs). **a** Crystal attachment to the tubular walls detected by polarized light optical microphotography of hematoxylin and eosin-stained renal cortex sections (magnification, × 800). **b** Crystal attachment to the tubular walls detected by scanning electron microscopy (SEM) of the crystal ultrastructure. **c** Energy-dispersive X-ray spectroscopy (EDX) of the mineral components on the surface of SEM-detected crystal deposits. The EDX spectrum shows calcium as the main component of the deposits

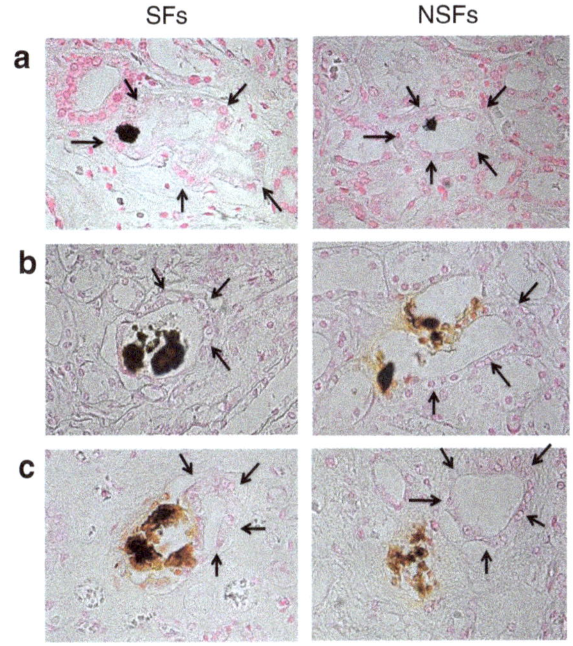

Fig. 2 Microscopic observation of Pizzolato-stained calcium oxalate crystal deposits in the renal cortex, medulla, and papilla of stone formers (SFs) and non-stone formers (NSFs). **a** In the renal cortex, the crystals were located in the tubular lumen and attached to the walls. **b** In the medullary region, the crystal-attached tubular epithelial cells were abraded and crystal transmigration into the interstitium was observed. (**c**) In the papillary region, almost all the crystals were detected in the interstitium. Arrows indicate tubules with crystal deposits

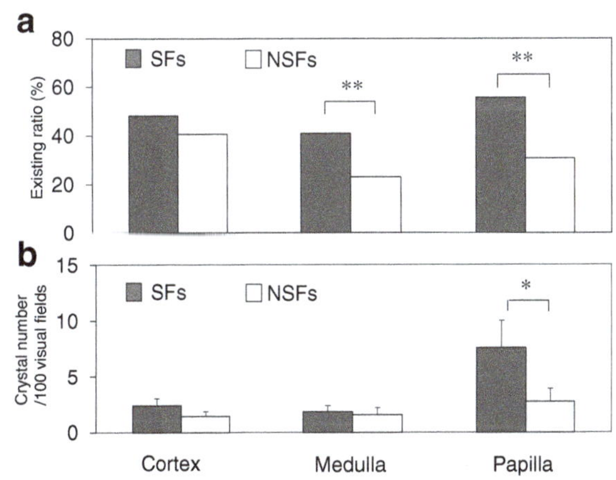

Fig. 3 Comparison of the crystal distribution in the renal cortex, medulla, and papilla between stone formers (SFs) and non-stone formers (NSFs). **a** The existing ratios (number of kidneys with crystal formation/whole kidneys). **b** The crystal numbers per 100 visual fields (magnification, × 100). Data represent means (standard deviation); $^*P < 0.05$ and $^{**}P < 0.01$ indicates statistically significant differences by repeated-measures analysis of variance

the papilla of SFs and relatively high *CD68* expression level in NSFs suggest some important roles of macrophages in kidney stone prevention. The OPN, SOD, and CD68 expression levels were similar to those indicated in previous basic studies: SFs had increased OPN expression in the renal tubular cells, tubular-cell injury by oxidative stress, and reduced migration of renal macrophages. In particular, the significantly lower THP expression level in SFs indicates that THP has a crucial role as a kidney stone-preventive factor in humans.

On the basis of our results, we hypothesize the phenomena of human renal intratubular crystal processing. First, crystal nidi are generated in the tubular lumen of the renal cortex because of a urinary supersaturated condition [2, 3]. Some oxidative stresses, such as anemia or smoking, and renal tubular-cell injuries cause collapse of mitochondria and microvilli with decreased SOD expression [16–18]. Consecutively, OPN expression increases and THP downregulation induces crystal-cell interaction and the adaptation of aggregated crystals to the tubular epithelium [26]. Thereafter, the tubular epithelium disintegrates via apoptosis and crystal clusters transmigrate to the renal interstitium via the regenerating epithelium [32]. Tubular-cell injury increases the expression of MCP-1 or various chemokines, in turn inducing monocytes, their transmigration to the renal interstitium, and their differentiation into macrophages [20]. The interstitial crystals can then be removed by macrophages.

These calcification processes, including epithelial-cell injury via oxidative stress, the participation of OPN via inflammation, macrophage activity with phagocytosis, and processing and conversion of foam cells into calcified tissue, are similar to the processes of atherosclerosis formation [34]. SFs tended to have higher levels of aortic calcification. These outcomes suggest a new approach to kidney stone formation involving similar biomolecular processes to those involved in metabolic syndrome that are not related to kidney stone disease because of hyperuricemia, decreased urinary pH, or hypocitraturia caused by metabolic syndrome [35–37].

Multivariate analysis indicated that the presence of renal papillary crystals was significantly and independently related to stone formation. This result represents all of the relationships discussed above. These findings suggest the possibility that the process of kidney stone formation depends on some renoprotective abilities related to the processing of crystals formed in the renal parenchyma, especially the renal papilla.

This study has some limitations that should be discussed. We could not clarify how cancer background,

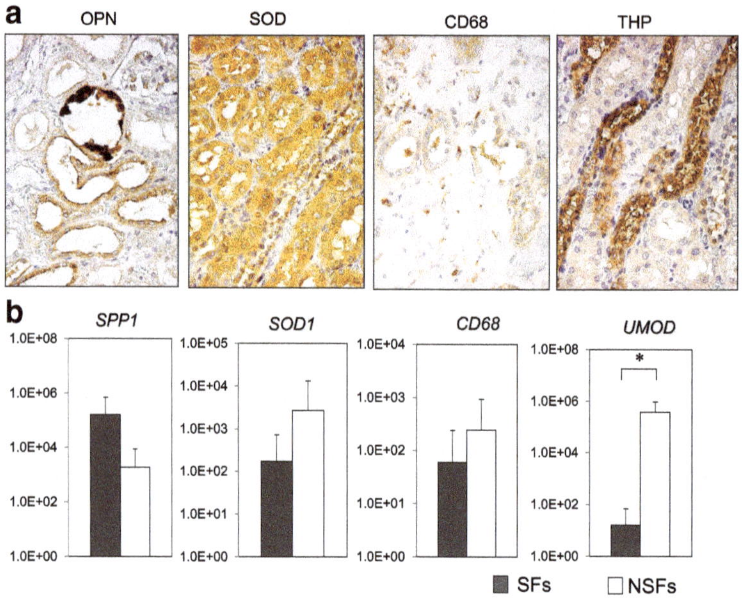

Fig. 4 Kidney stone-related gene and protein expressions in stone formers (SFs) and non-stone formers (NSFs). **a** Immunohistochemistry (magnification, × 100) for osteopontin (OPN), superoxide dismutase (SOD), CD68, and Tamm–Horsfall protein (THP). **b** mRNA expression levels of the secreted phosphoprotein-1 gene (*SPP1*), *SOD1*, *CD68*, and uromodulin gene (*UMOD*) detected by quantitative polymerase chain reaction (qPCR). The glyceraldehyde 3-phosphate dehydrogenase gene was used as the internal control. Data represent means (standard deviation). $^{*}P < 0.05$ indicates statistically significant differences by the Mann-Whitney *U*-test

involving environmental and genetic factors, affected "true" kidney stone formation. Furthermore, because this study was conducted retrospectively, detailed analysis of stone component and urinary biochemistry could not be performed. Moreover, Randall's plaques were not detectable in the study sample.

Conclusions

We identified similar phenomena to those detected in previous basic studies, such as crystal-cell interactions, increased OPN expression, decreased SOD and THP expression, and macrophage involvement in the human renal parenchyma. The new findings of this study were crystal formation in patients without kidney stones, crystal transmigration to the papillary interstitium, and crystal processing at the renal papilla regardless of stone formation. SFs may have reduced ability to eliminate renal parenchymal crystals than NSFs (especially in the papilla region), with associated gene expression changes.

Table 7 Multivariate analysis for relationships between extracted factors and kidney stone formation

	OR (95% CI) For stone formers	*P*-value*
Smoking (+)	1.95 (0.40–9.92)	0.4037
RBC (≤ 4.6 × 10^6/μL)	0.30 (0.03–2.38)	0.2518
Ht (≤ 48%)	1.28 (0.17–12.01)	0.8135
Urinary RBC (≤ 4.3/μL)	1.52 (0.28–8.29)	0.6211
Urinary bacteria (≤ 0.99 × 10^3/μL)	4.46 (0.90–29.08)	0.0687
Renal papillary crystals (+)	5.55 (1.08–37.18)	0.0395
UMOD (existing ratio < 0.001)	4.15 (0.67–37.96)	0.1313

$^{*}P < 0.05$ indicates a statistically significant difference. *OR* odds ratio, *CI* confidence interval, *RBC* red blood cell, *Ht* hematocrit, *UMOD* uromodulin

Abbreviations

CaOx: Calcium oxalate; CT: Computed tomography; EDX: Energy-dispersive X-ray spectroscopy; GAPDH: Glyceraldehyde 3-phosphate dehydrogenase; H&E: Hematoxylin and eosin; Ht: Hematocrit; IHC: Immunohistochemistry; IL-6: Interleukin-6; KSF: Kidney stone formation; MCP-1: Monocyte chemotactic protein-1; NSF: Non-stone former; OPN: Osteopontin; PBS: Phosphate-buffered saline; qRT-PCR: Quantitative reverse transcription-polymerase chain reaction; RBC: Red blood cell; RCC: Renal cell carcinoma; SEM: Scanning electron microscopy; SF: Stone former; SOD: Superoxide dismutase; SPP1: Secreted phosphoprotein-1; THP: Tamm-Horsfall protein; UMOD: Uromodulin; WBC: White blood cell

Acknowledgments

We thank N. Kasuga and M. Noda for administrative assistance.

Authors' contributions

AO carried out the data collection, performed the statistical analysis, and drafted the manuscript. RU, TS, and KT performed sample staining and image analysis. RA, KM, TK participated in the study design and statistical analysis. KK and TY coordinated the project. All authors read and approved the final manuscript.

References

1. Chaussy C, Brendel W, Schmiedt E. Extracorporeally induced destruction of kidney stones by shock waves. Lancet. 1980;2:1265–8.

2. Werness PG, Brown CM, Smith LH, Finlayson B. EQUIL2: a BASIC computer program for the calculation of urinary saturation. J Urol. 1985;134:1242–4.
3. Tiselius HG. An improved method for the routine biochemical evaluation of patients with recurrent calcium oxalate stone disease. Clin Chim Acta. 1982; 122:409–18.
4. Daudon M, Traxer O, Conort P, Lacour B, Jungers P. Type 2 diabetes increases the risk for uric acid stones. J Am Soc Nephrol. 2006;17:2026–33.
5. Taylor EN, Stampfer MJ, Curhan GC. Obesity, weight gain, and the risk of kidney stones. JAMA. 2005;293:455–62.
6. Randall A. The origin and growth of renal calculi. Ann Surg. 1937;105:1009–27.
7. Evan AP, Lingeman JE, Coe FL, Parks JH, Bledsoe SB, Shao Y, et al. Randall's plaque of patients with nephrolithiasis begins in basement membranes of thin loops of Henle. J Clin Invest. 2003;111:607–16.
8. Evan A, Lingeman J, Coe FL, Worcester E. Randall's plaque: pathogenesis and role in calcium oxalate nephrolithiasis. Kidney Int. 2006;69:1313–8.
9. Coe FL, Evan AP, Worcester EM, Lingeman JE. Three pathways for human kidney stone formation. Urol Res. 2010;38:147–60.
10. Kohri K, Suzuki Y, Yoshida K, Yamamoto K, Amasaki N, Yamate T, et al. Molecular cloning and sequencing of cDNA encoding urinary stone protein, which is identical to osteopontin. Biochem Biophys Res Commun. 1992;184:859–64.
11. Okada A, Nomura S, Higashibata Y, Hirose M, Gao B, Yoshimura, et al. Successful formation of calcium oxalate crystal deposition in mouse kidney by intraabdominal glyoxylate injection. Urol Res. 2007;35:89–99.
12. Okada A, Nomura S, Saeki Y, Higashibata Y, Hamamoto S, Hirose M, et al. Morphological conversion of calcium oxalate crystals into stones is regulated by osteopontin in mouse kidney. J Bone Miner Res. 2008;23:1629–37.
13. Okada A, Yasui T, Hamamoto S, Hirose M, Kubota Y, Itoh Y, et al. Genome-wide analysis of genes related to kidney stone formation and elimination in the calcium oxalate nephrolithiasis model mouse: detection of stone-preventive factors and involvement of macrophage activity. J Bone Miner Res. 2009;24:908–24.
14. Yasui T, Fujita K, Asai K, Kohri K. Osteopontin regulates adhesion of calcium oxalate crystals to renal epithelial cells. Int J Urol. 2002;9:100–8.
15. Evan AP, Coe FL, Rittling SR, Bledsoe SM, Shao Y, Lingeman JE, et al. Apatite plaque particles in inner medulla of kidneys of calcium oxalate stone formers: osteopontin localization. Kidney Int. 2005;68:145–54.
16. Itoh Y, Yasui T, Okada A, Tozawa K, Hayashi Y, Kohri K. Preventive effects of green tea on renal stone formation and the role of oxidative stress in nephrolithiasis. J Urol. 2005;173:271–5.
17. Hirose M, Tozawa K, Okada A, Hamamoto S, Shimizu H, Kubota Y, et al. Glyoxylate induces renal tubular cell injury and microstructural changes in experimental mouse. Urol Res. 2008;36:139–47.
18. Hirose M, Yasui T, Okada A, Hamamoto S, Shimizu H, Itoh Y, et al. Renal tubular epithelial cell injury and oxidative stress induce calcium oxalate crystal formation in mouse kidney. Int J Urol. 2010;17:83–92.
19. Okada A, Yasui T, Fujii Y, Niimi K, Hamamoto S, Hirose M, et al. Renal macrophage migration and crystal phagocytosis via inflammatory-related gene expression during kidney stone formation and elimination in mice; detection by association analysis of stone-related gene expression and microstructural observation. J Bone Miner Res. 2010;25:2701–11.
20. Umekawa T, Chegini N, Khan SR. Oxalate ions and calcium oxalate crystals stimulate MCP-1 expression by renal epithelial cells. Kidney Int. 2002;61:105–12.
21. Mo L, Huang HY, Zhu XH, Shapiro E, Hasty DL, Wu XR. Tamm-Horsfall protein is a critical renal defense factor protecting against calcium oxalate crystal formation. Kidney Int. 2004;66:1159–66.
22. Yasui T, Itoh Y, Bing G, Okada A, Tozawa K, Kohri K. Aortic calcification in urolithiasis patients. Scand J Urol Nephrol. 2007;41:419–21.
23. Pizzolato P. Histochemical recognition of calcium oxalate. J Histochem Cytochem. 1964;12:333–6.
24. Kohri K, Yasui T, Okada A, Hirose M, Hamamoto S, Fujii Y, et al. Biomolecular mechanism of urinary stone formation involving osteopontin. Urol Res. 2012;40:623–37.
25. Taguchi K, Hamamoto S, Okada A, Unno R, Kamisawa H, Naiki T, et al. Genome-wide gene expression profiling of Randall's plaques in calcium oxalate stone formers. J Am Soc Nephrol. 2017;28:333–47.
26. Słojewski M, Czerny B, Safranow K, Drozdzik M, Pawlik A, Jakubowska K, et al. Does smoking have any effect on urinary stone composition and the distribution of trace elements in urine and stones? Urol Res. 2009;37:317–22.
27. Puddu P, Puddu GM, Cravero E, De Pascalis S, Muscari A. The emerging role of cardiovascular risk factor-induced mitochondrial dysfunction in atherogenesis. J Biomed Sci. 2009;16:112.
28. Nemoto T, Yokota N, Keane WF, Rabb H. Recombinant erythropoietin rapidly treats anemia in ischemic acute renal failure. Kidney Int. 2001;59:246–51.
29. Sahin G, Acikalin MF, Yalcin AU. Erythropoietin resistance as a result of oxalosis in bone marrow. Clin Nephrol. 2005;63:402–4.
30. Ciftçioğlu N, Vejdani K, Lee O, Mathew G, Aho KM, Kajander EO, et al. Association between Randall's plaque and calcifying nanoparticles. Int J Nanomedicine. 2008;3:105–15.
31. Bergsland KJ, Coe FL, Gillen DL, Worcester EM. A test of the hypothesis that the collecting duct calcium-sensing receptor limits rise of urine calcium molarity in calcium kidney stone formers. Am J Physiol Renal Physiol. 2009; 297:F1017–23.
32. Vervaet BA, Verhulst A, Dauwe SE, De Broe ME, D'Haese PC. An active renal crystal clearance mechanism in rat and man. Kidney Int. 2009;75:41–51.
33. Boonla C, Hunapathed C, Bovornpadungkitti S, Poonpirome K, Tungsanga K, Sampatanukul P, et al. Messenger RNA expression of monocyte chemoattractant protein-1 and interleukin-6 in stone-containing kidneys. BJU Int. 2008;101:1170–7.
34. Scatena M, Liaw L, Giachelli CM. Osteopontin: a multifunctional molecule regulating chronic inflammation and vascular disease. Arterioscler Thromb Vasc Biol. 2007;27:2302–9.
35. Sakhaee K, Maalouf NM. Metabolic syndrome and uric acid nephrolithiasis. Semin Nephrol. 2008;28:174–80.
36. Cupisti A, Meola M, D'Alessandro C, Bernabini G, Pasquali E, Carpi A, et al. Insulin resistance and low urinary citrate excretion in calcium stone formers. Biomed Pharmacother. 2007;61:86–90.
37. Khan SR, Canales BK. Unified theory on the pathogenesis of Randall's plaques and plugs. Urolithiasis. 2015;43:109–23.

3

Systemic analysis of urinary stones from the Northern, Eastern, Central, Southern and Southwest China by a multi-center study

Rui-hong Ma[1*], Xiao-bing Luo[1], Qin Li[2] and Hai-qiang Zhong[1]

Abstract

Background: To provide some basis for the prevention of urinary stones in general population, we did a systemic analysis of urinary stones from Northern, Eastern, Central, Southern and Southwest China by a multi-center study.

Methods: A total of 11,157 urinary stones from Northern, Eastern, Central, Southern and Southwest China were obtained and analyzed by Fourier transform infrared spectroscopy. Combined with scanning electron microscopy and X-ray energy spectrometer, urinary stones were classified into different types. Furthermore, the correlation between stone types and clinical characteristics, as well as their regional distribution were elucidated.

Results: Calcium oxalate stones were the most common type in each region, followed by calcium oxalate-calcium phosphate mixed stones, uric acid stones and calcium phosphate stones. The distribution of calcium oxalate stones were highest prevalence in Southwest China (67.9%, $P < 0.05$), followed by Eastern and Northern China. Anhydrous uric acid stones, with a constituent ratio of 19.3% in Southern China, and 13.7% in Central China, were significantly higher than that in other regions ($P < 0.05$). Elements analysis indicated varieties among stone types as well as distribution regions. Moreover, the clinical characteristics were highly correlated with stone types and anatomical locations but not their distribution regions.

Conclusions: The material and elements composition of urinary stones among different regions showed some varieties. Calcium oxalate stone has the highest constituent ratio in Southwest China, while anhydrous uric acid stone has the highest constituent ratio in Southern China. Moreover, the clinical characteristics were highly correlated with stone types and anatomical locations but not their distribution regions.

Keywords: Urinary stones, Fourier transform infrared spectroscopy, Scanning electron microscopy, X-ray energy spectrometer, Calcium oxalate stones, Uric acid stones, Regional distribution

Background

Urinary stone disease, also known as urolithiasis, is one of the leading afflictions worldwide. The incidence differs with geographic distribution. In general, as described in detail previously [1, 2], the average prevalence is higher in western countries (5–9% in Europe, and 13% in North America) than the eastern (1–5% in Asia). While in Saudi Arabia, nearly 20% people suffer from it. In China, the disease approximately affects 4% of population and increases steadily during the recent 20 years, due to high calories intake from dietary and lack of exercise in lifestyle [3–5]. Therefore, effective prevention strategy and precise treatment are needed to alleviate the burden caused by high prevalence of urolithiasis.

Urolithiasis cause undoubtedly considerable burden on public health worldwide not only by its high prevalence but also for the recurrence rate. A report in Germany indicated that about 40% of patients suffered from recurrent urolithiasis once or more, and even over 10%

* Correspondence: olive5327@163.com
[1]The Department of Clinical Laboratory, The Sixth People's Hospital of Nansha, Xingye Road No. 7, Dagang Town, Nansha, Guangzhou 511470, People's Republic of China
Full list of author information is available at the end of the article

underwent five or more stone episodes [6]. Therefore, it is important to clearly define the etiology and establish an effective prevention program on urinary stones [7]. As the composition of urinary stone may provide some clue for the formation process, stone analysis is important in determining the possible etiology of urinary stones. Moreover, there exists a wide geographic variation in proportion for different stone types. The phenomenon is demonstrated well in the United States but still limited in China [8, 9]. Therefore, in the present study, we did a systemic analysis of urinary stones from Northern, Eastern, Central, Southern and Southwest China by a multi-center study to describe the commons and differences of stone composition, major and trace elements as well as clinical characteristics.

Methods

Ethics statement

The sample collection procedures were explained to all patients. Written informed consent was obtained from all patients. The principles outlined in the Declaration of Helsinki of 1975 (revised in 1983 and 1989) were followed throughout the study period. The study was approved by both the Ethics Committee of The Sixth People's Hospital of Nansha, Guangzhou (reference number is No: 20130821057P) and the Ethics Committee of The Kingmed Diagnostics Center of Guangzhou (KM20130149).

Subjects and specimens

Urinary stones from 11,157 urolithiasis patients were collected from department of the urinary surgery in The Sixth People's Hospital of Nansha, Guangzhou, and the Kingmed Diagnostics Center of Guangzhou during September 2013 to September 2017. The patients consisted of 7437 males, ranged from 18 to 95 years old, the mean age was 49.61 ± 14.40 (*Mean* ± *S.D*) years, and 3720 females, ranged from 20 to 88 years old, the mean age was 49.31 ± 13.23 (*Mean* ± *S.D*) years. The age of the two groups had no statistically significant difference.

China's regional division

Northern China includes: Beijing, Tianjin, Hebei, Shanxi, Inner Mongolia provinces; Eastern China includes: Shanghai, Shandong, Jiangsu, Anhui, Jiangxi, Zhejiang, Fujian provinces; Central China includes: Hubei, Hunan, Henan; Southern China includes: Guangdong, Guangxi, Hainan provinces; Southwest China includes: Chongqing, Sichuan, Guizhou, Yunnan, Tibet provinces.

The recruitment of the urinary lithiasis patients

Of the above patients, 844 from Northern China, including 646 males, with average age of 45.58 ± 13.45, and 198 females, with average age of 43.16 ± 14.87; 2149 from Eastern China, including 1277 males, with average age of 47.07 ± 13.19, and 872 females, with average age of 46.95 ± 12.56; 713 from Central China, including 463 males, with average age of 49.65 ± 14.36, and 250 females, with average age of 48.98 ± 13.11; 6423 from Southern China, including 4339 males, with the average of 50.50 ± 14.75, and 2084 females, with the average age of 50.31 ± 13.38; 1028 from Southwest China, including 712 males, with the average of 46.85 ± 14.00, and 316 females, with the average age of 47.92 ± 13.09. The proportion of males and females from each region is slightly different, with a higher proportion of males in Northern China, and a lower in Eastern China. The age has some differences among different regions, with older age in Southern China and Central China, and younger age in Northern China.

Systemic classification of urinary stones

A total of 11,157 urinary stones were classified into different types with systemic classification combing using FTIR spectroscopy, SEM and X-ray energy spectrometer, the procedure has been detailed in our previous work [7].

Comparison of stone composition and clinical characteristics in patients with different regions

Urinary lithiasis patients were divided into five groups according to the regions, such as Northern China, Eastern China, Central China, Southern China and Southwest China, and urinary stones were divided into five groups according to the composition, such as calcium oxalate stones, calcium phosphate stones, uric acid stones, calcium oxalate-calcium phosphate mixed stones and other kinds of stone group. Others consisted of magnesium ammonium phosphate, cystine, brushite, urate stones and some subtypes of mixed stones that were minority. Stone composition and clinical characteristics in different regions were compared and analyzed.

Statistic methods

Age was analyzed using One-Way ANOVA and presented as mean ± SD, while the ratio of male and female, and the ratio with different types of stones as well as from different anatomical locations or regions were analyzed using a chi square test. LSD and the partitions of the chi square methods were used for multiple comparisons using IBM SPSS Statistics 24 software. $P < 0.05$ was regarded as statistically significant.

Results

Urinary stone composition were distinct in different regions of China

Calcium oxalate (whewellite and weddellite) stones were the most common in each region, followed by calcium oxalate-calcium phosphate mixed, anhydrous uric acid and calcium phosphate stones. The distribution of calcium oxalate stones were highest prevalence in Southwest China (67.9%, *P* < *0.05*), followed by Eastern and Northern China. Anhydrous uric acid stones, with a constituent ratio of 19.3% in Southern China, and 13.7% in Central China, were significantly higher than that in Northern, Eastern and Southwest China (*P* < *0.05*). The constituent ratio of calcium phosphate stones (about 5%) among different regions had no statistical differences (*P* > *0.05*). The stone type constitution in the five regions of China was shown in Table 1.

Element composition and distribution in each type of urinary stone

Besides the main elements (Italic), each type of stone still contains a small amount of metal and non-metallic elements, which had some varieties among stone types as well as regions. For calcium oxalate stones, besides the main elements carbon, oxygen, calcium, they still contain some sodium, kalium, magnesium, chlorine, aluminum, phosphorus, niobium, hafnium, sulphur, etc. For calcium phosphate stones, in addition to carbon, oxygen, calcium, phosphorus, they still contain some sodium, kalium, magnesium, chlorine, aluminium, niobium, fluorine, zinc, technetium, hafnium, chrome, etc.; and for those anhydrous uric acid stones, in addition to carbon, oxygen, nitrogen, they still had some sodium, calcium, aluminium, chlorine. Urinary stones from Southern China usually contained some zinc, and those from Southwest China usually contained some silicon, which seems more complex and diverse compared with other regions (Table 2). Mapping analysis of element distribution in general stones with X-ray energy spectrometer showed that for those calcium oxalate stones with micro dishes of calcium phosphate and calcium oxalate-calcium phosphate mixed stones, calcium oxalate crystals were always distributed in the outer layer while calcium phosphate crystals were in the core (Fig. 1a, b). Moreover, for those calcium phosphate stones, usually with a small amount of ammonium magnesium phosphate crystals scattered in the profile (Fig. 1c). Uric acid stones, mixed with micro or macro dishes of calcium oxalate crystals, displayed inconsistent crystal distribution characteristics. In some of the uric acid stones, uric acid crystals were shown in the outer layer and calcium oxalate crystals were in the core. Calcium oxalate crystals in the outer layer while uric acid crystals in the center were also found in some kind of uric acid stones. Besides, uric acid crystals mixed with calcium oxalate crystals in circular layers were observed in uric acid stones (Fig. 2). Mapping analysis of element distribution in micro field with magnification of 3000 times showed that there was only calcium distribution in calcium oxalate crystals, and both calcium and phosphorus distribution in calcium phosphate crystals and calcium oxalate-calcium phosphate mixed crystals, with a consistent distribution in calcium phosphate crystals and inconsistent distribution in calcium oxalate-calcium phosphate mixed crystals. Calcium was distributed in both calcium oxalate and calcium phosphate crystals; phosphorus was distributed in calcium phosphate crystals (Fig. 3). Moreover, there was only nitrogen distribution in uric acid crystals, and both nitrogen and calcium distribution in uric acid-calcium oxalate mixed crystals (Fig. 4).

The clinical characteristics of each type of urinary stone

Urinary stones were divided as upper urinary stones (kidney and ureteral stones) and lower urinary stones (bladder and urethral stones) according to the anatomical location. In our current studies, we did correlation analysis on 9073 urinary stones and clinical characteristics of these patients. Interestingly, the clinical characteristics were highly correlated with stone types and anatomical locations but not their regions. As shown in Table 3, 7448 cases were upper urinary stones while 1625 were lower urinary stones, and the ratio were 4.6:1. Among the patients with upper urinary stones, 4523 were males, accounting for 60.7%, while those with lower urinary stones, 1504 were males, accounting for 92.6%, which had statistically significant difference (*P* < *0.05*). It was indicated in the present study that calcium oxalate stone was the main stone type of upper urinary stones, constituting 60.6%, while uric acid stone was that of lower urinary stones, constituting 43.0% (*P* < *0.05*). Patients with calcium oxalate stones were mainly males between the ages of 30 and 60, accounting for 49.4%, while those with calcium phosphate stones were mainly

Table 1 Distribution of stone types in five regions of China

Stone type/regions	Calcium oxalate	Calcium phosphate	Uric acid	Calcium oxalate-calcium phosphate mixed	Other types	Total
Northern	485 (57.5%)	42 (5.0%)	52 (6.2%)	183 (21.7%)	82 (9.7%)	844 (100%)
Eastern	1360 (63.3%)	121 (5.6%)	123 (5.7%)	490 (22.8%)	55 (2.6%)	2149 (100%)
Central	377 (52.9%)	36 (5.0%)	98 (13.7%)	177 (24.8%)	25 (3.5%)	713 (100%)
Southern	3317 (51.6%)	359 (5.6%)	1242 (19.3%)	1221 (19.0%)	284 (4.4%)	6423 (100%)
Southwest	698 (67.9%)	48 (4.7%)	60 (5.8%)	188 (18.3%)	34 (3.3%)	1028 (100%)
Total	6237 (55.9%)	606 (5.4%)	1575 (14.1%)	2259 (20.2%)	480 (4.3%)	11,157 (100%)

Table 2 Element composition in each type of urinary stone with different regions

Stone type/ region	Calcium Oxalate	Calcium Phosphate	Uric Acid	Calcium Oxalate-Calcium Phosphate Mixed
Northern	*C, O, Ca*, Na,Cl,Mg,Al,P,Nb,Tc	*C, O, Ca, P*, Na,Mg,F,Cl,Nb,Tc,Hf,Cr	*C, O, N*, Ca	*C, O, Ca, P*, Na,Mg,K,F,Cl,Al,Nb
Eastern	*C, O, Ca*,Na,Cl,Mg,Al,P,K,Nb,Tc,Br	*C, O, Ca, P*, Na,Mg,K,Al,Cl,Nb,Tc,Hf	*C, O, N*,Na,Al,Cl,Ca	*C, O, Ca, P*, Na,Mg,K,F,Cl,Al,Nb,Tc,Hf,Fe
Central	*C, O, Ca*,Na,Al, Mg,P	*C, O, Ca, P*, Na,Mg,Nb	*C, O, N*,Ca	*C, O, Ca, P*, Na,Mg,F,Cl,Nb,Tc
Southern	*C, O, Ca*,Na,Cl,Mg,Al,P,K,F,Si,Nb,Tc,Hf,Zn	*C, O, Ca, P*, Na,Mg,Nb, Tc,Hf, Zn,F	*C, O, N*,Al,Ca	*C, O, Ca, P*, Na,Mg,F,Cl,Al,Nb,Tc,Hf,Zn
Southwest	*C, O, Ca*, Na,Cl,Mg,Al,P,K,Nb,Tc,Zn,S,Fe,Si	*C, O, Ca, P*, Na,Mg,K,F,Cl, Nb, Tc,Si	*C, O, N*,Al,Cl,Ca,Si	*C, O, Ca, P*, Na,Mg,F,Cl,Al,Nb, Tc,Si

The italics are the main elements of corresponding stone types

females between the ages of 30 and 60, accounting for 42.1%, and those with uric acid stones were mainly elder males over the age of 60, accounting for 45.8%, the difference was statistically significant ($P < 0.05$). Calcium phosphate stones and calcium oxalate-calcium phosphate mixed stones were mainly from upper urinary tract. Patients with calcium oxalate-calcium phosphate mixed stones were males or females, the ratio tend to 1, while those with magnesium ammonium phosphate and urate stones were mainly females, and those with brushite and cystine stones were mainly males (not list in the table).

Discussion

Urolithiasis, a common urological disease with multiple etiologies, has been a public burden to the world. In the last few decades, urolithiasis has been steadily increased [6, 10]. The present data indicated that the highest incidence of urinary stones occurred in 40–49 years old males and 50–59 years old females respectively. Urinary stones can be classified as metabolic stones (calcium oxalate and some uric acid or urate) and infectious stones (struvite, apatite or a mixture of the two), males are more likely to have metabolic stones, while females, with a high probability of urinary tract infections than men, are more prone to infectious stones [11]. The present data showed that patients with calcium oxalate stones and uric acid stones were mainly males, while those with calcium phosphate stones and magnesium ammonium phosphate (struvite) stones were mainly females.

The present data showed calcium oxalate stone was the most frequent stone type in all age groups, with high frequency between the ages of 30 and 60 years, and relatively low frequency in the younger and elderly. As previously detailed [12], the intake of oxalate and calcium in the diet has an important effect on urinary oxalate excretion, which also play a major role in the formation of calcium oxalate stone. Increased intake of dietary oxalate lead to an increase of urinary oxalate excretion, and decreasing dietary oxalate lowers urinary oxalate excretion [13]. Dietary calcium has a bidirectional effect on urinary oxalate excretion, Borghi's study showed the low-calcium (10 mmol/day) group presented a higher relapse of calcium oxalate stones than the normal-calcium (30 mmol/day) group [14]. The high percentage of calcium oxalate stone in Southwest China may be originated from water quality, soil and the local dietary structure. It was supposed that the major contributing factor maybe the increase of Ca^{2+}/Mg^{2+} ratio (in meq) in drinking water [15]. Additionally, the high calcium-content in local plants grown on karst soils along with the high ingestion of oxalate food may lead to the high incidence of calcium oxalate stones [15]. In China, karst soils mainly distributes in Southwest of China (Chongqing, Sichuan, Guizhou, Yunnan) [16], with a consistent distribution with calcium oxalate stones, which presents the highest constituent ratio in the Southwest among all areas of China. Meanwhile, calcium oxalate- calcium phosphate mixed stones account for a large proportion. In our opinion, it is difficult to manage urinary stones as stone recurrence is common because residual stone fragment contain bacteria and become the core of recurrent stone [11]. Furthermore, a previous research showed urinary tract infection was closely related to the existence of amorphous carbonated calcium phosphate (or whitlockite) and carbonated apatite [17]. Other research indicated that for recurrent stones, the admixed $CaOx/CaPO_4$ stones were converted from pure $CaPO_4$ more commonly than from pure CaOx stone [18]. Therefore, we conclude that calcium oxalate-calcium phosphate mixed or calcium oxalate stones with $CaPO_4$ in the core, the infectious factors maybe first involved in the stone process, and a considerable proportion of which may be recurrent stones.

Uric acid stones has a prevalence of about 10% among all stones [19], but this percentage become extremely high in those patients with gout [20]. Consistent with other reports [21], we found that uric acid stones increased with older age, elder males over the age of 60 accounted for 45.8% of total uric acid stones in the present study. UA urolithiasis is a complex disease that is affected by many factors. Diseases relevant with aging, such as obesity, insulin resistance and diabetes, are also associated with low urinary pH and UA stone formation [22–24]. Furthermore, as previously described [25], persistent acidic urine ($pH \leq 5.5$) is considered to be the

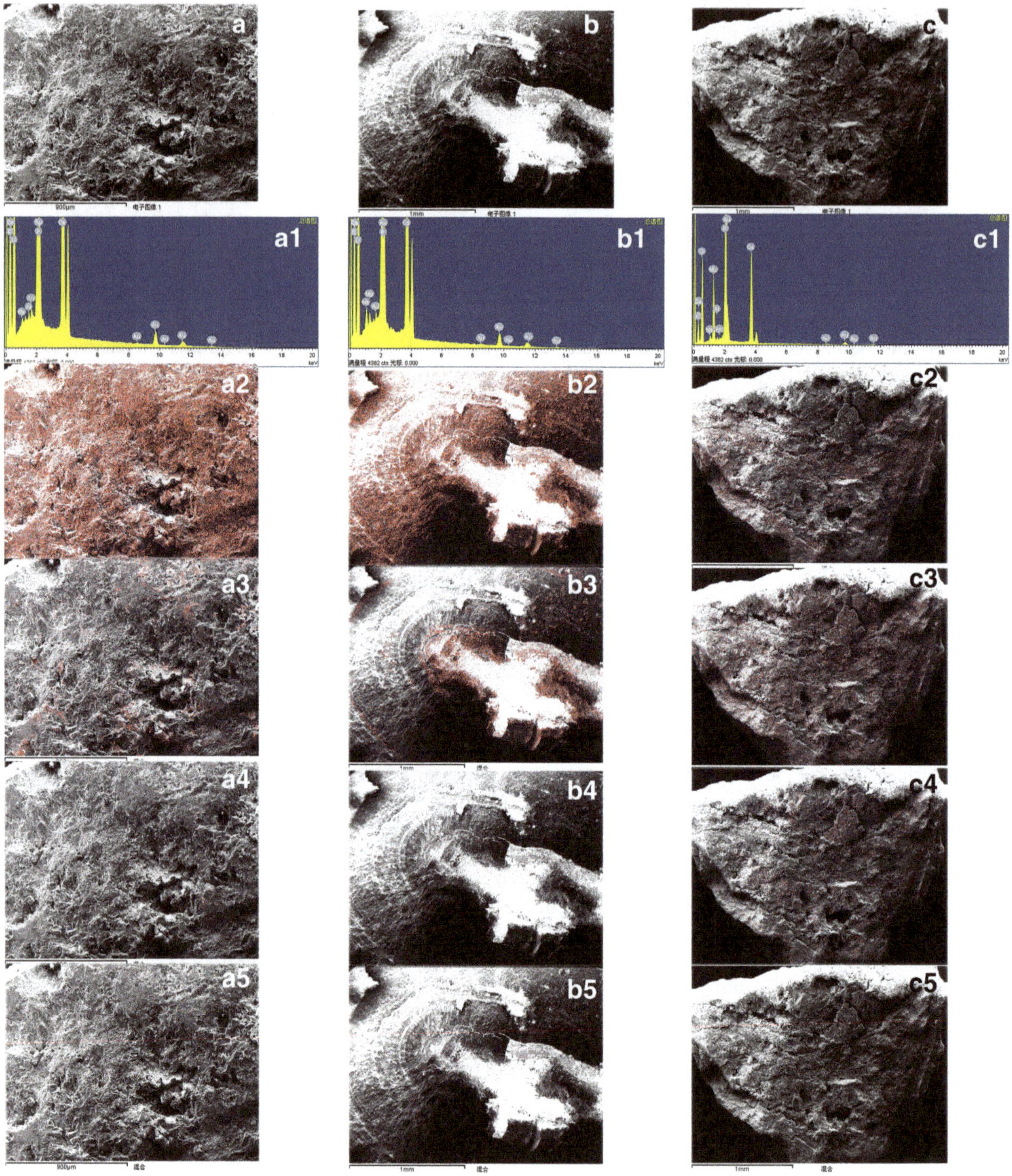

Fig. 1 Element distribution in general stones (the red dot represented element distribution). **a** calcium oxalate stones with micro dishes of calcium phosphate: calcium oxalate crystals were distributed in the outer layer and profile, with micro dishes of calcium phosphate crystals in the core. A1.The energy spectrum, A2. Calcium distribution, A3. Phosphorus distribution, A4. Magnesium distribution, A5. Natrium distribution; **b** calcium oxalate-calcium phosphate mixed stones: calcium oxalate crystals were distributed in the outer layer, calcium phosphate crystals were in the core. B1. The energy spectrum, B2. Calcium distribution, B3. Phosphorus distribution, B4. Aluminum distribution, B5. Natrium distribution; **c** Calcium phosphate stones: a small amount of ammonium magnesium phosphate crystals were scattered in the profile. C1. The energy spectrum, C2. Calcium distribution, C3. Phosphorus distribution, C4. Magnesium distribution, C5. Aluminum distribution

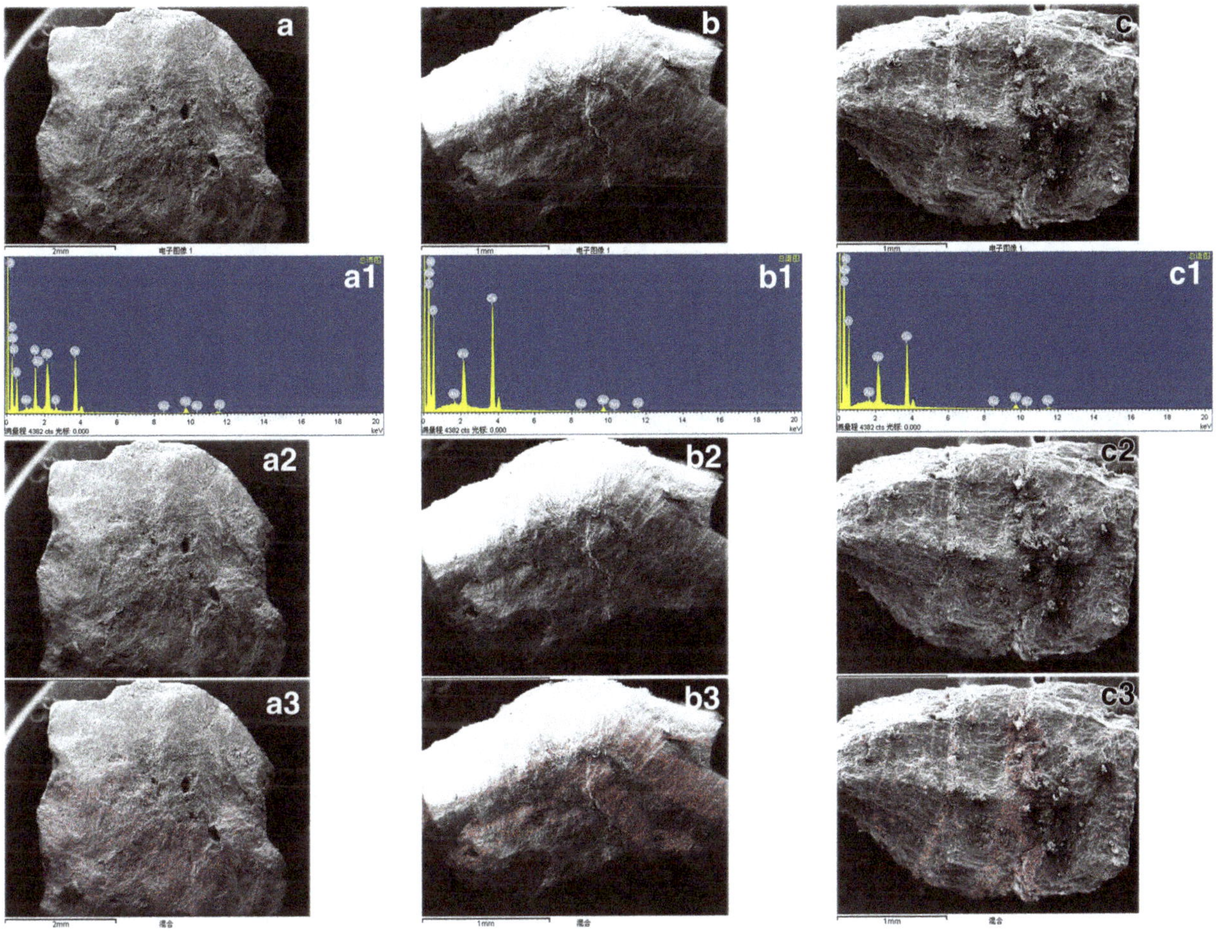

Fig. 2 Element distribution in general stones: uric acid stones mixed with some calcium oxalate crystals (the red dot represented element distribution). **a** Uric acid- calcium oxalate mixed stones: uric acid crystals were distributed in the outer layer, and calcium oxalate crystals in the core. A1. The energy spectrum, A2. Nitrogen distribution, A3. Calcium distribution; **b** Calcium oxalate - uric acid mixed stones: calcium oxalate crystals were distributed in the outer layer, and uric acid crystals in the core. B1. The energy spectrum, B2. Nitrogen distribution, B3. Calcium distribution; **c** Uric acid stones mixed with micro dishes of calcium oxalate crystals: uric acid crystals were distributed in circular layer, and calcium oxalate crystals were scattered between the layers: C1. The energy spectrum, C2. Nitrogen distribution, C3. Calcium distribution

most important risk factor for the formation of UA stones. Additionally, environmental factors may have a prominent influence on the composition of urinary stones. As reported [26], climate and diet play a crucial role in the formation of UA stones. Hot and dry climate increases fluid losses with reduced urinary volume and decreased urinary pH. Consistent with these, our studies showed the incidence of UA stone in Southern China was the highest, followed by Central, Northern, Eastern and Southwest in China. For those uric acid-calcium oxalate mixed stones, some research indicated that patients with this kind of mixed stones presented with metabolic abnormalities that promote both CaOx and UA stone formation [27, 28]. We supposed that the process of uric acid crystals deposition and that of calcium oxalate crystals deposition may promote each other, whichever occurred first, the formation process probably accelerate when the other emerged. Therefore, uric acid and calcium oxalate crystals may be distributed in the core or outer layer or in circular layers.

There were other epidemiologic surveys in other countries. A study in the United States indicated that the prevalence of urinary stones in Southeast was almost twice of that in Northwest, which was ascribed to climatologic factors [29]. Moreover, another research based on five U.S. metropolitan areas further confirmed the strongest association between high temperature and kidney stones [30]. Furthermore, a multi-center analysis in Germany also showed significant regional differences in urinary stone distribution: a higher rate of uric acid stones in Southern Germany was supposed to be associated with their diets based on more red meat, and the higher incidence of infectious stones in Eastern Germany maybe due to lower standard medical care and infections [19].

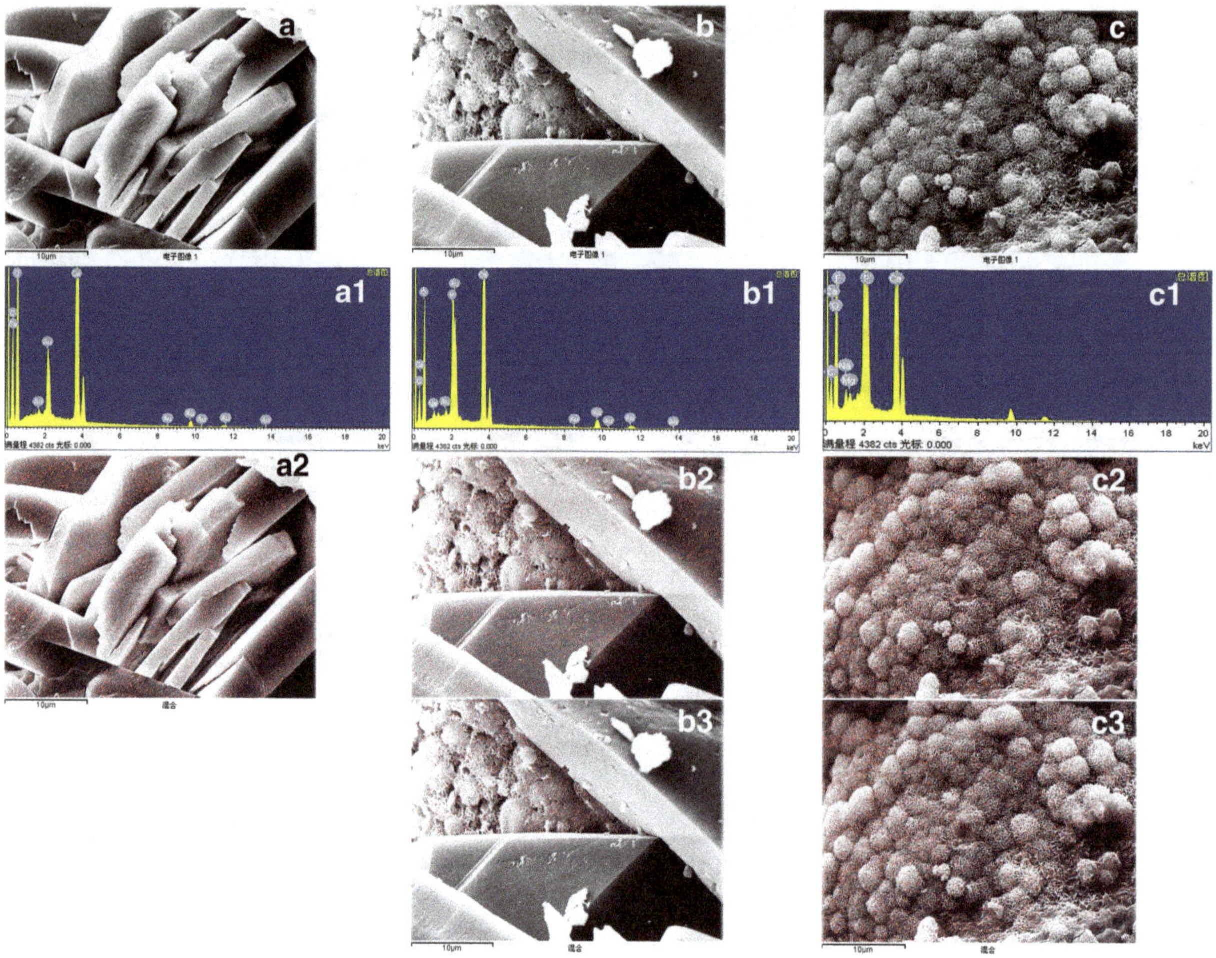

Fig. 3 Calcium and phosphorus distribution in calcium oxalate and calcium phosphate crystals (the red dot represented element distribution). **a** calcium oxalate crystals: A1. The energy spectrum, A2. Calcium distribution; **b** Calcium oxalate- calcium phosphate mixed crystals: B1. The energy spectrum, B2. Calcium distribution, B3. Phosphorus distribution; **c** Calcium phosphate crystals: C1. The energy spectrum, C2. Calcium distribution, C3. Phosphorus distribution

As reported, urinary stone form in multiphase steps, apart from the specific conditions like molar concentrations, pH, temperature, etc., different types of trace elements may also affect the crystallization process [31]. In the present study, X-ray energy spectrometer analysis indicated that besides the major elements of urinary stones, other minor elements, such as Na, Cl, Mg, Al, K, Fe, Zn, S, F, Nb, Tc, Hf, Cr and Si were also detected. According to the present study and the previous reports, we found they might play an important part in the urinary stone formation. What is the role of different elements? A study showed sodium concentration was marginally associated with increased risk of stone formation in elder participants (mean age of 61 years) with a history of kidney stone [32]. Nevertheless, the relationship between the sodium content and the risk of formation urinary stone is still under limited studies. Magnesium is also essential to stone formation. One study suggested an oral of 500 mg magnesium oxide each day may inhibit the crystallization of CaO_X stones in normal volunteers [33], yet a research on rats implied that strict restriction of dietary magnesium may promote stone formation [34]. Potassium was also known as a lithogenesis inhibitor, a randomized trial demonstrated that potassium citrate can prevent the formation of new stones in idiopathic hypocitraturic calcium nephrolithiasis patients [35]. Aluminum is a non-essential element for human. One study showed that a positive correlation between aluminum level in the urine and stones, as well as between urine and hair, suggesting aluminum probably play a role in stone formation [36]. Another study indicated that Al^{3+} affected crystal growth of calcium phosphate at physiologic concentration, but evidence for the inhibitory role in calcium phosphate stone growth was insufficient [37]. Sulphur is an essential nonmetal element existing in all the cells of human body, and

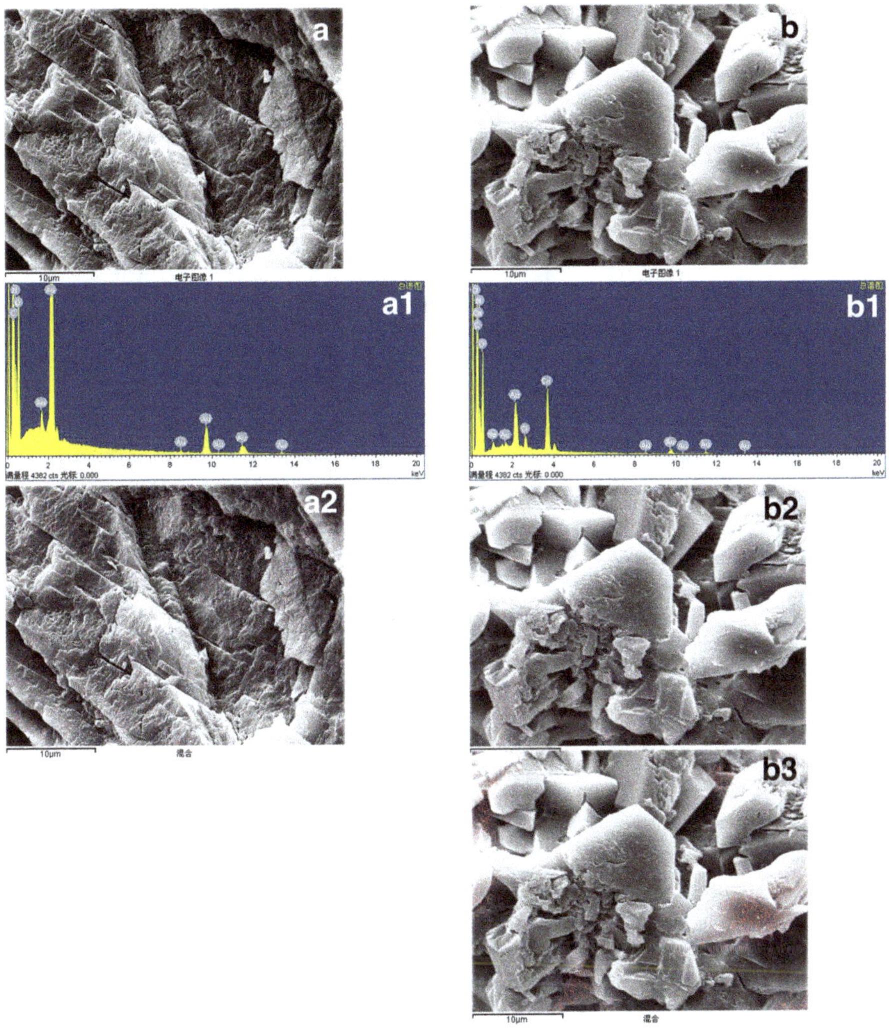

Fig. 4 Nitrogen and calcium distribution in uric acid and uric acid- calcium oxalate mixed crystals (the red dot represented element distribution). **a** Uric acid crystals: A1. The energy spectrum, A2. Nitrogen distribution; **b** Uric acid- calcium oxalate mixed crystals: B1. The energy spectrum, B2. Nitrogen distribution, B3. Calcium distribution

mainly obtained from sulfur-containing proteins in diet. The effects of sulphur on urinary stone formation are almost unknown, but yet a report indicated animal protein-induced hypercalciuria result in the presence of nonresorbable calcium sulfate in the tubular lumen, which may further lead to sulfate production and stone formation [38]. Moreover, the effects of zinc on urinary stone formation was controversial. One research suggested a positive correlation of dietary zinc intake and the risk of kidney stone [39], another showed zinc acts as an inhibitor on the formation of calcium oxalate stone [40]. Silicon may be an essential element for human. A previous research showed silicon plays an essential part in the metabolism of calcium and magnesium [41]. Furthermore, another research indicated ingestion of trisilicate may result in the formation stone entirely or partially composed of silica [42]. Nevertheless, how silicon make an effect on urinary stone formation is still unclear. In the present study, sodium, magnesium, potassium presented a scattered distribution in the profile of urinary stones, while aluminum was more concentrated in the interior than the crust of the stones and usually accompanied with calcium phosphate crystals, which suggest that aluminum may play a role in the early phase of lithogenesis.

Conclusions

The systemic analysis of urinary stones from the Northern, Eastern, Central, Southern and Southwest China by a multi-center study indicated that the material and elements composition of urinary stones among different regions had some difference. Calcium oxalate stone has the highest constituent ratio in Southwest China, while anhydrous uric acid stones have a highest constituent

Table 3 Clinical characteristics of patients with each type of stone

Stone type		Calcium Oxalate		Calcium Phosphate		Uric Acid		Calcium oxalate-calcium phosphate mixed		Other rare type		Total
	No	4995		489		1398		1831		360		9073
	Rate (%)	55.05%		5.39%		15.41%		20.18%		3.97%		100%
	Age (years) & gender	Male	Female	Male	Female	Male	Female	Male	Female	Male	Female	
Upper urinary stones	< 20	48	18	0	6	0	0	12	6	0	6	96
	20~29	174	87	18	33	2	2	105	54	18	2	495
	30~39	546	204	18	71	46	8	213	120	21	15	1262
	40~49	909	432	24	60	132	40	258	225	48	29	2157
	50~59	753	522	51	62	168	80	183	189	42	48	2098
	60~69	396	273	24	29	95	78	72	75	15	33	1090
	> = 70	99	57	0	6	25	23	2	23	6	9	250
	Total	2925	1593	135	267	468	231	845	692	150	142	7448
Lower urinary stones	< 20	3	3	3	0	3	2	0	0	2	3	19
	20~29	3	3	0	1	10	1	42	12	0	0	72
	30~39	45	1	15	9	15	3	27	6	0	3	124
	40~49	87	2	9	1	33	3	36	3	9	3	186
	50~59	126	6	15	3	78	23	60	3	6	3	323
	60~69	108	3	15	1	205	3	54	2	12	3	406
	> = 70	87	0	12	3	315	5	48	1	21	3	495
	Total	459	18	69	18	659	40	267	27	50	18	1625
Total		3384	1611	204	285	1127	271	1112	719	200	160	9073

ratio in Southern China. It was confirmed that composition of urinary stones has wide geographic variation and the formation of which was associated with environmental factors (water quality and soil) as well as dietary structure, weather and climate. Moreover, the clinical characteristics were highly correlated with stone types and anatomical locations but not their regions. Furthermore, different type of urinary stones presented distinct elemental composition and distribution, and some minor element may play an important role in the formation of urinary stones. These findings would be meaningful to prevent stone occurrence and recurrence in general population from different areas of China in future.

Abbreviations

CaOx: Calcium oxalate; FTIR: Fourier transform infrared spectroscopy; SEM: Scanning electron microscopy; UA: Uric acid

Acknowledgments

We are grateful to Chun-yu Qi, Ming-quan Chen in the Urinary Surgery Department of our hospital and Yong Liu, Qi-jun Huang in the KingMed Dignostics Center of Guangzhou for kindly providing the specimens. We thank our colleagues in the Urinary Surgery Department and the operating room for their enthusiastic help, and the leaders of our hospital for their support.

Authors' contributions

Conceived and designed the experiments or acquisition of data: RHM, XBL, QL and HQZ. Performed the experiments: RHM, XBL, HQZ. Analyzed the data: RHM, XBL, HQZ. Contributed reagents/materials/analysis tools: QL. Wrote the paper or involved in drafting the manuscript: RHM, XBL, HQZ. Critical revision of the manuscript: QL. All authors read and approved the final manuscript.

Author details

[1]The Department of Clinical Laboratory, The Sixth People's Hospital of Nansha, Xingye Road No. 7, Dagang Town, Nansha, Guangzhou 511470, People's Republic of China. [2]The Department of Pulmonary, Critical Care and Sleep, Yale School of Medicine, New Haven, USA.

References

1. Ramello A, Vitale C, Marangella M. Epidemiology of nephrolithiasis. J Nephrol. 2000;S(3):S45–50.
2. Alaya A, Nouri A, Belgith M, Saad H, Jouini R, Najjar MF. Changes in urinary stone composition in the Tunisian population: a retrospective study of 1,301 cases. Ann Lab Med. 2012;32(3):177–83.
3. Zeng Q, He Y. Age-specific prevalence of kidney stones in Chinese urban inhabitants. Urolithiasis. 2013;41:91–3.
4. Romero V, Akpinar H, Assimos DG. Kidney stones: a global picture of prevalence, incidence, and associated risk factors. Rev Urol. 2010;12:e86–96.
5. Ning X, Zhan C, Yang Y, Yang L, Tu J, Gu H, et al. Secular trends in prevalence of overweight and obesity among adults in rural Tianjin, China from 1991 to 2011: a population-based study. PLoS One. 2014;9:e116019.
6. Hesse A, Brandle E, Wilbert D, Kohrmann KU, Alken P. Study on the prevalence and incidence of urolithiasis in Germany comparing the years 1979 vs. 2000. Eur Urol. 2003;44:709–13.
7. Ma RH, Luo XB, Li Q, Zhong HQ. The systematic classification of urinary stones combine-using FTIR and SEM-EDAX. Int J Surg. 2017;41:150–61.
8. Lieske JC, Rule AD, Krambeck AE, Williams JC, Bergstralh EJ, Mehta RA, et al. Stone composition as a function of age and sex. Clin J Am Soc Nephrol. 2014;9:2141–6.
9. Scales CD Jr, Smith AC, Hanley JM, Saigal CS. Prevalence of kidney stones in the United States. Eur Urol. 2012;62:160–5.

10. Trinchieri A, Coppi F, Montanari E, Del Nero A, Zanetti G, Pisani E. Increase in the prevalence of symptomatic upper urinary tract stones during the last ten years. Eur Urol. 2000;37:23–5.
11. Rosenstein I, Osborn RS, Hopewell JP, Hamilton-Miller JM, Brumfitt W. Bacteriological and crystallographical analysis of urinary calculi: aid to patient management. J R Soc Med. 1984;77(6):478–82.
12. Holmes RP, Knight J, Assimos DG. Lowering urinary oxalate excretion to decrease calcium oxalate stone disease. Urolithiasis. 2016;44(1):27–32.
13. Lieske JC, Tremaine WJ, De Simone C, O'Connor HM, Li X, Bergstralh EJ, et al. Diet, but not oral probiotics, effectively reduces urinary oxalate excretion and calcium oxalate supersaturation. Kidney Int. 2010;78:1178–85.
14. Borghi L, Schianchi T, Meschi T, Guerra A, Allegri F, Maggiore U, et al. Comparison of two diets for the prevention of recurrent stones in idiopathic hypercalciuria. N Engl J Med. 2002;346:77–84.
15. Yang Y, Deng Y, Wang Y. Major geogenic factors controlling geographical clustering of urolithiasis in China. Sci Total Environ. 2016;571:1164–71.
16. Li D, Wen L, Jiang S, Song T, Wang K. Responses of soil nutrients and microbial communities to three restoration strategies in a karst area, Southwest China. J Environ Manag. 2018;207:456–64.
17. Carpentier X, Daudon M, Traxer O, Jungers P, Mazouyes A, Matzen G, et al. Relationships between carbonation rate of carbapatite and morphologic characteristics of calcium phosphate stones and etiology. Urology. 2009; 73(5):968–75.
18. Mandel N, Mandel I, Fryjoff K, Rejniak T, Mandel G. Conversion of calcium oxalate to calcium phosphate with recurrent stone episodes. J Urol. 2003; 169(6):2026–9.
19. Knoll T, Schubert AB, Fahlenkamp D, Leusmann DB, Wendt-Nordahl G, Schubert G. Urolithiasis through the ages: data on more than 200, 000 urinary stone analyses. J Urol. 2011;185(4):1304–11.
20. Marchini GS, Sarkissian C, Tian D, Gebreselassie S, Monga M. Gout, stone composition and urinary stone risk: a matched case comparative study. J Urol. 2013;189:1334.
21. Daudon M, Doré JC, Jungers P, Lacour B. Changes in stone composition according to age and gender of patients: A multivariate epidemiological approach. Urol Res. 2004;32:241–7.
22. Maalouf NM, Sakhaee K, Parks JH, Coe FL, Adams-Huet B, Pak CY. Association of urinary pH with body weight in nephrolithiasis. Kidney Int. 2004;65:1422–5.
23. Abate N, Chandalia M, Cabo-Chan AV Jr, Moe OW, Sakhaee K. The metabolic syndrome and uric acid nephrolithiasis: novel features of renal manifestation of insulin resistance. Kidney Int. 2004;65:386–92.
24. Daudon M, Traxer O, Conort P, Lacour B, Jungers P. Type 2 diabetes increases the risk for uric acid stones. J Am Soc Nephrol. 2006;17:2026–33.
25. Ordon M, Andonian S, Blew B, Schuler T, Chew B, Pace KT. CUA guideline: management of ureteral calculi. Can Urol Assoc J. 2015;9(11–12):E837–51.
26. Trinchieri A, Montanari E. Prevalence of renal uric acid stones in the adult. Urolithiasis. 2017;45(6):553–62.
27. Alvarez Arroyo MV, Traba ML, Rapado A. Hypocitraturia as a pathogenic risk factor in the mixed (calcium oxalate/uric acid) renal stones. Urol Int. 1992; 48(3):342–6.
28. Friedlander JI, Moreira DM, Hartman C, Elsamra SE, Smith AD, Okeke Z. Comparison of the metabolic profile of mixed calcium oxalate/uric acid stone formers to that of pure calcium oxalate and pure uric acid stone formers. Urology. 2014;84(2):289–94.
29. Soucie JM, Thun MJ, Coates RJ, McClellan W, Austin H. Demographic and geographic variability of kidney stones in the United States. Kidney Int. 1994;46(3):893–9.
30. Tasian GE, Pulido JE, Gasparrini A, Saigal CS, Horton BP, Landis JR, et al. Daily mean temperature and clinical kidney stone presentation in five U.S. metropolitan areas: a time-series analysis. Environ Health Perspect. 2014; 122(10):1081–7.
31. Wilson EV, Bushiri MJ, Vaidyan VK. Characterization and FTIR spectral studies of human urinary stones from southern India. Spectrochim Acta A Mol Biomol Spectrosc. 2010;77(2):442–5.
32. Curhan GC, Willett WC, Speizer FE, Stampfer MJ. Twenty-four-hour urine chemistries and the risk of kidney stones among women and men. Kidney Int. 2001;59:2290–8.
33. Kato Y, Yamaguchi S, Yachiku S, Nakazono S, Hori J, Wada N, et al. Changes in urinary parameters after oral administration of potassium-sodium citrate and magnesium oxide to prevent urolithiasis. Urology. 2004;63:7–11 discussion 11–12.
34. Kasaoka S, Kitano T, Hanai M, Futatsuka M, Esashi T. Effect of dietary magnesium level on nephrocalcinosis and growth in rats. J Nutr Sci Vitaminol (Tokyo). 1998;44:503–14.
35. Barcelo P, Wuhl O, Servitge E, Rousaud A, Pak CY. Randomized double-blind study of potassium citrate in idiopathic hypocitraturic calcium nephrolithiasis. J Urol. 1993;150:1761–4.
36. Słojewski M, Czerny B, Safranow K, Jakubowska K, Olszewska M, Pawlik A, et al. Microelements in stones, urine, and hair of stone formers: a new key to the puzzle of lithogenesis? Biol Trace Elem Res. 2010;137:301–16.
37. Meyer JL, Angino EE. The role of trace metals in calcium urolithiasis. Investig Urol. 1977;14:347–50.
38. Heilberg IP, Goldfarb DS. Optimum nutrition for kidney stone disease. Adv Chronic Kidney Dis. 2013;20:165–74.
39. Tang J, McFann K, Chonchol M. Dietary zinc intake and kidney stone formation: evaluation of NHANES III. Am J Nephrol. 2012;36:549–53.
40. Atakan IH, Kaplan M, Seren G, Aktoz T, Gül H, Inci O. Serum, urinary and stone zinc, iron, magnesium and copper levels in idiopathic calcium oxalate stone patients. Int Urol Nephrol. 2007;39:351–6.
41. Najda J, Gmiński J, Drózdz M, Danch A. The action of excessive, inorganic silicon (Si) on the mineral metabolism of calcium (ca) and magnesium (mg). Biol Trace Elem Res. 1993;37:107–14.
42. Haddad FS, Kouyoumdjian A. Silica stones in humans. Urol Int. 1986;41:70–6.

4

A rare case of primary malignant fibrous histiocytoma: A sarcoma of the kidney

Forough Ebrahimtabar[1], Hamid Shafi[2*], Mohammad Ranaee[3] and Mohammad Mehdi Darzi[2]

Abstract

Background: Primary malignant fibrous histiocytoma of the kidney (MFH) is an extremely rare tumor which is indistinguishable from its' mimics in particular renal cell carcinoma (RCC) by clinical features and preoperative imaging evaluation. Due to its high predilection to local recurrence and distant metastases, early diagnosis has great value.

Case presentation: Herein, we describe a 62 year-old man with a 3-month history of abdominal discomfort and a palpable right loin mass whom computerized tomography (CT) showed a large heterogeneous solid mass in the right kidney. With the suspicious to RCC; the patient underwent radical nephrectomy. However, histopathological report revealed pleomorphic-storiform malignant fibrous histiocytoma. Immunohistochemistry study was also confirmed the diagnosis of MFH. Six month follow up showed no evidence of any recurrence.

Conclusions: The therapeutic options for MFH differ from other renal tumors, hence histopathology and immunohistochemistry studies are required to establish a definite diagnosis of the disease. Despite of progress made in clinical studies and advances in diagnostic modalities, early diagnosis of MFH has not achieved yet. Further studies and accumulated experience with renal MFH are required to determine the approach to prolong survival in selected cases along with management and prognostic factors of such tumors.

Keywords: Malignant fibrosis histiocytoma, Sarcoma, Kidney, Immunohistochemistry

Background

Primary malignant fibrous histiocytoma (MFH) is a rare mesenchymal-derived sarcoma that belongs to a group of soft tissue malignancies with fibroblastic and histiocytic differentiation [1–3]. Although MFH is a rare disease, it has been classically defined as the most common type of renal sarcoma occurring more frequently in late adult population [4–6]. MFH is commonly found in the extremities and abdomen, but rarely in retroperitoneum with the primeval involvement of Kidney [7, 8]. Generally it is known as a poor prognostic disease with a great tendency to distant metastasis and a high rate of recurrence (> 50%) [7–11]. There are no definite clinical and radiological signs for early diagnosis of MFH [9, 12, 13]. Due to its low 5-year survival (14%) [7], early diagnostic finding can be incredibly beneficial. To the best of our knowledge, it's the first case of renal MFH reported from Iran. Clinical manifestation of this case raised our suspicious to RCC due to its non-specified features of tumor such as hematuria that commonly seen in cases of RCC. Hereby, the clinical course of this case, histological study and management of primary renal malignant fibrous histiocytoma is discussed.

Case report

A 62 year-old man presented with a 3-month history of obscure abdominal discomfort accompanied by sensation of mass in his right loin. He also complained from voiding difficulty and frequency. Physical examination confirmed the presence of a large, mobile and non-tender mass in the right flank. His past medical history was uneventful. Hematological tests showed leukocytosis (12.9×10^3 μL) with thrombocytosis (664×10^3 μL), elevated erythrocyte sedimentation rate (87 mm/hr) along with increased C-reactive protein level (86.2 mg/L). Urine analysis showed a number of RBC (15–16/hpf) in urine, explaining the microscopic hematuria. Tumor markers test revealed a raised prostate specific antigen level (PSA = 4.195 ng/ml). Serum biochemistry and chest X-ray were unremarkable. Ultrasound

* Correspondence: dr_hamidshafi@yahoo.com
[2]Department of Urology, Faculty of Medicine, Babol University of Medical Sciences, School of Medicine, Babol, Iran
Full list of author information is available at the end of the article

examination demonstrated a hypervascular encapsulated Solid cystic tumor (114 × 108 × 97 mm) in the lower zone of the right kidney. Mild hydronephrosis was seen as a result of the tumor compression. Computerized tomography (CT) also detected a large heterogeneous solid mass (131 × 129 mm) in the lower-mid portion of the right kidney with the extension to the hilum causing renal parenchymal destruction. The mass adhered to inferior vena cava (IVC) without the invasion of tumor to the IVC or thrombosis. There was no involvement of adjacent structures. In addition, a non-specific calcified nodule (12 mm) was disclosed next to the upper pole of the right kidney. The preoperative metastatic work-up showed no abnormalities. With the great suspicious to RCC, the patient underwent right nephrectomy via thoracoabdominal approach.

During hospitalization, hematological and biochemical tests were evaluated again. The levels of the erythrocyte sedimentation rate, white blood count and platelet count were all normalized. However, the laboratory data showed that creatinine level briskly increased to 4 mg/dl without oliguria. After nephrology consult and appropriate measures, the patient was discharged 7 days postoperatively in a satisfactory condition and with the following laboratory data: urea = 55.4 mg/dl, BUN = 25.9 mg/dl, creatinine = 2.25 mg/dl, glomerular filtration rate = 32 ml/min. To date, 6 months after surgery, the patient is alive with no evidence of disease recurrence.

Considering to pathological study, nephrectomy specimen was grossly 21 × 16.5 × 11 cm in size and consisted of a huge tumor attached to the kidney with the prerenal fat. The cut incision disclosed a relative hypervascular tumor with almost soft consistency arising from medial portion of upper pole to lower lobe with the extra-renal extension. The tumor was mostly separated from renal parenchyma with a definite border except some upper parts of the tumor which were admixed to the renal parenchyma. There was no evidence of adrenal gland or pericolic fat on the surface of tumor and the tumor did not invade into the perinephric tissue.

Microscopic examination showed a mesenchymal tumor with different patterns, including uniformed to sometimes pleomorphic nuclei spindle cells in a storiform arrangement embedded in variant amount of fibrous stroma (Fig. 1 (a)). Most part of the tumor was occupied by pleomorphic and atypical histiocytic cells arranged in a cartwheel or storiform pattern. Mononuclear to multinucleated giant cells were presented with bizarre-shaped hyperchromatic nucleus and frequent mitotic activity (Fig. 2 (a)). Areas of myxoid change and hyalinization along with aggregates of lymphocytes were also seen throughout the lesion. The tumor was not extended to pelvic, renal vessels and ureter segment. Immunohistochemical analysis revealed strong reactivity for CD68 (Fig. 2 (a)), vimentin and CD34 (Fig. 2 (b)), but the tumor was negative for CD10, Pan-cytokeratin (Fig. 2 (d)), S100 protein, desmin and H.coldesmon. Based on histological and immunohistological studies, a diagnosis of pleomorphic malignant fibrous histiocytoma was established.

Discussion and conclusions

Renal MFH is a rarely seen mesenchymal malignant tumors comprising 1–3% of the kidney malignant tumors and about 6% of all primary renal sarcomas [12, 14, 15]. It was first established by O'Brien and Stout in 1964 with the name of malignant fibrous xanthoma [1]. MFH occurs most commonly during 6th–7th decade of life with equal sex distribution [11, 16]. The most predilection site of MFH is the extremities, followed by body trunk and retroperitoneum [7, 17]. There are also infrequent sites, such as prostate [18], spermatic cord [19], bladder [20, 21], and kidney [4, 7]. The most frequent symptoms encountered are abdominal or flank pain, palpable mass and weight loss [3, 22–24]. Although hematuria is known as a common symptom of RCC, it rarely can be an evidence of

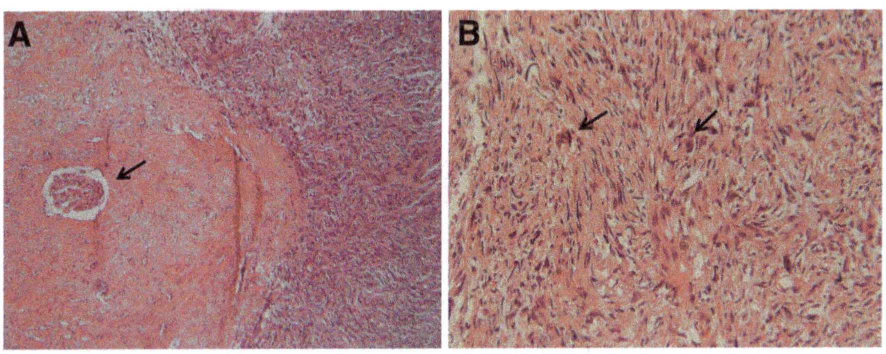

Fig. 1 Microscopic appearance of renal sarcoma. (**a**) The tumor composed of pleomorphic spindle cells with storiform pattern which attached to kidney parenchyma (the arrow shows the glomeruli of kidney). (**b**) Frequent atypical mitosis of spindle cells has shown in this figure (haematoxylin-eosin, original magnification (**a**) 40X, (**b**) 100X)

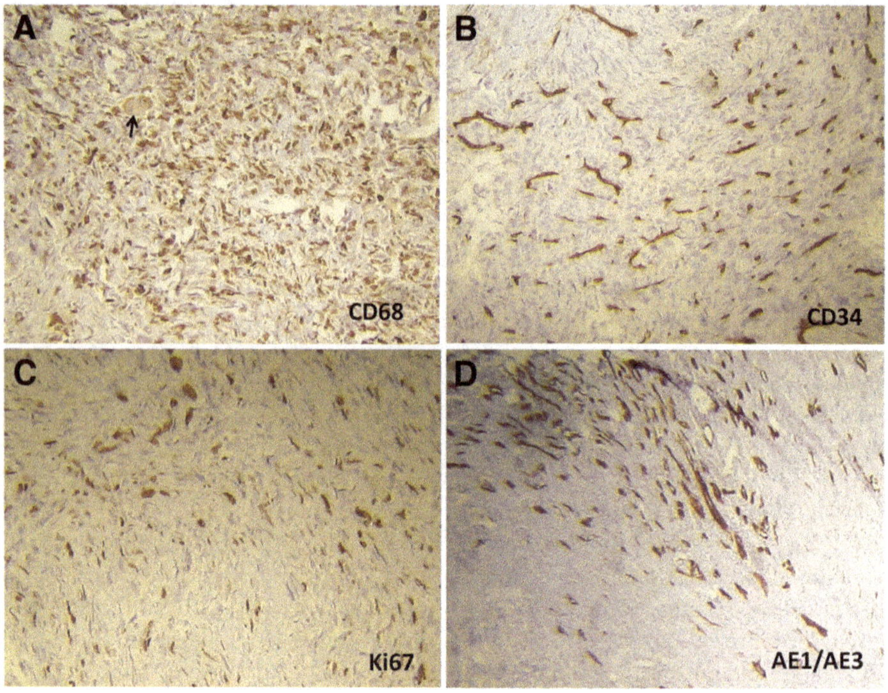

Fig. 2 Immunohistochemistry (IHC) findings. (**a**) Tumor cells was positive for CD68 and multinucleated giant cell was observed in this Fig. (**b**) CD34 was negative in the tumor but positive in the vessel walls. (**c**) Ki67 was examined as a proliferation marker of tumor cells. (**d**) AE1/AE3 was negative in the tumor but positive in the kidney tubules. (IHC, original magnification 100X)

MFH [9, 24, 25]. A review of literature yielded only one case presented without any symptoms and found out incidentally via ultrasonography [24].

Nonspecific symptoms and indefinite radiological features make MFH indistinguishable from its preoperatively differential diagnosis specially RCC [3]. The diagnosis mostly depends on postoperative histology with the assistance of immunohistochemistry [24–26]. Regarding the histopatalogical studies, MFH as a mesenchymal tumor typically surrounded by a pseudocapsule. In many cases this can be found in the form of local recurrence and it's difficult to be recognized macroscopically [27]. Specific findings suggestive of sarcoma rather than RCC include its potency to growth without lymph nodes involvement and its origination which mostly arise from capsule or perisinuous region [28]. Because renal MFH mostly arise from the capsule, hematuria can be found rarely. In our case, we found microscopic hematuria regarding to his urinalysis examination which raised our suspicious to RCC. Further studies are necessary to find out definite diagnostic and therapeutic approaches for this type of kidney sarcoma.

Histologically, MFH is divided to five types, including storiform-pleomorphic, myxoid, giant cells, inflammatory and angiomatoid [9, 29, 30], among which the storiform-pleomorphic type is the most usual and commonly high grade variant of MFH [24, 31]. MFH is characterized by typical immunepositivity for CD68, vimentin and alfa-1-antitrypsin that can differentiate it from other renal sarcomas [29] and among these markers, CD68 has become as a specific histological marker for confirming MFH [32]. Our case was also consistent with storiform arrangement of spindle cells admixed with mononuclear to multinucleated giant cells and histiocytic cells known as a histological hallmark of MFH [33] and the diagnosis was confirmed by immunohistological staining. This pleomorphic undifferentiated sarcoma portends a poor prognosis with a high risk of recurrence and distal metastases. Metastases can particularly occur in lung, lymph node, liver and bone [9, 10, 31]. Rate of metastases correlates with depth of the tumor, size, inflammatory component and myxoid change [16, 34]. Myoxid type is recognized as a high grade variant, often presented with low metastatic tendency. Therefore because of its favorable prognosis, it seems to be essential to distinct this entity from other non-myoxid types of MFH [31, 33] .

According to the literatures, most of the cases underwent radical nephrectomy as a choice of primarily treatment which is usually followed by radiotherapy, chemotherapy [12, 25, 31] and immunotherapy [35, 36]. However the success of these modalities for preventing local recurrence or distant metastases were not satisfactory, among which 25% of patients die within 1 year [7, 37]. The few reported cases of renal MFH with details are summarizedin Table 1.

Table 1 Details of survival, prognosis and other related factors of MFH cases from 2006-2017

Author	Year	Management	Chemo/radio	Pathology	immune histochemistry	Survival (months/ years)	Metastasis & recurrence
Gil-Julio H et al., [9]	2012	Partial nephrectomy	------------------	pleomorphic MFH (with an abundant giant-cell population)	CD_{68} +	After a 41-month follow-up period, she was alive	During follow up period, there was no evidence of recurrence
Pathrose G et al., [16]	2015	Radical nephrectomy& splenectomy	---------	Inflammatory subtype of MFH (pleomorphic spindle cells, interspersed with foamy histiocytes)	CD_{68} + anti α1 antichymotrysin+	------------------------	------------------------
Ghosh A et al., [22]	2008	Radical nephrectomy	------------------	Inflammatory subtype of MFH (xanthoma cells with atypical histiocytes, mononuclear and multinu-Cleated giant cells)	Vimentin+	The patient died, 11 months after surgery	local recurrence, and pulmonary metastasis
Chen Y et al., [25]	2014	radical nephrectomy	The patient refused further treatment	MFH	Vimentin+, CD_{68} +	she remains alive, 78 months after first operation	9-month after surgery, a metastatic focus was found near to the abdominal aorta, however 12 and 18 months after first surgery, the metastases had disappeared (CT scan examination).
Gogus C et al., [26]	2013	Radical nephrectomy& resection of colon	Poly-chemotherapy (Adriblastina, Holoxan, Uromitexan, and radiotherapy)	MFH penetrated the capsule (Spindle-shaped fibroblastic cells in collagenous stroma)	CD10++, vimentin ++ and CD68++. α1-antitrypsin+ and α1-antichymotrypsin +	she died within the first postoperative year	Five months after operation, she was found with multiple metastases. recurrence and omental metastases were observed.
Bairwa S et al., [30]	2017	radical nephrectomy	chemotherapy	MFH (pleomorphic spindle and multinucleated polygonal cells with storiform pattern admixed with some inflammatory cells)	vimentin+	the patient died within 6 months due to recurrence.	There was evidence of recurrence (side of metastasis was not exactly mentioned).
Singh SK et al., [36]	2006	The tumors were found to be non-resectable, so biopsies only were taken.	----------------	Neutrophilic infiltrate, scattered spindle cells and foam cells	CD68+, CD34+	he died due to the disease within 1 month.	--
Cormio L et al., [37]	2014	Radical nephrectomy	Adjuvant radiotherapy (50 Gy in 25 sessions)	MFH (pleomorphic, and multinucleated cells, admixed with inflammatory cells)	Vimentin+	five years after surgery, she was alive	no evidence of disease recurrence.
Hsiao PJ et al., [42]	2016	exploratory laparotomy (the tumor was not completely removed at first. 6 months later, whole tumor resected by En bloc method)	neo-adjuvant chemotherapy with 4 cycles (mesna, doxorubicin, ifosfamide, dacarbazine).	MFH (spindle cells in a storiform pattern and polygonal or rounded cells)	vimentin+	>5 years without recurrence.	The patient survives without tumor recurrence.

Gil-Julio et al' reported a case with conservative treatment underwent partial nephrectomy without additional radiotherapy or chemotherapy modalities and survived after 41-month of follow-up period [9]. *Cormio* et al' case report showed a conflicting result of a 68 year-old woman whom received adjuvant radiotherapy with considerable long-term survival consequence (72 months after surgery) as well as *Hsiao PJ* et al' whose patient was alive more than 5 five years after neo-adjuvant chemotherapy [37, 38]. On the other hand, *Göğüş* et al' report revealed recurrence and metastases after five months postoperatively, and the patient died within the first postoperative year despite of polychemotherapy [26]. Therefore, the role of adjuvant radio or chemotherapy have not been found to be of obvious benefit and most of the patients succumbing to the local recurrence within the first year post radical nephrectomy [11, 25]. Our case received adjuvant chemotherapy without evidence of recurrence during 6 months follow up. Due to the poor prognosis of MFH disease and its tendency for metastasis, it is recommended that to follow up cases for longer periods.

Some case studies provide evidence of synchronization of renal MFH with transitional cell carcinoma of bladder or contralateral renal cell carcinoma [39, 40]. Therefore, it is important to be aware of other synchronous renal tumor through our work-ups.

In conclusion, malignant fibrous histiocytoma (MFH) term has implied as a rare aggressive tumor with a short term survival and poor prognosis [41, 42]. Due to the nonspecific symptoms and indefinite radiological signs, preoperative diagnosis of MFH is almost impossible which depends on postoperative histopathology. Radical nephrectomy is referred as the best choice of treatment. Adjuvant chemotherapy or radiotherapy have usually used which may not alter the poor prognosis of the disease [33]. It still needs more experience and additional case reports to early detection of the tumor related to the therapeutic consequence and prognosis.

Abbreviations

CT: computed tomography; IVC: inferior vena cava; MFH: malignant fibrous histiocytoma; RCC: renal cell carcinoma

Acknowledgements

The authors wish to thank Dr. A. Firouzjaee, head of the Department of Pathology, Rohani Hospital, for kindly reviewing the slides of the primary tumor in case.

Authors' contributions

FE did conception and design of the study, acquisition of data, interpretation of data and drafted the manuscript. HS made substantial contributions to conception and revising it critically for important intellectual content. MR performed the histological examination of the kidney and revised the pathological section of study. MMD was involved in the operation of the case and acquisition of data. All authors read and approved the final manuscript.

Author details

[1]Faculty of Medicine, Babol University of Medical Sciences, Babol, Iran. [2]Department of Urology, Faculty of Medicine, Babol University of Medical Sciences, School of Medicine, Babol, Iran. [3]Department of Pathology, School of Medicine, Babol University of Medical Sciences, Babol, Iran.

References

1. O'Brien JE, Stout AP. Malignant fibrous xanthomas. Cancer. 1964;17:1445–55.
2. Weiss S, Goldblum JR. Enzinger and Weiss's Soft Tissue Tumors. St Louis, MO: Mosby. Inc; 2001.
3. Kollias G, Giannopoulos T. Primary malignant fibrous histiocytoma of the kidney: report of a case. J Urol. 1987;138(2):400–1.
4. Papadopoulos I, Rudolph P. Primary renal malignant fibrous histiocytoma: case report. Urol Int. 1999;63(2):136–8.
5. Chen KT. Malignant fibrous histiocytoma of the kidney. J Surg Oncol. 1984; 27(4):248–50.
6. Zagars GK, Mullen JR, Pollack A. Malignant fibrous histiocytoma: outcome and prognostic factors following conservation surgery and radiotherapy. Int J Radiat Oncol Biol Phys. 1996;34(5):983–94.
7. Kim SJ, Ahn BC, Kim SR, Kim YB, Joo HJ, Lee KB, et al. Primary malignant fibrous histiocytoma of the kidney. Yonsei Med J. 2002;43(3):399–402.
8. Froehner M, Manseck A, Haase M, Hakenberg OW, Wirth MP. Locally recurrent malignant fibrous histiocytoma: a rare and aggressive genitourinary malignancy. Urol Int. 1999;62(3):164–70.
9. Gil-Julio H, Vazquez-Alonso F, Puche-Sanz I, Fernandez-Sanchez AJ, Cozar-Olmo JM. Conservative treatment of malignant fibrous histiocytoma of the kidney: a case report. Curr Urol. 2012;6(1):46–9.
10. Sugihara T, Fujimura T, Kume H, Homma Y. Successful treatment of metastatic malignant fibrous histiocytoma of the kidney. Urol Int. 2010;85(1): 118–20.
11. Tarjan M, Cserni G, Szabo Z. Malignant fibrous histiocytoma of the kidney. Scand J Urol Nephrol. 2001;35(6):518–20.
12. Kitajima K, Kaji Y, Morita M, Okuda Y, Sugimura K. Malignant fibrous histiocytoma arising from the renal capsule. Magn Reson Med Sci. 2003;2(4): 199–202.
13. Mellas S, Bouchikhi AA, Tazi MF, Khallouk A, Elammari JE, El Fassi MJ, et al. Primary pleomorphic undifferentiated sarcoma-a rare renal localization: A case report. Case Rep Urol. 2012;2012:862493.
14. Farrow GM, Harrison Jr EG, Utz DC. Sarcomas and sarcomatoid and mixed malignant tumors of the kidney in adults—part II. Cancer. 1968;22(3):551-5.
15. Muretto P, Lemma E, Grianti C, Staccioli MP, Fabbretti G, Sbarbati A. Inflammatory malignant fibrous histiocytoma of the kidney: an immunohistochemical and ultrastructural study. Tumori. 1985;71(2):147–53.
16. Pathrose G, John NT, Manojkumar R. A rare case of malignant fibrous histiocytoma/ pleomorphic undifferentiated sarcoma of the kidney. J Clin Diagn Res. 2015;9(1):Pd27–9.
17. Kearney MM, Soule EH, Ivins JC. Malignant fibrous histiocytoma: a retrospective study of 167 cases. Cancer. 1980;45(1):167.
18. Zhang G, Chen KK, Manivel C, Fraley EE. Sarcomas of the retroperitoneum and genitourinary tract. J Urol. 1989;141(5):1107–10.
19. Glazier DB, Vates TS, Cummings KB, Pickens RL. Malignant fibrous histiocytoma of the spermatic cord. J Urol. 1996;155(3):955–7.
20. Stearns MM, Mitchell AD, Powell NE, Wood WG, Mebust WK. Fibrous histiocytoma of the bladder. J Urol. 1976;115(1):114–5.
21. Karol JB, Eason AA, Tanagho EA. Fibrous histiocytoma of bladder. Urology. 1977;10(6):593–5.
22. Ghosh A, Dwivedi US, Kumar A. Inflammatory malignant fibrous histiocytoma of kidney: a case report. Pathol Res Pract. 2008;204(11):857–61.
23. Resorlu M, Karatag O, Uysal F, Ozturk M. Malignant fibrous histiocytoma in a patient presenting with urinary system symptoms. Rev Assoc Med Bras (1992). 2017;63(11):950–2.
24. Ptochos A, Karydas G, Iosifidis N, Tyrothoulakis E, Papazafiriou G, Kehagia-Koutoufari T. Primary renal malignant fibrous histiocytoma. A case report and review of the literature. Urol Int. 1999;63(4):261–4.
25. Chen Y, Rao D, Zhu H, Yu H, Yang S. Primary malignant fibrous histiocytoma of the renal pelvis: a 78-month follow-up case report. OncoTargets and therapy. 2014;7:1.
26. Gogus C, Gokce MI, Suer E, Tulunay O, Safak M. Primary malignant fibrous histiocytoma of the kidney: report of a case and literature review. Turk J Urol. 2013;39(3):194–7.
27. Russo P, Brady MS, Conlon K, Hajdu SI, Fair WR, Herr HW, Brennan MF. Adult urological sarcoma. J Urol. 1992 Apr;147(4):1032.

28. Shirkhoda A, Lewis E. Renal sarcoma and sarcomatoid renal cell carcinoma: CT and angiographic features. Radiology. 1987 Feb;162(2):353.
29. Rosenberg AE. Malignant fibrous histiocytoma: past, present, and future. Skelet Radiol. 2003;32(11):613–8.
30. Fu DL, Yang F, Maskay A, Long J, Jin C, Yu XJ, et al. Primary intestinal malignant fibrous histiocytoma: two case reports. World J Gastroenterol. 2007;13(8):1299–302.
31. Karki B, Xu YK, Wu YK, Zhang WW. Primary malignant fibrous histiocytoma of the abdominal cavity: CT findings and pathological correlation. World J Radiol. 2012;4(4):151–8.
32. Bairwa S, Sangwaiya A, Ansari M, Jindal A, Singla S, Yadav A. Malignant fibrous histiocytoma arising from renal capsule: an extremely rare entity. Indian J Pathol Microbiol. 2017;60(3):402–4.
33. Raghavaiah NV, Mayer RF, Hagitt R, Soloway MS. Malignant fibrous histiocytoma of the kidney. J Urol. 1980;123(6):951–3.
34. Weiss SW, Enzinger FM. Myxoid variant of malignant fibrous histiocytoma. Cancer. 1977;39(4):1672–85.
35. Mauri D, Panou C, Valachis A, Kamposioras K, Tsali L. Tyrosine kinase inhibitors in treatment of fibrous histiocytoma. Exp Oncol. 2009;31:60–1.
36. Singh SK, Mandal AK, Agarwal MM, Das A. Primary renal inflammatory malignant fibrous histiocytoma: a diagnostic challenge. Int J Urol. 2006; 13(7):1000–2.
37. Cormio L, Sanguedolce F, Massenio P, Di Fino G, Lucarelli G, Mancini V, et al. Long-term results of radical surgery and adjuvant radiotherapy in a case of primary malignant fibrous histiocytoma of the kidney. The Open Urology & Nephrology Journal. 2014;7(1).
38. Hsiao PJ, Chen GH, Chang YH, Chang CH, Chang H, Bai LY. An unresectable retroperitoneal malignant fibrous histiocytoma: a case report. Oncol Lett. 2016 Apr 1;11(4):2403–7.
39. Lopez JI, Angulo JC, Flores N, Toledo JD. Malignant fibrous histiocytoma of the renal capsule and synchronous transitional cell carcinoma of the bladder. Pathol Res Pract. 1996;192(5):468–71 discussion 72-3.
40. Singh EO, Barrett DM, Adams VI. Synchronously occurring malignant fibrous histiocytoma of the kidney with contralateral renal cell carcinoma. J Urol. 1982;128(3):586–8.
41. Goodman AJ, Greaney MG. Malignant fibrous histiocytoma of the bladder. Br J Urol. 1985;57(1):106–7.
42. Kyriakos M, Kempson RL. Inflammatory fibrous histiocytoma. An aggressive and lethal lesion. Cancer. 1976;37(3):1584–606.

5

Hand-assisted living-donor nephrectomy: A retrospective comparison of two techniques

Jeannette D. Widmer[2*], Andrea Schlegel[1], Philipp Kron[1], Marc Schiesser[3], Jens G. Brockmann[4] and Markus K. Muller[1,2]

Abstract

Background: Living-donor nephrectomy (LDN) is challenging, as surgery is performed on healthy individuals. Minimally invasive techniques for LDN have become standard in most centers. Nevertheless, numerous techniques have been described with no consensus on which is the superior approach. Both hand-assisted retroperitoneoscopic (HARS) and hand-assisted laparoscopic (HALS) LDNs are performed at Zurich University Hospital. The aim of this study was to compare these two surgical techniques in terms of donor outcome and graft function.

Method: Retrospective single-center analysis of 60 consecutive LDNs (HARS $n = 30$; HALS $n = 30$) from June 2010 to May 2012, including a one-year follow-up of the recipients.

Results: There was no mortality in either group and little difference in the overall complication rates. Median warm ischemia time (WIT) was significantly shorter in the HARS group. The use of laxatives and the incidence of postoperative vomiting were significantly greater in the HALS group. There was no difference between right- and left-sided nephrectomies in terms of donor outcome and graft function.

Conclusions: Both techniques appear safe for both donors and donated organs. The HARS technique is associated with a shorter WIT and a reduced incidence of postoperative paralytic ileus. Therefore, we consider HARS LDN a valuable alternative to HALS LDN.

Background

For patients with end-stage renal disease, kidney transplantation is the only treatment to improve their survival, and it quickly enhances their quality of life [1, 2]. During the last several decades, living-donors have become the primary source of donor kidneys for transplantation [3]. As well as expanding the donor organ pool, living-donor kidneys allow preemptive transplantation, and surgery can be efficiently planned with both the donor and the recipient in optimum medical condition. Hence, the outcome of living-donor kidney transplantation is superior to transplantation of deceased donor kidneys in terms of improved long-term recipient survival, quality of life, early graft function and better graft survival [4–6]. However, living-donor nephrectomy (LDN) remains a surgical challenge in terms of minimizing postoperative complications as it is performed on healthy individuals. Therefore, the most important goal is ensuring the safety and well-being of the voluntary donor [7–9]. The surgical technique must result in the least possible risk of morbidity without compromising the functional outcome of grafts.

The first laparoscopic donor nephrectomy was performed in 1995 by Kavoussi and Ratner [10] and became a well-established technique due to many advantages, including less postoperative pain, a shorter hospital stay and better cosmetics, when compared to open surgical approaches [11, 12]. In contrast, the prolonged warm ischemia time (WIT) has been highlighted as the major disadvantage [13, 14]. A compromise was found in the hand-assisted laparoscopic (HALS) donor nephrectomy technique, which was first described by Wolf et al. in 1998 [15]. This approach shortens the WIT compared to a purely laparoscopic nephrectomy. Further advantages

* Correspondence: jeannette.widmer@gmx.net
[2]Department of Surgery, Kantonsspital Frauenfeld, 8500 Frauenfeld, Switzerland
Full list of author information is available at the end of the article

include tactile feedback, easier and rapid control of bleeding by digital pressure and more rapid kidney recovery [16, 17]. Injuries to the bowel and/or other organs are more likely by a transperitoneal approach due to its nature of abdominal access [18]. In 2001, Wadström et al. combined the advantages of HALS nephrectomy and the retroperitoneoscopic approach favored by urologists and introduced the hand-assisted retroperitoneoscopic (HARS) LDN technique [19]. Direct access to the kidneys without entering the peritoneal cavity obviates bowel injury and is associated with shorter operating time, shorter WIT, less blood loss and a shorter length of hospital stay compared to HALS LDN [20, 21].

The aim of this study was to compare these two surgical techniques in terms of donor outcome and graft function.

Methods

Donors

All donors undergoing HARS or HALS LDNs at the University Hospital of Zurich between June 2010 and May 2012 and the corresponding recipients were identified. A preoperative work-up was carried out according to our standard donor protocol (conformable to the Amsterdam forum guidelines [22]). Indications and results were discussed by the donor kidney board, which is a panel of transplant surgeons, nephrologists, transplantation coordinators, and immunology and psychology experts who meet on a weekly basis. The decision of which donor kidney to retrieve was based first on functional investigations. In the case of functional differences of less than 3%, anatomical considerations guided surgical decision-making. The guiding principle was to leave the better, greater-functioning organ with the donor. The choice of surgical technique depended on the preference of the lead surgeon. All donors received standard postoperative analgesia plus on-demand medication. Donors were followed-up with in our surgical outpatient clinic at 3 months after surgery.

Surgical procedure

For both techniques, the donor was placed in the contralateral flank position with slight hip flexion, thereby extending the ipsilateral flank.

HARS technique: A Pfannenstiel incision was made to introduce the hand-port (GelPort™, Applied Medical Resources Corporation). The retroperitoneal space was created by blunt dissection. The introduction of the first trocar (camera) in the lateral upper abdomen was guided by the surgeon's hand, followed by insufflation of carbon dioxide up to 12 cm H_2O. One or two additional working trocars were placed under direct vision in the medial lower abdomen. Identification and dissection of the kidney, ureter and vascular structures were performed by hand and with an endoscopic device (Harmonic Ultrasonic Shears, Ethicon). Following complete dissection of all structures, the ureter was clipped and transected distally, and the renal vein and artery were accurately exposed and then divided by a stapler device. The kidney was recovered through the open hand-port.

HALS technique: A periumbilical camera port was introduced into the abdominal cavity, followed by insufflation of carbon dioxide up to 15 cm H_2O. Two or three additional working trocars were placed in the lateral upper and lower abdomen under direct vision. Before clipping the ureter and dividing the renal vein and artery, the hand-port was introduced through a Pfannenstiel incision. After full mobilization, the kidney was extracted through the open hand-port.

Abdominal closure for both techniques was performed in a standard fashion. Drains were not routinely placed.

Recipients

All renal grafts were placed extraperitoneally into the iliac fossa. The immunosuppressive regimen was determined preoperatively depending on immunological and donor-specific risk stratification. Postoperative care was undertaken by the surgical lead. Recipients were followed-up regularly with by the Department of Nephrology at the University Hospital of Zurich.

Data collection

Demographic and clinical data were retrospectively obtained from the clinical information system, which maintains all patients' data electronically. The following parameters from donors and recipients were retrieved: preoperative renal retention parameters, BMI, blood group, and HLA status. Operative time (OT), WIT and organ site were noted. Kidney function (creatinine, GFR) before and after surgery were recorded for both donors and recipients. Delayed graft function (DGF) was defined as the use of dialysis in the first postoperative week [23]. In terms of postoperative parameters, the time to first bowel movement, laxative use, postoperative vomiting, use of analgesics and length of hospital stay were recorded. Complications were routinely ranked using the Clavien-Dindo classification, a five-grade therapy-based system in which higher grades reflect more severe complications [24]. In this study, the Comprehensive Complication Index (CCI), a new scale to better quantify postoperative morbidity, was also applied [25]. All complications arising from a single case and ranked by the Clavien-Dindo classification were summarized and expressed on a scale of 0 to 100. The calculation was made using the CCI® calculator (www.assessurgery.com). The CCI score allows quantification of all complications after a surgical procedure, while the Clavien-Dindo classification describes only the most severe complication. Donors were followed-up until 90 days after surgery.

Statistical analysis

Data analysis was performed using SPSS 21 (SPSS Inc., Chicago IL, USA). All data values presented are median values with an interquartile range (IQR) unless otherwise stated. A bivariate analysis was carried out comparing selected variables in the HALS and HARS cohorts. Differences in continuous variables between groups were tested for statistical significance using the Mann-Whitney U test. For comparison of proportions Fisher's exact tests was used. *P* values < 0.05 were considered statistically significant.

Availability of data and materials

The datasets used and/or analyzed during the current study are available from the corresponding author on reasonable request.

Results

Donor

Demographic and clinical data

A total of 60 live kidney donors were included in the study ($n = 30$ HARS, $n = 30$ HALS). The demographic and clinical characteristics of the kidney donors are summarized in Table 1. There was no relevant difference between the two groups.

Perioperative data

The median OT did not differ considerably between groups (Table 2). Conversion to laparotomy was never required. In the HARS group, 16 (53.3%) patients underwent right-sided donor nephrectomy, compared to 12 (40%) in the HALS group. There was no relevant difference between right- and left-sided nephrectomies within the two groups with regard to postoperative renal function. There was a trend for the OT to be shorter in both groups for right-sided nephrectomies, but these differences did not reach statistical significance (HARS: 132 min versus 145 min, $p = 0.15$; HALS: 140 min versus 180 min, $p = 0.06$).

Median WIT was significantly shorter in the HARS group than in the HALS group (120 s versus 150 s, $p = 0.008$). There was no relevant difference in WIT for left-sided compared to right-sided organ harvest for both surgical techniques.

Table 1 Demographic and clinical characteristics of kidney donors

	HARS ($n = 30$)	HALS ($n = 30$)	*p*-value
Age (years)	56 (17)	50 (18)	0.268
Female	21 (70)	19 (63.3)	0.784
BMI (kg/m^2)	24.8 (4.4)	25.5 (3.8)	0.765
Art. hypertension	4 (13.3)	5 (16.6)	1.000
Right-sided donation	16 (53.3)	12 (40)	0.437

Values are median and IQR, frequencies are in absolute numbers and %

Table 2 Donors' intra- and postoperative data

	HARS ($n = 30$)	HALS ($n = 30$)	*p*-value
OT overall (min)	140 (34)	170 (47)	0.060
- OT right-sided (min)	132 (40)	140 (52)	0.315
- OT left-sided (min)	145 (75)	180 (28)	0.197
WIT (sec)	120 (49)	150 (16)	0.008
- WIT of right kidneys (sec)	120 (38)	150 (23)	0.208
- WIT of left kidneys (sec)	120 (60)	150 (4)	0.017
First bowel movement (d)	2.1 (0)	2.4 (1)	0.385
Use of laxatives	19 (63.3)	27 (90)	0.030
Vomiting [a]	4 (13.3)	7 (23.3)	0.506
- plus laxatives	1/4	7/7	0.010
Length of hospital stay (d)	6 (3)	6 (3)	0.062
Creatinine (umol/l)			
- Preoperative	69 (16)	69 (14)	0.646
- Postoperative	99 (28)	102 (26)	0.794
- Follow-up	104 (23)	100 (21)	0.556

OT operative time, *WIT* warm ischemia time
Values are median and IQR, frequencies are in absolute numbers and %
[a]vomiting after 24 h and 7 days postoperatively

The demand for postoperative analgesia was similar between groups. Median time to first bowel movement after surgery did not differ between the HARS and HALS groups. However, there was a significant difference in the use of laxatives: 19 (63.3%) donors in the HARS group received laxatives compared to 27 (90%) in the HALS group. In the HARS group, 4 (13.3%) patients experienced at least one episode of postoperative emesis (24 h - 7 days) compared to 7 (23.3%) in the HALS group. All HALS donors experiencing emesis required laxatives, while this was the case for only one donor in the HARS group.

It is institutional policy that donors can decide how long they would like to stay in the hospital following surgery, and their wishes are accommodated. However, the median length of hospital stay did not differ between the two groups. The median creatinine preoperatively, before discharge, and during 3 months of follow-up did not differ between the two groups.

Minor complications (grade 0-II)

Postoperative courses were uneventful in 22 (73.3%) donors in the HARS group and 18 (60%) in the HALS group (Table 3).

Two (6.6%) Grade I complications occurred in each group, including incisional pain, lumbago and shoulder ache. They all could be eased by either subcutaneous infiltration of local anesthetics or oral analgesia and

Table 3 Donor complications according to the Clavien-Dindo score and CCI within 90 days

	HARS (n = 30)	HALS (n = 30)	p-value
Clavien-Dindo Score			
Grade I	2 (6.6)	2 (6.6)	0.672
Grade II	3 (10)	6 (20)	
Grade IIIb	3 (10)	4 (13.3)	
None	22 (73.3)	18 (60)	
CCI			
Overall	6.16 (11.26)	10.36 (15.28)	0.245
Right-sided LDN	6.83 (12.25)	8.18 (11.97)	0.775
Left-sided LDN	5.39 (9.96)	11.70 (16.98)	0.307

Values are mean and SD, frequencies are in absolute numbers and %

physiotherapy. All Grade I complications corresponded to a CCI of 8.7 points.

Three (10%) Grade II complications occurred in the HARS group, including seroma, hematoma and a new onset of arterial hypertension. All complications required medical treatment with antibiotics combined with frequent wound hygiene or antihypertensive drugs and corresponded to a CCI of 20.9 points. Within the HALS group, six (20%) Grade II complications were observed, including newly diagnosed arterial hypertension, fever of unknown origin and wound seroma. All complications could be treated by drug therapy and corresponded to a CCI of 20.9 points except a donor with two postoperative complications (Grade I and Grade II), whose CCI totaled 22.6 points.

Major complications (grade III-V)

Three donors in the HARS group underwent surgical evacuation of subcutaneous hematoma in the area of the Pfannenstiel incision (Grade IIIb). The CCI was 33.7 points in all three cases. Four Grade IIIb complications occurred in the HALS group. Two subcutaneous hematomas required operative evacuation. One subcutaneous infection had to be treated surgically, followed by vacuum-assisted wound closure. One of those donors additionally underwent subcutaneous infiltration of local anesthetic (Grade I) due to persistent incisional pain. In that donor, the CCI was 34.8 points. The others corresponded to a CCI of 33.7 points. In addition, one donor underwent three surgical revisions (two subcutaneous evacuations of hematoma and one exploratory laparotomy) for a severe hemorrhage. During the exploratory laparotomy, laceration of the spleen and the small bowel mesentery was found. Treatment consisted of a splenectomy and mesenteric suture. The same donor developed a hypertensive crisis during postoperative monitoring in the ICU that required intravenous antihypertensive medication. The sum of complications in this donor resulted in a CCI of 58.4 points. High-grade complications, i.e., single- or multi-organ failure (Grade IVa or IVb) as well as donor death (Grade V) did not occur in either group.

Recipients

Demographic and clinical data

The recipients' detailed preoperative characteristics are shown in Table 4. In the HARS group, 20 (66%) recipients underwent dialysis for a median of 8 months prior to transplantation; 14 had hemodialysis and 6 had peritoneal dialysis. In the HALS group, 23 (77%) recipients were dialyzed preoperatively for a median of 10 months, with 22 by hemodialysis and 1 by peritoneal dialysis.

Perioperative data

There were no relevant differences between the two groups in the median serum creatinine level and creatinine clearance before discharge and at 1 year after transplantation.

Survival and graft function

The recipients' one-year survival rate was 93.3% in the HARS group and 100% in the HALS group. The one-year graft survival rate was also comparable in both groups (90% versus 93.3%). In the HARS group, 29 recipients (96.6%) had an immediate or delayed onset of diuresis compared to all recipients (100%) in the HALS group (Table 4).

Table 4 Demographic and clinical characteristics of recipients' data

	HARS (n = 30)	HALS (n = 30)	p-value
BMI (kg/m^2)	23.9 (5.8)	25.6 (5.4)	0.174
Preoperative Dialysis	20 (3.3)	23 (76.6)	0.567
- Hemodialysis	14 (46.6)	22 (73.3)	
- Peritoneal Dialysis	6 (20)	1 (3.3)	
First Kidney-Tx	24 (80)	29 (96.6)	0.103
Retransplantation	6 (20)	1 (3.3)	0.103
AB0-Incompatibility	5 (16.6)	5(16.6)	1.000
HLA			
- 0-2 mismatches	3	5	0.819
- 3-4 mismatches	12	15	0.604
- 5-6 mismatches	15	10	0.294
OT (min)	106 (39)	120 (20)	0.271
DGF/PNF	4	1	0.353
- PNF	1	0	
Creatinine (umol/l)			
- Before discharge	110 (47)	108 (41)	0.996
- After one year	118 (31)	115 (37)	0.605

Values are median and IQR, frequencies are in absolute numbers and %, *Tx* Transplantation, *DGF* delayed graft function, *PNF* primary non-function

The patient with primary non-function in the HARS group developed multiple complications, starting with an acute vascular rejection from the very beginning. In the further course a dehydrating diarrhea due to a pseudomembranous colitis occurred, followed by intestinal bleeding necessitating a hemicolectomy, and finally sepsis and multiple organ failure. The patient died 14 weeks after transplantation.

There were three cases of DGF in the HARS group and one in the HALS group. One of the DGF patients in the HARS group developed a subcutaneous hematoma postoperatively, which led to a hemodynamic instability and required two units of blood prior to the occurrence of diuresis. The second patient with DGF had a perforation of the cecum due to ischemic colitis, necessitating an ileocecal resection. The patient developed a burst abdomen postoperatively because of an abscess in the renal graft bed. The kidney, which worked perfectly before the ileoceacal resection, did not recover from this septic burst and was explanted 4 months after transplantation. The third recipient suffered from a very severe diarrhea postoperatively resulting in a metabolic derailment, which led to a temporary loss of kidney function. This recipient later developed necrotizing pancreatitis, resulting in permanent loss of graft function and the development of multiple organ failure 6 weeks after transplantation, and died. The DGF patient in the HALS group underwent immediate surgical revision due to bleeding from the venous anastomosis. Temporary hemodialysis was required, and the kidney did partially recover; the GFR was 21 ml/min at the one-year follow-up, but dialysis was not yet needed.

Discussion

There are two different approaches for hand-assisted donor nephrectomy: transabdominal and retroperitoneal. Evidence of the superiority of either technique is lacking. This analysis has shown equivalent donor outcomes after both techniques in terms of postoperative kidney function and complications. The overall WIT was significantly shorter for kidneys recovered by the retroperitoneal approach despite similar operating times for the two surgical techniques. There does, however, seem to be a trend for a shorter OT using the HARS approach. Laxatives were used significantly more often in the HALS group, and concurrent vomitus was observed in all of these patients, suggesting that the transabdominal technique has a greater effect on bowel function. Finally, both left and right nephrectomies appear to be safe and feasible with both surgical techniques.

The first LDN was performed in 1954 with an open approach [26], which remained the gold standard for more than 40 years. In 1995, a purely laparoscopic technique to procure kidneys from living-donors was pioneered [10]. Wolf et al. [15] described the HALS donor nephrectomy in 1998 for the first time, followed by Wadström et al. [19], who introduced the HARS nephrectomy 3 years later. Various advantages soon became obvious, such as the ability to use tactile feedback, easier and rapid control of bleeding by digital pressure, better exposure and dissection of structures, and more rapid kidney recovery [16]. Studies of HALS or HARS procedures describe superiority compared to purely laparoscopic nephrectomies with regard to OT and WIT [18]. Therefore, the laparoscopic approach with or without hand-assistance has become the gold standard at most kidney transplant centers [27].

Postoperative donor complication rates range from 0 to more than 40% in different reports, depending on how authors classify adverse events after a nephrectomy [20, 28–30]. Our analysis defined complications according to the Clavien-Dindo classification as well as to the CCI [24, 25]. The latter is a new scale to measure surgical morbidity and is not yet routinely used in clinical practice. Therefore, we were interested in its applicability to living kidney donors as well as in how it compares to the Clavien-Dindo classification. First, there were no mortalities or life-threatening complications except for one donor who required an emergency relaparotomy and splenectomy. There were no conversions from laparoscopic to open surgery. We found no relevant differences in graft survival and function between the two groups at the one-year follow-up. DGF occurred in three (10%) recipients transplanted with a kidney recovered by the retroperitoneal approach and in one (3.3%) patient with a kidney harvested by the transperitoneal approach. DGF as well as PNF (primary non-function, defined as permanent loss of allograft function starting immediately after transplantation) certainly are very important indicators for graft function and should not be neglected. In this regard the definition of DGF is crucial. We defined DGF as needed dialysis within the first week after transplantation [23]. In the literature, the frequency of DGF varies from 0 to 10% in living-donor transplantation, indicating that the presented results are within the expected range [28, 31, 32]. We hypothesized that the graft functions were delayed or not existing due to complications in the recipient. Either there was a hemodynamic instability postoperatively due to a subcutaneous bleeding, a sepsis because of a cecal perforation during the first week after transplant surgery, a severe diarrhea postoperatively which led to a metabolic derailment followed by a secondary anuria, an acute vascular rejection or a bleeding from the venous anastomosis. But still, contributing factors during the donor kidney harvesting cannot be totally ruled out. The overall donor complication rate according to the Clavien-Dindo classification during follow-up tended to be higher, though not significantly, in the HALS group for in-hospital minor adverse events. However, Dols et al. [21] reported in a randomized controlled trial an increased incidence for high-grade complications in HALS compared to HARS nephrectomy patients. On the other hand, Ruszat et al. [20] documented overall complication rates of 20% for the retroperitoneoscopic and 15% for the hand-assisted transabdominal approach. Interestingly, these complication rates were significantly lower than those for purely laparoscopic nephrectomies (42.9%). Analysis of the CCI of our donors showed higher scores in the HALS group compared to the HARS group, although these differences did not reach statistical significance. The CCI better represents the severity of adverse events than does the Clavien-Dindo Score. In our opinion, the new CCI scoring system is applicable and yields more information about overall complications following donor nephrectomy.

There was no relevant difference in the OT between the two techniques in our analysis, although there was a trend for a longer OT in the HALS group, mirroring other published results [21]. A key difference between the two techniques that may affect the OT is the timing of when the surgeon installs the hand-port and inserts his/her hand. In the HARS technique, hand assistance is part of the procedure from the very beginning, while in the HALS technique, hand assistance is only used for dissecting the vascular structures and for recovery of grafts. Whether this influences the recorded time of the operation remains speculative. OT is an important consideration, as there is sufficient evidence that both renal function and organ perfusion are compromised by the duration of pneumoperitoneum [33, 34]. The WIT was significantly shorter in our study for kidneys that were recovered by the retroperitoneal approach. Given the various definitions of WIT that exist, it is difficult to compare WITs across different studies. It has been previously reported that the WIT in the HARS technique is shorter than in the HALS technique [20, 35]. The differences in the WIT measured in our study did not translate into differences in delayed graft function, graft loss or renal function. This is consistent with previously published results [31].

Our study indicates for the first time that patients undergoing HALS procedures require significantly more laxatives compared to those undergoing HARS procedures. All of the donors in the HALS group who vomited after 24 h postoperatively required laxatives in contrast to only 25% in the HARS group. This is perhaps not surprising, but it confirms the hypothesis that patients undergoing transperitoneal nephrectomies are more frequently afflicted with a paralytic ileus. Still, other factors (e.g. OT) may have influenced these results. Matas et al. compared morbidity rates among open, hand-assisted laparoscopic and pure laparoscopic nephrectomies [7]. Bowel obstruction also occurred significantly more often in the hand-assisted laparoscopic group then in the others. Other studies showed more serosa and splenic lesions in transperitoneal approaches [18].

There is repeated discussion concerning the preference for right or left donor nephrectomies. Most centers favor left kidneys for donation because of the longer renal vein, which makes implantation less demanding. On the other hand, some surgeons prefer the right kidney because it is easier to retrieve. A recent Meta-Analysis demonstrate a significant difference in terms of OT in favor of right-sided HALS nephrectomies [36]. In our study, there was a trend for a shorter OT in both groups for right-sided nephrectomies, although these differences did not reach statistical significance. A shorter OT for the right kidney can be expected due to the lower position of the right kidney and generally no adrenal, lumbar or genital veins draining into the right renal vein. There is also less need for colonic dissection and no risk of lacerating the spleen. Our OTs for right- and left-sided nephrectomies in both groups are shorter overall when compared to results of other similar studies [16, 37]. Eventually, the OT depends on the experience of the performing surgeon. The donor complication rates were comparable and did not show a relevant difference between right- and left-sided kidney donations.

An obvious limitation of our study is the small number of patients and, therefore, the low statistical power. The retrospective nature of the study is also a limitation. Only two surgeons carried out the donor procedures and patients were not randomized for the type of surgery performed. Hence, the procedures were always performed in the same way, and because both consultant surgeons were experienced, the results did not vary over time. The fact that the hand assistance in the two groups was at different time points during the procedure limits the direct comparison of the two groups. Recipient surgery in most of the cases was performed by just one of the two surgeons. Therefore, recipient surgery does not bias the presented results.

With respect to donor safety, surgeons should apply the surgical technique they are best trained in and feel most comfortable with. Future training of new surgeons should include various techniques to give them the confidence to use the best surgical approach to match individual circumstances and to be versatile enough to change procedures if research determines the superiority of one procedure. Furthermore, long-term follow-up is urgently needed because information about outcome (e.g., late complications caused by abdominal adhesions) over a longer time period in both groups is scarce.

Conclusion

There were no mortalities or intraoperative challenges leading to conversion in either donor group. In agreement with the current literature, it was demonstrated that HARS and HALS approaches for LDN are safe and feasible for renal graft recovery on either side. Neither of the two techniques provided clear evidence of superiority. And we found no relevant difference in graft function after 1 year postoperatively. However, given that the WIT is significantly shorter and the incidence of postoperative paralytic ileus is less frequent in the HARS group, we suggest that this technique might be preferred for living related kidney organ donors. Further advantages might be found for more complex patients, such as obese donors or donors with previous abdominal surgery.

Abbreviations

BMI: Body mass index; CCI: Comprehensive complication index; DGF: Delayed graft function; GFR: Glomerular filtration rate; HALS: Hand-assisted laparoscopic; HARS: Hand-assisted retroperitoneoscopic; LDN: Living-donor nephrectomy; OT: Operative time; WIT: Warm ischemia time

Authors' contributions

JW carried out the research design, wrote the paper, collected, analyzed and interpreted data. AS helped carrying out the research design, revised the paper critically, analyzed and interpreted data. PK collected and interpreted data. MS was one of the performing surgeons. JGB helped carrying out the research design, drafting the manuscript. He was one of the performing surgeons. MKM gave final approval of the version to be published, helped analyzing and interpreting data. All authors read and approved the final manuscript.

Author details

[1]Division of Visceral and Transplantation Surgery, University Hospital, Zurich, Switzerland. [2]Department of Surgery, Kantonsspital Frauenfeld, 8500 Frauenfeld, Switzerland. [3]Department of Surgery, Kantonsspital St. Gallen, St. Gallen, Switzerland. [4]Department of Surgery, Kidney and Pancreas Transplantation, King Faisal Specialist Hospital, Riyadh, Kingdom of Saudi Arabia.

References

1. Reese PP, Shults J, Bloom RD, Mussell A, Harhay MN, Abt P, et al. Functional status, time to transplantation, and survival benefit of kidney transplantation among wait-listed candidates. Am J Kidney Dis Off J Natl Kidney Found. 2015;66(5):837–45.
2. Biancone L, Cozzi E, López-Fraga M, Nanni-Costa A. Long-term outcome of living kidney donation position paper of the European committee on organ transplantation (CD-P-TO), Council of Europe. Transpl Int Off J Eur Soc Organ Transplant. 2015.
3. Bundesamt für Gesundheit - Zahlen und Fakten [Internet]. [cited 2014 Aug 14]. Available from: https://www.bag.admin.ch/bag/de/home/service/zahlen-fakten/zahlen-fakten-zu-transplantationsmedizin/zahlen-fakten-zur-spende-und-transplantation-von-organen.html#925789694.
4. Hariharan S, Johnson CP, Bresnahan BA, Taranto SE, McIntosh MJ, Stablein D. Improved graft survival after renal transplantation in the United States, 1988 to 1996. N Engl J Med. 2000;342(9):605–12.
5. Branco F, Cavadas V, Rocha A, Vidinha J, Osório L, Martins L, et al. Living versus cadaveric-donor renal transplant recipients: a comparison on sexual function. Transplant Proc. 2013;45(3):1066–9.
6. Gozdowska J, Zatorski M, Torchalla P, Białek Ł, Bojanowska A, Tomaszek A, et al. Living-donor versus deceased-donor kidney transplantation: comparison of psychosocial consequences for recipients. Transplant Proc. 2016;48(5):1498–505.
7. Matas AJ, Bartlett ST, Leichtman AB, Delmonico FL. Morbidity and mortality after living kidney donation, 1999-2001: survey of United States transplant centers. Am J Transplant Off J Am Soc Transplant Am Soc Transpl Surg. 2003;3(7):830–4.
8. Morgan BR, Ibrahim HN. Long-term outcomes of kidney donors. Curr Opin Nephrol Hypertens. 2011;20(6):605–9.
9. Muzaale AD, Massie AB, Wang M-C, Montgomery RA, McBride MA, Wainright JL, et al. Risk of end-stage renal disease following live kidney donation. JAMA. 2014;311(6):579–86.
10. Ratner LE, Ciseck LJ, Moore RG, Cigarroa FG, Kaufman HS, Kavoussi LR. Laparoscopic live donor nephrectomy. Transplantation. 1995;60(9):1047–9.
11. Fonouni H, Mehrabi A, Golriz M, Zeier M, Müller-Stich BP, Schemmer P, et al. Comparison of the laparoscopic versus open live donor nephrectomy: an overview of surgical complications and outcome. Langenbeck's Arch Surg. 2014;399(5):543–51.
12. Nicholson ML, Elwell R, Kaushik M, Bagul A, Hosgood SA. Health-related quality of life after living donor nephrectomy: a randomized controlled trial of laparoscopic versus open nephrectomy. Transplantation. 2011;91(4):457–61.
13. Chin EH, Hazzan D, Edye M, Wisnivesky JP, Herron DM, Ames SA, et al. The first decade of a laparoscopic donor nephrectomy program: effect of surgeon and institution experience with 512 cases from 1996 to 2006. J Am Coll Surg. 2009;209(1):106–13.
14. Altinel M, Akinci S, Gunes ZE, Olcucuoglu E, Gonenc F, Yazicioglu AH. Open versus laparoscopic donor nephrectomy: perioperative parameters and graft functions. Transplant Proc. 2011;43(3):781–6.
15. Wolf JS, Tchetgen MB, Merion RM. Hand-assisted laparoscopic live donor nephrectomy. Urology. 1998;52(5):885–7.
16. Minnee RC, Bemelman F, Kox C, Surachno S, Ten Berge IJM, Bemelman WA, et al. Comparison of hand-assisted laparoscopic and open donor nephrectomy in living donors. Int J Urol Off J Jpn Urol Assoc. 2008;15(3):206–9.
17. Yuan H, Liu L, Zheng S, Yang L, Pu C, Wei Q, et al. The safety and efficacy of laparoscopic donor nephrectomy for renal transplantation: an updated meta-analysis. Transplant Proc. 2013;45(1):65–76.
18. Özdemir-van Brunschot DMD, Koning GG, van Laarhoven KCJHM, Ergün M, van Horne SBCE, Rovers MM, et al. A comparison of technique modifications in laparoscopic donor nephrectomy: a systematic review and meta-analysis. PLoS One. 2015;10(3):e0121131.
19. Wadström J, Lindström P. Hand-assisted retroperitoneoscopic living-donor nephrectomy: initial 10 cases. Transplantation. 2002;73(11):1839–40.
20. Ruszat R, Sulser T, Dickenmann M, Wolff T, Gürke L, Eugster T, et al. Retroperitoneoscopic donor nephrectomy: donor outcome and complication rate in comparison with three different techniques. World J Urol. 2006;24(1):113–7.
21. Dols LFC, Kok NFM, d'Ancona FCH, Klop KWJ, Tran TCK, Langenhuijsen JF, et al. Randomized controlled trial comparing hand-assisted Retroperitoneoscopic versus standard laparoscopic donor nephrectomy. Transplantation. 2013.
22. Delmonico FL, Dew MA. Living donor kidney transplantation in a global environment. Kidney Int. 2007;71(7):608–14.
23. Mallon DH, Summers DM, Bradley JA, Pettigrew GJ. Defining delayed graft function after renal transplantation: simplest is best. Transplantation. 2013; 96(10):885–9.
24. Clavien PA, Barkun J, de Oliveira ML, Vauthey JN, Dindo D, Schulick RD, et al. The Clavien-Dindo classification of surgical complications: five-year experience. Ann Surg. 2009;250(2):187–96.
25. Slankamenac K, Graf R, Barkun J, Puhan MA, Clavien P-A. The comprehensive complication index: a novel continuous scale to measure surgical morbidity. Ann Surg. 2013;258(1):1–7.
26. Murray JE, Tilney NL, Wilson RE. Renal transplantation: a twenty-five year experience. Ann Surg. 1976;184(5):565–73.
27. Klop KWJ, Dols LFC, Kok NFM, Weimar W, Ijzermans JNM. Attitudes among surgeons towards live-donor nephrectomy: a European update. Transplantation. 2012;94(3):263–8.
28. Baron PW, Ben-Youssef R, Ojogho ON, Kore A, Baldwin DD. Morbidity of 200 consecutive cases of hand-assisted laparoscopic living donor nephrectomies: a single-center experience. J Transp Secur. 2012;2012:121523.
29. Bachmann A, Wyler S, Wolff T, Gürke L, Steiger J, Kettelhack C, et al. Complications of retroperitoneoscopic living donor nephrectomy: single center experience after 164 cases. World J Urol. 2008;26(6):549–54.
30. Lentine KL, Lam NN, Axelrod D, Schnitzler MA, Garg AX, Xiao H, et al. Perioperative complications after living kidney donation: a National Study. Am J Transplant Off J Am Soc Transplant Am Soc Transpl Surg. 2016;16(6):1848–57.
31. Lucas SM, Liaw A, Mhapsekar R, Yelfimov D, Goggins WC, Powelson JA, et al. Comparison of donor, and early and late recipient outcomes following hand assisted and laparoscopic donor nephrectomy. J Urol. 2013;189(2):618–22.
32. Minnee RC, Bemelman WA, Donselaar-van der Pant KA, Booij J, ter Meulen S, ten Berge IJM, et al. Risk factors for delayed graft function after hand-assisted laparoscopic donor nephrectomy. Transplant Proc 201042(7):2422–2426.

33. Demyttenaere S, Feldman LS, Fried GM. Effect of pneumoperitoneum on renal perfusion and function: a systematic review. Surg Endosc. 2007;21(2):152–60.
34. Wever KE, Bruintjes MHD, Warlé MC, Hooijmans CR. Renal perfusion and function during pneumoperitoneum: a systematic review and meta-analysis of animal studies. PLoS One. 2016;11(9):e0163419.
35. Klop KWJ, Kok NFM, Dols LFC, Dor FJMF, Tran KTC, Terkivatan T, et al. Can right-sided hand-assisted retroperitoneoscopic donor nephrectomy be advocated above standard laparoscopic donor nephrectomy: a randomized pilot study. Transpl Int. 2014;27(2):162–9.
36. Wang K, Zhang P, Xu X, Fan M. Right versus left laparoscopic living-donor nephrectomy: a meta-analysis. Exp Clin Transplant Off J Middle East Soc Organ Transplant. 2015;13(3):214–26.
37. Tsoulfas G, Agorastou P, Ko D, Hertl M, Elias N, Cosimi AB, et al. Laparoscopic living donor nephrectomy: is there a difference between using a left or a right kidney? Transplant Proc. 2012;44(9):2706–8.

6

Early post-operative serum albumin level predicts survival after curative nephrectomy for kidney cancer

Yongquan Tang[1†], Zhihong Liu[2†], Jiayu Liang[2], Ruochen Zhang[3], Kan Wu[2], Zijun Zou[4], Chuan Zhou[2], Fuxun Zhang[2] and Yiping Lu[2*]

Abstract

Background: Previous studies have shown that albumin-related systemic inflammation is associated with the long-term prognosis of cancer, but the clinical significance of an early (≤ 7 days) post-operative serum albumin level has not been well-documented as a prognostic factor in patients with renal cell cancer.

Methods: We retrospectively included patients hospitalized for kidney cancer from January 2009 to May 2014. First, the receiver operating characteristic analysis was used to define the best cut-off of an early post-operative serum albumin level in determining the prognosis, from which survival analysis was performed.

Results: A total of 329 patients were included. The median duration of follow-up was 54.8 months. Patients with an early post-operative serum albumin level < 32 g/L had a significantly shorter median recurrence-free survival (RFS; 49.1 versus 56.5 months, $P = 0.001$) and median overall survival (OS; 52.2 versus 57.0 months, $P = 0.049$) than patients with an early post-operative serum albumin level ≥ 32 g/L. After adjusting for age, BMI, tumor stage, post-operative hemoglobin concentration, and pre-operative albumin, globulin, and hemoglobin levels, multivariate Cox regression showed that an early post-operative serum albumin level < 32 g/L was an independent prognostic factor associated with a decreased RFS (HR = 3.60; 95% CI,1.05–12.42 [months], $P = 0.042$) and decreased OS (HR = 9.95; 95% CI, 1.81–54. 80 [months], $P = 0.008$).

Conclusion: An early post-operative serum albumin level < 32 g/L is an independent prognostic factor leading to an unfavorable RFS and OS. Prospective trials and further studies involving additional patients are warranted.

Keywords: Kidney cancer, Survival, Hypoalbuminemia, Radical resection

Background

Kidney cancer is one of the most common malignancies involving the urogenital system [1]. The most important treatment for kidney cancer is surgical resection, but post-operative recurrences are common, especially for stage II and above. A number of risk factors have been reported; however, prognostication remains difficult [2, 3]. Notably, new prognostic factors have been described in recent years [4–7].

Several studies have reported that the early post-operative neutrophil-to-lymphocyte ratio may be a long-term prognostic factor for some cancers, including pancreatic, prostate, and bladder cancers [8–10]. This association may result from the potential anti-tumor effect of acute inflammation. Albumin is commonly used to evaluate nutritional status, but a recent study has shown that albumin is also involved in the inflammatory/stress reaction [11]. McMillan and colleagues [12] reported that the serum albumin level was positively correlated with the C-reactive protein level in 40 patients with lung or gastrointestinal cancer. Bozzetti

* Correspondence: yiping_luuro@163.com
[†]Yongquan Tang and Zhihong Liu contributed equally to this work.
[2]Department of Urology, Institute of Urology, West China Hospital, Sichuan University, Chengdu, China
Full list of author information is available at the end of the article

and colleagues [13] first reported the phenomenon of frequent hypoalbuminemia status in the early period after extensive surgery. Based on our previous data, the serum albumin level was < 35 g/L in > 50% of patients following curative nephrectomy ($P < 0.05$), then always recovered to the pre-operative level within 2 weeks. Some researchers have concluded that early post-operative hypoalbuminemia is associated with the pre-operative serum albumin level, age, and extent of surgery [12], while other studies have shown that post-operative hypoalbuminemia may lead to unfavorable short-term prognoses, such as acute kidney injury [13, 14], unbalanced substance metabolism [15–17], and surgical site infections [18, 19]. Such findings suggest that albumin has a role in immune-inflammatory reactions [11, 20].

Recent studies have revealed that albumin-related systemic inflammation is associated with the long-term prognosis in patients with advanced gastrointestinal cancer [11, 21, 22]. Cai and colleagues [23] found that hypoalbuminemia 3–5 weeks after initiation of tyrosine kinase inhibitors is independently associated with a significantly decreased progression-free survival (PFS) and overall survival (OS) in patients with advanced kidney cancer. Furthermore, when combined with the Memorial Sloan-Kettering Cancer Center (MSKCC) risk model, hypoalbuminemia improves the efficiency in predicting recurrence-free survival (RFS) and OS [23]. The current retrospective study determined the potential association between early (≤ 7 days) post-operative hypoalbuminemia with long-term prognosis after resection of kidney cancer.

Methods

Study population

In this retrospective single-center study we reviewed the electronic medical records of inpatients with kidney cancer who were admitted to the Department of Urology at West China Hospital of Sichuan University (Sichuan, China) between January 2009 and May 2014. All of the patients underwent curative surgery. The inclusion criteria included the following: > 18 years of age; a pathologic diagnosis of kidney cancer; and negative surgical margins. Negative surgical margin was defined as macroscopic evidence on surgical report or microscopic evidence on histopathologic report. The exclusion criteria were as follows: incomplete resection; history of other life-threatening diseases within 5 years before or after surgery; adjuvant or neoadjuvant treatment; and distant metastasis, with the exception of the adrenal gland. The study conformed to the Declaration of Helsinki and was approved by the Ethics Committee of West China Hospital.

Objectives

We primarily assessed the prognostic value of early post-operative hypoalbuminemia with respect to RFS and OS in the curative resection of kidney cancer. We then determined the optimal cut-off point of the early post-operative serum albumin level in predicting the prognosis of kidney cancer. RFS was defined as the date of surgery to the date of recurrence, and OS was measured from the date of surgery to the date of death. For patients without a recurrence or who did not die, survival was censored at the date of the last follow-up evaluation. To distinguish confounding factors, subgroup analyses were performed.

Data collection

All data were obtained from medical records. The follow-up project adhered to the National Comprehensive Cancer Network (NCCN) clinical practice guidelines for kidney cancer [24]. Data were collected by two well-trained researchers. Any discrepancies in data interpretation were resolved by consensus of all authors. The data collected included demographic characteristics, date and type of surgery, clinical-pathologic TNM stage at the time of surgery, histopathologic characteristics, and date of recurrence and/or death if available or date of the last follow-up. TNM stage referred to the tumor size (T), local lymph node involvement (N), and remote metastasis (M), and was assessed according to imaging studies, surgical records, and histopathologic reports. TNM stage and anatomic stage/prognostic groups were also guided by the 2018 NCCN guidelines for kidney cancer [24]. Cancer recurrence was defined as unequivocal radiologic or biopsy evidence of emerging local or distant tumor lesions. In addition, we collated serum albumin, globulin, and hemoglobin data obtained pre- and post-operatively.

Statistics

All statistical analyses were carried out using Stata 14.0 (Stata Corp, College Station, TX, USA). The receiver operating characteristic (ROC) curve analysis was performed to determine the optimal cut-off point for the post-operative serum albumin level for use in the post-operative prognosis. Based on the cut-off point, we divided the patients into two groups, then survival curves were created using the Kaplan-Meier method and compared using the log-rank test. Gender, age, body mass index (BMI), stage, type of surgery, and pathologic pattern for both groups of patients were compared and tested one-by-one. Four-fold or R × C table data were analyzed with a chi-square test. The median of data with a non-normal distribution was designated as the average and analyzed with the Wilcoxon rank-sum test. The mean of data with a normal distribution was designated as the average and analyzed with a t-test [25]. A factor was entered into multivariate Cox regression analysis if a statistical difference existed in both groups of patients. The hazard ratio (HR) was adopted as the measurement. A P value < 0.05 indicated statistical significance.

Results

Patients and disease characteristics

A total of 694 patients were available in the database; 329 patients met the inclusion criteria. Among the 329 patients, 64% were male and the median age at the time of surgery was 56 years (range, 22–84 years). The median duration of follow-up was 54.8 months (range, 5.2–96.4 months). The mean pre- and post-operative serum albumin levels were 42.2 and 34.1 g/L, respectively ($P = 0.000$). ROC curve analyses showed that the optimal post-operative serum albumin cut-off level was 32 g/L (area under the curve [AUC] = 0.71) in predicting tumor recurrence (Fig. 1a) and 31 g/L (AUC = 0.80) in predicting death (Fig. 1b). Thus, we used 32 g/L as the cut-off point for grouping comparisons. A total of 99 patients had a serum albumin level < 32 g/L and 230 patients had a serum albumin level ≥ 32 g/L. The patient characteristics and laboratory test results for both groups are presented in Table 1. Age, BMI, tumor stage, post-operative hemoglobin concentration, and pre-operative albumin, globulin, and hemoglobin levels were statistically different (Table 1).

Survival analysis

No patients were lost to follow-up. The mean duration of follow-up in both groups was similar [58.5 (albumin < 32 g/L) and 59.9 (albumin ≥32 g/L) months, respectively; $P > 0.05$]. During follow-up, 30 patients (30.3%) had tumor recurrences and 24 patients (24.2%) did not survive in the group of patients with a post-operative serum albumin level < 32 g/L. Only 20 patients (8.7%) had tumor recurrences and 8 patients (3.5%) did not survive in the group of patients with a post-operative serum albumin level ≥ 32 g/L. The median RFS of patients with a post-operative serum albumin level < 32 g/L was significantly less than patients with a post-operative serum albumin level ≥ 32 g/L (49.1 and 56.5 months, respectively; $P = 0.001$). The median OS of patients with a post-operative serum albumin level < 32 g/L was also significantly less than patients with a post-operative serum albumin level ≥ 32 g/L (52.2 and 57.0 months, respectively; $P = 0.049$). The group survival curves are shown in Fig. 2. The log-rank test revealed that the differences in group survival curves was significant ($P = 0.000$) for RFS (Fig. 2a) and OS (Fig. 2b).

Multivariate cox regression

Based on difference testing, age, BMI, tumor stage, post-operative hemoglobin concentration, and pre-operative albumin, globulin, and hemoglobin levels were entered into multivariate Cox regression analysis. An early post-operative serum albumin level < 32 g/L was shown to have an independent impact on the decreased RFS (HR = 3.60; 95% CI,1.05–12.42 [months]; $P = 0.042$) and OS (HR = 9.95; 95% CI, 1.81–54.80 [months]; $P = 0.008$). In addition, tumor stage was also an independent prognostic factor (Table 2). Therefore, subgroup analysis was performed based on tumor stage.

Sub-group analysis of stages II and III kidney cancer

The survival curves of patients grouped by tumor stage and relevant log-rank testing showed significant differences between stages I and II, and stages III and IV for RFS and OS, but not between stages II and III. Furthermore, after excluding patients with stages I and IV, the two groups had similar TNM stage distributions ($P = 0.995$). Survival analysis and log-rank testing showed that patients with a post-operative serum albumin level < 32 g/L had a significantly decreased RFS ($P = 0.036$) and decreased OS ($P = 0.012$) compared to patients with a post-operative

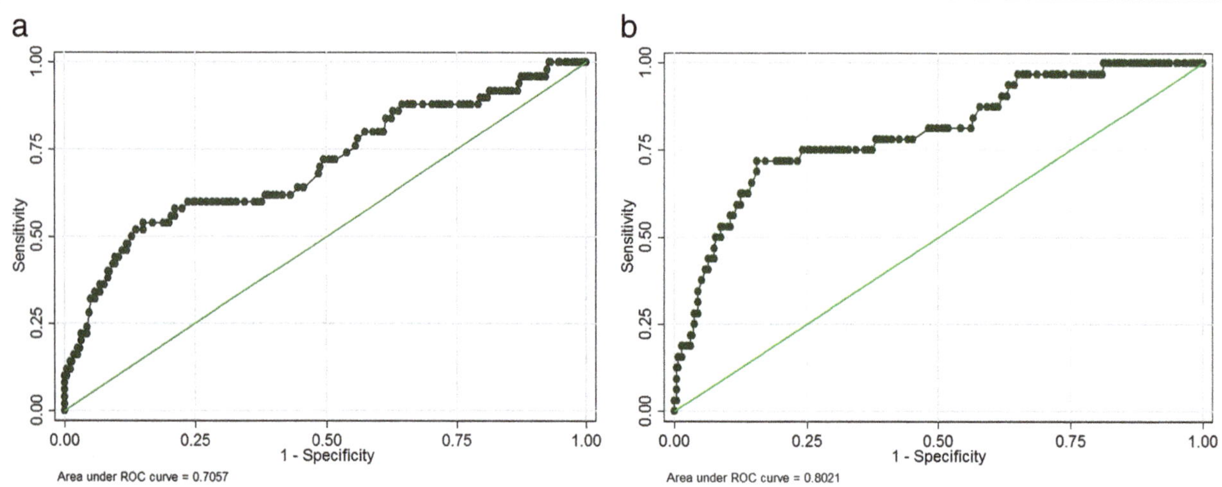

Fig. 1 Receiver operating characteristic (ROC) analysis to predict the best cutoff point of early post-operative serum albumin level in predicting recurrence (**a**) and death (**b**) and to calculate the area under the curve (AUC)

Table 1 The baseline and clinic-pathologic characteristics of patients grouped by post-operative serum albumin level

Variable	Serum albumin < 32 g/L (n = 99)	Serum albumin ≥ 32 g/L (n = 230)	P
Gender (%)			0.229
Male	59 (60)	153 (67)	
Female	40 (40)	77 (33)	
Age, y, median(range)	63 (22–82)	53 (24–84)	0.000*
BMI, Kg/m^2, mean ± SD	22.19 ± 0.38	23.84 ± 0.37	0.007*
Symptom (none/local/system)	(90/9/0)	(211/19/0)	0.805
ECOG-PS (0/1/2/3/4/5)	88/11/0/0/0	213/17/0/0/0	0.267
Stage (%)			0.000*
I	46 (46)	192 (83)	
II	18 (18)	13 (6)	
III	29 (29)	21 (9)	
IV	6 (6)	4 (2)	
Pathological type (%)			0.208
ccRCC	88 (89)	214 (93)	
nccRCC	11 (11)	16 (7)	
Type of surgery (%)			0.149
Radical nephrectomy	73 (74)	151 (66)	
Partial nephrectomy	26 (26)	79 (34)	
Fuhrman grade (%)			0.074
1–2	52 (53)	145 (63)	
3–4	47 (47)	85 (37)	
Preoperative, mean ± SD			
Alb, g/L	39.42 ± 0.43	43.43 ± 0.20	0.000*
Glb, g/L	29.20 ± 0.58	26.09 ± 0.25	0.000*
Hgb, g/L	128.09 ± 2.12	138.24 ± 1.06	0.000*
Post-operative, mean ± SD			
Alb, g/L	36.43 ± 0.19	28.77 ± 0.34	0.000*
Glb, g/L	24.27 ± 0.54	24.16 ± 0.24	0.834
Hgb, g/L	106.81 ± 1.78	123.71 ± 1.15	0.000*

*Significant
BMI body mass index, *SD* standard deviation, *ECOP-PS* Eastern Cooperative Oncology Group-performance status, *ccRCC* clear cell renal cell carcinoma, *nccRCC* non-clear cell renal cell carcinoma, *Alb* albumin, *Glb* globulin, *Hgb* hemoglobin

serum albumin level ≥ 32 g/L. Multivariate Cox regression analysis also showed that a early post-operative serum albumin level < 32 g/L was an independent prognostic factor associated with decreased RFS (HR = 6.76; 95% CI, 1.07–42.60; $P = 0.042$) and OS (HR = 26.92; 95% CI, 1.52–477.30; $P = 0.025$).

Sub-group analysis based on other factors

The histopathologic type of RCC is an important prognostic factor. Clear cell renal cell carcinoma (ccRCC) is the most common histopathologic type of kidney cancer. There were 88 (89%) and 214 (93%) patients in the post-operative serum albumin levels < 32 g/L and ≥ 32 g/L, respectively. Survival analysis and log-rank testing showed that ccRCC patients with a post-operative serum albumin level < 32 g/L had a significantly decreased RFS ($P = 0.00$) and decreased OS ($P = 0.00$) than patients with a post-operative serum albumin level ≥ 32 g/L.

The type of surgical procedure is another important factor determining prognosis in patients with kidney cancer, especially in patients who undergo partial or radical nephrectomies. Of 329 patients, 224 and 105 underwent radical and partial nephrectomies, respectively. Log-rank testing showed that patients who underwent radical nephrectomies with post-operative serum albumin levels < 32 g/L had a significantly decreased RFS ($P = 0.00$) and decreased OS ($P = 0.00$) than patients with a post-operative serum albumin level ≥ 32 g/L. The RFS and OS among patients who underwent partial nephrectomies with a post-operative serum albumin level < 32 g/L were not significantly different compared with patients who had a post-operative serum albumin ≥32 g/L ($P = 0.15$ and 0.76, respectively).

Discussion

Despite radical resection of kidney cancer, local recurrence or distant metastasis is commonplace [26–28]. With the exception of known prognostic factors, such as tumor stage, pathologic type, and type of surgical procedure, other potential prognostic factors warrant further elucidation [2, 3, 29, 30]. In this retrospective study we report for the first time that an early post operative serum albumin level is another long-term prognostic factor after radical resection of kidney cancer.

To prevent confounding factors as much as possible, we excluded patients who had incomplete tumor resections, other life-threatening diseases, and adjuvant and/or neoadjuvant treatment. We excluded patients without serum protein and cell testing post-operatively, but it is unlikely that bias was introduced because no guidelines specify laboratory testing early after surgery without an indication. In our medical center, all radical surgeries for kidney cancer were performed by well-trained clinicians. To ensure a sufficient duration of follow-up, we only included patients who underwent surgery prior to May 2014. Approximately 42% of the enrolled patients had a duration of follow-up > 5 years and 94% of the enrolled patients had a duration of follow-up > 3 years. The median duration of follow-up was nearly 5 years, and no patients were lost to follow-up.

The serum albumin level nearly returned to the pre-operative level in all patients who had repeat serum protein testing. A decrease in the serum albumin level may primarily result from exudation into the extravascular space and attenuation by perioperative bleeding and

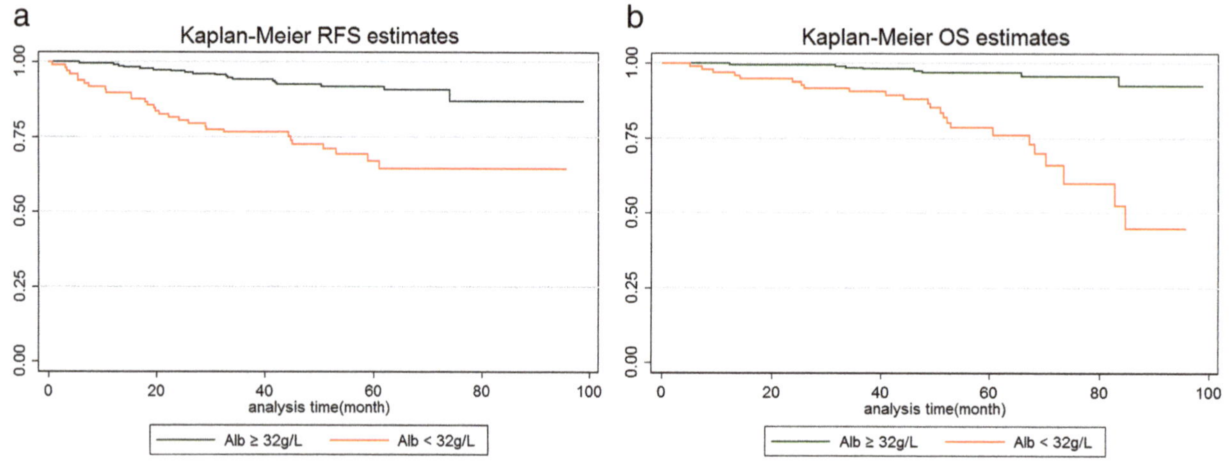

Fig. 2 Recurrence-free survival (RFS) (**a**) and overall survival (OS) (**b**) curves of patients with early post-operative serum albumin level ≥32 g/L versus < 32 g/L

fluid transfusion [11, 31]. We found a significant decrease in the hemoglobin concentration early after surgery coincident with the decrease in serum albumin level; however, the post-operative serum albumin level was significantly decreased compared with the serum albumin level regulated by the hemoglobin concentration (34.1 versus 37.0 g/L, $P = 0.00$), as follows: regulated serum albumin level ÷ pre-operative albumin level = post-operative hemoglobin concentration ÷ pre-operative hemoglobin concentration. This decrease is regarded as extravascular exudation. When the post-operative serum albumin level and extravascular exudation were entered into Cox regression, the results showed that the post-operative serum albumin level had a close association with RFS (HR = 0.85, $P = 0.000$) and OS (HR = 0.82, $P = 0.000$), unlike the association between extravascular exudation and RFS (HR = 1.00, $P = 0.113$) and OS (HR = 0.99, $P = 0.116$).

Table 2 Effect of early post-operative plasma albumin level on recurrence-free survival and overall survival in multivariate Cox regression analyses adjusted by gender, age, body mass index (BMI), tumor stage and some other laboratory indexes

	Recurrence-free survival			Overall survival		
	HR	95% CI	*P*	HR	95% CI	*P*
Age	0.99	0.95–1.03	0.573	1.00	0.96–1.04	0.980
BMI	0.99	0.88–1.12	0.892	0.97	0.85–1.11	0.684
Stage	1.51	1.03–2.21	0.034*	1.40	0.90-2.17	0.136
Preoperative						
Alb	0.99	0.86–1.13	0.866	0.99	0.83–1.18	0.906
Glb	1.09	0.99–1.19	0.055	1.08	0.99–1.19	0.094
Hgb	1.01	0.98–1.05	0.420	1.00	0.96–1.05	0.816
Post-operative						
Alb < 32 g/L	3.60	1.05–12.42	0.042*	9.95	1.81-54.80	0.008*
Hgb	1.00	0.97-1.04	0.966	1.02	0.98–1.06	0.418

*Significant
HR hazard ratio, *CI* confidence interval, *Alb* albumin, *Glb* globulin, *Hgb* hemoglobin

For patients who underwent pathologic-complete resection of kidney cancer, we entered other universally-accepted prognostic factors before survival analysis, including gender, age, nutritional status (BMI), tumor stage, pathologic type, Fuhrman grade, and type of surgical procedure. Survival analysis showed that patients who had an early post-operative serum albumin level < 32 g/L had a significantly decreased RFS and OS. Although patients in the group of patients with a lower post-operative albumin level were older, had a lower BMI, and more than stage III cancer and some laboratory values differed, multivariate Cox regression analysis admitted all of these factors, and the results showed that an early post-operative serum albumin level < 32 g/L was an independent risk factor for a decreased RFS and OS. Positive results were obtained, even when patients were confined to stages II and III. In contrast, the log rank test did not reveal significant differences in RFS ($P = 0.360$) and OS ($P = 0.814$) between stages II and III in our patients. Sub-group analysis showed an association between the post-operative serum albumin level and long-term prognosis based on patients with ccRC who underwent radical nephrectomies versus partial nephrectomies; however, only 26 patients with a post-operative serum albumin level < 32 g/L underwent partial nephrectomies. Indeed, the negative result may reflect the limited sample size.

Limited by the potential retrospective bias, the prognostic value of an early post-operative serum albumin level warrants more high-quality studies for further elucidation. Based on good category power (AUC = 0.71–0.8), an early post-operative serum albumin level deserves more attention in predicting prognosis after radical resection of kidney cancer, especially combined with other prognostic factors. The mechanisms underlying the association remain unclear. In addition, whether or not transfusion of albumin leads to decreased tumor recurrence and death after resection of kidney cancer should be investigated.

Conclusion

In patients after curative resection of kidney cancer, this retrospective study revealed that an early post-operative serum albumin level < 32 g/L is an independent risk factor associated with a decreased RFS and decreased OS. Prospective trials and further research in additional patients are needed.

Abbreviations

HR: Hazard Ratio; MSKCC: Memorial Sloan-Kettering Cancer Center; NCCN: National Comprehensive Cancer Network; OS: Overall Survival; RFS: Recurrence-free Survival; ROC: Receiver Operating Characteristic

Acknowledgements

Not applicable

Authors' contributions

YT and ZL contributed primarily to the conception and design, acquisition of data and analysis, interpretation of data and manuscript drafting; JL and RZ participated in the design, acquisition of data and analysis, interpretation of data and manuscript drafting. KW and ZZ involved in collecting data and drafting the manuscript; CZ and FZ have been involved in data analysis and manuscript drafting; YL mainly contributed to interpretation of data, revision in critical content, supervision and final approval of the version to be published. All authors have read and approved the manuscript, and ensure that this is the case.

Author details

[1]Department of Pediatric Surgery, West China Hospital, Sichuan University, No. 37 of Guoxue Xiang, Chengdu 610041, China. [2]Department of Urology, Institute of Urology, West China Hospital, Sichuan University, Chengdu, China. [3]Department of Urology, Fujian Provincial Hospital, Fuzhou, China. [4]Department of Urology, the Third Affiliated Hospital, Sun Yat-sen University, Guangzhou, China.

References

1. Wein AJ, Kavouss LR, Partin AW, Novick AC, Peters CA: CAMPBELL-WALSH Urology, 10th Edition. Saunders 2012.
2. Dall'Oglio MF, Ribeiro-Filho LA, Antunes AA, Crippa A, Nesrallah L, Goncalves PD, Leite KR, Srougi M. Microvascular tumor invasion, tumor size and Fuhrman grade: a pathological triad for prognostic evaluation of renal cell carcinoma. J Urol. 2007;178(2):425–8 discussion 428.
3. Goncalves PD, Srougi M, Dall'lio MF, Leite KR, Ortiz V, Hering F. Low clinical stage renal cell carcinoma: relevance of microvascular tumor invasion as a prognostic parameter. J Urol. 2004;172(2):470–4.
4. Rabjerg M. Identification and validation of novel prognostic markers in renal cell carcinoma. Dan Med J. 2017;64(10):B5339.
5. Ha YS, Chung JW, Chun SY, Choi SH, Lee JN, Kim BS, Kim HT, Kim TH, Byun SS, Hwang EC, et al. Impact of preoperative thrombocytosis on prognosis after surgical treatment in pathological T1 and T2 renal cell carcinoma: results of a multi-institutional comprehensive study. Oncotarget. 2017;8(38): 64449–58.
6. Errarte P, Beitia M, Perez I, Manterola L, Lawrie CH, Solano-Iturri JD, Calvete-Candenas J, Unda M, Lopez JI, Larrinaga G. Expression and activity of angiotensin-regulating enzymes is associated with prognostic outcome in clear cell renal cell carcinoma patients. PLoS One. 2017;12(8):e0181711.
7. Cai W, Zhong H, Kong W, Dong B, Chen Y, Zhou L, Xue W, Huang Y, Zhang J, Huang J. Significance of preoperative prognostic nutrition index as prognostic predictors in patients with metastatic renal cell carcinoma with tyrosine kinase inhibitors as first-line target therapy. Int Urol Nephrol. 2017; 49(11):1955–63.
8. Tsujita E, Ikeda Y, Kinjo N, Yamashita YI, Hisano T, Furukawa M, Taguchi KI, Morita M, Toh Y, Okamura T. Postoperative neutrophil-to-lymphocyte ratio as a predictor of long-term prognosis after pancreatectomy for pancreatic carcinoma: a retrospective analysis. Am Surg. 2017;83(6):610–6.
9. Jang WS, Cho KS, Kim MS, Yoon CY, Kang DH, Kang YJ, Jeong WS, Ham WS, Choi YD. The prognostic significance of postoperative neutrophil-to-lymphocyte ratio after radical prostatectomy for localized prostate cancer. Oncotarget. 2017;8(7):11778–87.
10. Kang M, Jeong CW, Kwak C, Kim HH, Ku JH. The prognostic significance of the early postoperative neutrophil-to-lymphocyte ratio in patients with urothelial carcinoma of the bladder undergoing radical cystectomy. Ann Surg Oncol. 2016;23(1):335–42.
11. Nazha B, Moussaly E, Zaarour M, Weerasinghe C, Azab B. Hypoalbuminemia in colorectal cancer prognosis: nutritional marker or inflammatory surrogate? World J Gastrointest Surg. 2015;7(12):370–7.
12. Critselis E, Panagiotakos DB, Machairas A, Zampelas A, Critselis AN, Polychronopoulos E. Postoperative hypoproteinemia in cancer patients following extensive abdominal surgery despite parenteral nutritional support. Nutr Cancer. 2011;63(7):1021–8.
13. Manning RD Jr. Effects of hypoproteinemia on renal hemodynamics, arterial pressure, and fluid volume. Am J Phys. 1987;252(1 Pt 2):F91–8.
14. Sang BH, Bang JY, Song JG, Hwang GS. Hypoalbuminemia within two postoperative days is an independent risk factor for acute kidney injury following living donor liver transplantation: a propensity score analysis of 998 consecutive patients. Crit Care Med. 2015;43(12):2552–61.
15. Shao M, Wang S, Parameswaran PK. Hypoalbuminemia: a risk factor for acute kidney injury development and progression to chronic kidney disease in critically ill patients. Int Urol Nephrol. 2017;49(2):295–302.
16. Zhang T, Deng Y, He P, He Z, Wang X. Effects of mild hypoalbuminemia on the pharmacokinetics and pharmacodynamics of dexmedetomidine in patients after major abdominal or thoracic surgery. J Clin Anesth. 2015;27(8): 632–7.
17. Miwa A, Morioka I, Hisamatsu C, Fujioka K, Morikawa S, Shibata A, Yasufuku M, Yokoyama N, Matsuo M. Hypoalbuminemia following abdominal surgery leads to high serum unbound bilirubin concentrations in newborns soon after birth. Neonatology. 2011;99(3):202–7.
18. Sullivan SA, Van Le L, Liberty AL, Soper JT, Barber EL. Association between hypoalbuminemia and surgical site infection in vulvar cancers. Gynecol Oncol. 2016;142(3):435–9.
19. Lee JI, Kwon M, Roh JL, Choi JW, Choi SH, Nam SY, Kim SY. Postoperative hypoalbuminemia as a risk factor for surgical site infection after oral cancer surgery. Oral Dis. 2015;21(2):178–84.
20. Critselis E, Panagiotakos DB, Machairas A, Zampelas A, Critselis AN, Polychronopoulos E. Risk and predictive factors of hypoalbuminemia in cancer patients following extensive abdominal surgery despite total parenteral nutritional support. Int J Food Sci Nutr. 2012;63(2):208–15.
21. Crumley AB, Stuart RC, McKernan M, McMillan DC. Is hypoalbuminemia an independent prognostic factor in patients with gastric cancer? World J Surg. 2010;34(10):2393–8.
22. McMillan DC, Watson WS, O'Gorman P, Preston T, Scott HR, McArdle CS. Albumin concentrations are primarily determined by the body cell mass and the systemic inflammatory response in cancer patients with weight loss. Nutr Cancer. 2001;39(2):210–3.
23. Cai W, Zhang J, Chen Y, Kong W, Huang Y, Huang J, Zhou L. Association of post-treatment hypoalbuminemia and survival in Chinese patients with metastatic renal cell carcinoma. Chin J Cancer. 2017;36(1):47.
24. NCCN: NCCN clinical practice guidelines in oncology, kidney Cancer (version 2. 2017). https://www.nccn.org/professionals/physician_gls/default.aspx#kidney.
25. KANG L, Jia H, Shibao Y, Jun M. Medical statistics, 6th edition: People's medical publishing house. 2013.
26. Shum CF, Bahler CD, Sundaram CP. Matched comparison between partial nephrectomy and radical nephrectomy for T2 N0 M0 tumors, a study based on the National Cancer Database. J Endourol. 2017;31(8):800–5.
27. Kunath F, Schmidt S, Krabbe LM, Miernik A, Dahm P, Cleves A, Walther M, Kroeger N. Partial nephrectomy versus radical nephrectomy for clinical localised renal masses. Cochrane Database Syst Rev. 2017;5:Cd012045.
28. Demir O, Bozkurt O, Celik S, Comez K, Aslan G, Mungan U, Celebi I, Esen A. Partial nephrectomy vs. radical nephrectomy for stage I renal cell carcinoma in the presence of predisposing systemic diseases for chronic kidney disease. Kaohsiung J Med Sci. 2017;33(7):339–43.
29. Tsukamoto T, Kumamoto Y, Miyao N, Yamazaki K, Takahashi A, Satoh M. Regional lymph node metastasis in renal cell carcinoma: incidence, distribution and its relation to other pathological findings. Eur Urol. 1990; 18(2):88–93.

30. Cheigh JS, Kim H, Stenzel KH, Tapia L, Sullivan JF, Stubenbord W, Riggio RR, Rubin AL. Systemic lupus erythematosus in patients with end-stage renal disease: long-term follow-up on the prognosis of patients and the evolution of lupus activity. Am J Kidney Dis. 1990;16(3):189–95.
31. Ryan AM, Hearty A, Prichard RS, Cunningham A, Rowley SP, Reynolds JV. Association of hypoalbuminemia on the first postoperative day and complications following esophagectomy. J Gastrointes Surg. 2007;11(10): 1355–60.

7

The application of barbed suture during the partial nephrectomy may modify perioperative results

Yifei Lin[1†], Banghua Liao[1†], Sike Lai[2], Jin Huang[3*], Liang Du[3*], Kunjie Wang[1*] and Hong Li[1]

Abstract

Background: Barbed sutures can avoid knot tying and speed the suture placement in the PN(partial nephrectomy). On account of the impact on clinical outcomes are ambiguous, this study is determined to identify the application of barbed suture during PN.

Methods: ClinicalTrials.gov, Cochrane Register of Clinical Studies, PubMed and EMBASE were searched for RCTs(randomized controlled trials) and cohort studies focusing on the comparison of barbed and traditional sutures in PN(last updated on Feb in 2015). According to Cochrane Library's suggestion, quality assessment was performed. Review Manager was applied to analyze all the data and sensitivity analyses were performed through omitting each study sequentially.

Results: Eight cohort studies and none of RCTs proved eligible (risk of bias: moderate to low,431 patients). Warm ischemia time(MD = – 6.55,95% CI -8.86 to – 4.24, $P < 0.05$) decreased statistically in the barbed suture group, as well as operative time(MD = – 11.29,95% CI -17.87 to-4.71, $P < 0.05$). Postoperative complications also reduced significantly(OR – 0.44, 95% CI 0.24 to0.80, $P < 0.05$). Unidirectional barbed suture resulted in fewer postoperative complications based on the subgroup analysis(OR = 0.48,95% CI 0.24 to 0.94, $P < 0.05$).

Conclusions: The barbed suture may be a useful surgical innovation which can modify perioperative results for surgeons and patients. Randomly-designed studies with longer follow up and larger sample sizes are in the need of to explore the applicability.

Keywords: Partial nephrectomy, Surgical technique, Systematic review

Background

Partial nephrectomy (PN) is regarded as the golden standard treatment for small-localized renal tumors currently [1]. With the development of the surgical technology, larger (until 7 cm and more) cases may also be the appropriate candidates. Type of resection, type of suture and the change of renal function usually play a significant role during the perioperative period of PN [2]. Generally, warm ischemia time (WIT), among many factors to predict renal function, is the only predictor that can be modified by the surgeon or surgical techniques [3–5]. Though several surgical and technological innovations have been invented to enhance the efficiency of renorrhaphy and decrease WIT, such as the application of hemostatic agents, or even the involvement of the robot assistance [6, 7], different approaches still had their own advantages and disadvantages.

Recently, an innovative of absorbable, the knotless barbed suture is applied for renal pelvicaliceal or/and parenchymal repair to diminish WIT in laparoscopic

* Correspondence: michael_huangjin@163.com; 125798620@qq.com; wangkj@scu.edu.cn
†Yifei Lin and Banghua Liao contributed equally to this work.
[3]West China Hospital, Sichuan University, Guoxuexiang 37, Chengdu 610041, Sichuan, China
[1]Department of Urology, Institute of Urology (Laboratory of Reconstructive Urology), West China Hospital, Sichuan University, Chengdu, Sichuan, People's Republic of China
Full list of author information is available at the end of the article

partial nephrectomy [8]. Initiated in 1964 [9], this approach has been first reported in gynaecological and plastic surgery previously [10]. And then some systematic reviews, in terms of radical prostatectomy [11–13], have confirmed equivalence of biocompatibility and tensile strength of knotless barbed suture compared to conventional sutures in urological field [14, 15].

Since partial nephrectomy was one of the earliest urological surgeries that adopted this advanced technology, various effects were reported. Nevertheless, the effect of length of intraoperative ischemia on renal function and life quality of patients after PN is a subject of significantly heated discussion. Thus, a meta-analysis and systematic review was carried out for a more validated result on the application of knotless barbed sutures in PN comparing with the conventional sutures.

Methods

Study selection

A comprehensive literature search, which addressed the topic of barbed suture in partial nephrectomy ("barbed" OR "knotless" AND "suturing" OR "suture") was performed. The databases includede Cochrane Register of Clinical Studies, MEDLINE, EMBASE and clinical trials registered in Clinicaltrials.gov. Available studies from inception to Feb. 21st, 2015 were evaluated for inclusion.

Randomized controlled trials (RCTs) or observational controlled studies reporting comparative outcomes of patients underwent partial nephrectomy using conventional suture or barbed suture were considered for inclusion. Excluded studies included patients using other materials to compare with barbed suture like mesh or staple rather than continues smooth sutures. Studies, including reviews, abstracts, overlapped studies and those published in languages other than English, were also excluded.

Data extraction and outcome measures

Search results were entered into a bibliographic software (EndNote X7) for further analysis. Two individual investigators (YL, SL) screened all titles and abstracts collected from the search strategy for relevance and full text review.. Extracted data included family name of the first author, publication year, original country, sample sizes, study design, and postoperative complications.

Warm ischemia time, operative time, estimated blood loss or change in hemoglobin level, perioperative blood transfusion, changes in renal function, hospital stay and postoperative complications were considered to be the main outcome measures for the meta-analysis. We also evaluated the heterogeneity of the outcomes to confirm the appropriateness of pooling studies.

Outcome definition

Operative time was defined as the total time of surgery. Warm ischemia time was determined from the minute of hilar clamping until the moment of unclamping which was the main procedure of partial nephrectomy. Estimated blood loss, change in hemoglobin level and perioperative blood transfusion were defined as the loss of blood during the surgery and it was generally acquired from the surgeons' operative reports or/and anesthesia records. After surgeries, postoperative complications of the suture and hospital stay were also recorded. We specially evaluated the postoperative complications based on the modified Clavien classification [16]. Renal function, including serum creatinine (sCr) and estimated glomerular filtration rate (eGFR), were measured using different measurement tools, for instance, CKD-Epi and RENAL nephrometry score system.

Quality assessment

Two authors (YL, SL) independently assessed the quality of each included study. Discrepancies were resolved by discussion and a consensus decision. For RCTs, the Cochrane risk of bias tools were used. Observational studies were evaluated using the Newcastle-Ottawa Scale to assess the risk of bias [17]. We included several categories for cohort studies: ascertainment of partial nephrectomy, representativeness of the barbed suture cohort, ascertainment of exposure to barbed suture, selection of the non-exposed cohort, demonstration that outcome of interest (i.e. warm ischemia time) was not reported at the beginning of study, comparability of study controls for important factors (e.g. adequate adjustment for confounders or matching for important confounding factors), assessment of outcome (e.g. adjudication and blinding assessment), and completeness of the follow up.

Statistical analysis

Results for each study were calculated using a fixed effects model. (random effects mode for high heterogeneity) The existence of statistical heterogeneity was evaluated through the χ^2 test and I^2 test. Pooled standardized mean difference (SMD) and mean difference (MD)are estimated to evaluate the continuous data, and the pooled odds ratios (ORs) were calculated for the evaluation of dichotomous data through Review Manager (Version 5.3). Sub group meta-analysis was performed based on different barbed suture (unidirectional and bidirectional barbed suture). Sensitivity analyses were also performed. $P < 0.05$ was considered significant.

Results

Study selection process and characteristics

A total of 8 cohort studies [18–25] (431 patients), and no RCTs proved eligible. A flow diagram of the detailed selection process is reported (Fig. 1). Table 1 shows the baseline characteristics and the results of all the eligible studies. All the data were comparable. Results of combined data comparing barbed suture versus conventional suture are presented in Table 2.

Low to moderate risk of bias were considered among all the included studies (Additional file 1: Table S1). Specifically, the participant population within a study was identified from a same clinical setting comparing barbed suture with control. Ascertainment of patients performed partial nephrectomy was based on surgical records. A total of 3 studies have adjusted important confounding factors by matching pairs (body mass index and operative approach). No loss to follow-up in all studies.

Warm ischemia time

Of the 8 cohort studies, 5 reported the warm ischemia time of partial nephrectomy [18–20, 22, 25] (Fig. 2a). Due to the fact that the heterogeneity is high among the WIT ($P = 0.09$, $I^2 = 50\%$), the random effects model was adopted instead of the fixed effects model. The pooling of raw data of these 283 cases suggested that patients with barbed suture versus conventional suture had a significantly shorter WIT. (MD = – 6.55, 95% CI -8.86 to – 4.24, $P < 0.00001$). Since Zondervan's study recruited both laparoscopic and open surgeries whereas others only focused on laparoscopic partial nephrectomy, it was excluded for a sensitivity analysis. Therefore, the newly pooled results (221 cases) with low heterogeneity ($I^2 = 0\%$,) indicated that

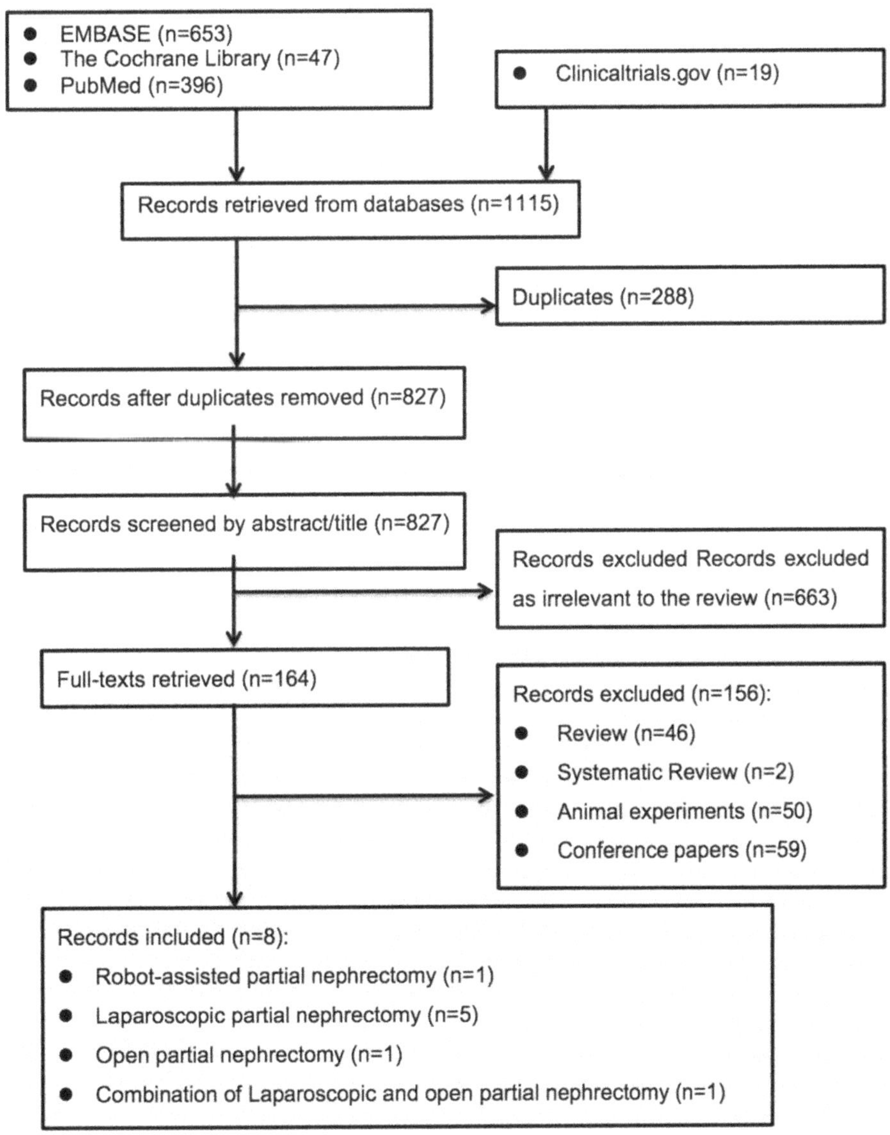

Fig. 1 Flow diagram of the detailed selection process

Table 1 Basic characteristics of all pooled studies in the meta-analysis

Author/ year	Surgery type	Country	Barbed type	Study design	Renorrhaphy type	Median follow up	Sample size	Age	BMI	Tumor size	RENAL/ PAUDA/ Charlson Score	Suture time(min ± SD or range)	Warm ischemia time(min ± SD or range)	Operative time(min ± SD or range)	Estimated blood loss(ml ± SD or range/ mmol/L ± SD or range)	Perioperative Blood transfusion (n)	Hospital stay (days)	Postoperative complications
							B/C	B/C	B/C	B/C	B/C	B/C	B/C	B/C	B/C	B/C	B/C	
Sammon 2011	RAPN	US	U	Prospective cohort study	2 layers	1 month/ 4.5 months	15/15	64 ± 11.3/ 61 ± 8.4	29.8 ± 5.8/34.7 ± 7.2	2.5 ± 0.9/2.8 ± 1.4	NR	NR	18.5 ± 5.3/ 24.7 ± 6.6	227.5 ± 66.7/275 ± 49.2	150 ± 119.3/ 150 ± 99.6	NR	2.0 ± 0.7/2.0 ± 1.3	Bleeding
Olweny 2012	LPN	US	U	Prospective cohort study	Sliding clips	NR	29/49	55.1 ± 13.0/ 55.1 ± 12.9	30.4 ± 6.0/29.9 ± 6.3	2.6 ± 1.2/2.7 ± 1.2	NR	NR	26.4 ± 8.3/ 32.8 ± 7.9	174 ± 35/ 178 ± 41	188 ± 205/255 ± 337	1/5	3.4 ± 1.3/3.6 ± 0.98	Urine leak, embolization, other
Zondervan 2012	OPN& LPN	Netherlands	U	Prospective cohort study	1 layer	1 week	31/31	58 (27–80)/ 60 (25–81)	26.5 (20–39.2)/26.5 (17.0–47.9)	3.0 (1.6–7.1)/3.1 (1.5–6.8)	3 (0–9)/2 (0–9)¶	NR	19.6 ± 7.5/ 21.8 ± 9.5	NR	1.6 (0.0–3.8)/1.9 (0.3–9.2)	1/5	not stated/ not stated	Bleeding,urinary fistula, lung embolism
Erdem 2013	LPN	Turkey	U	Retrospective cohort study	1 layer	NR	17/17	55 (29–80)/ 57 (32–78)	27.55 (19.53–31.25)/ 26.64 (21.25–30.43)	3.8 (2.2–6.3)/4.0 (2.0–6.5)	9 (6–13)/ 8 (6–12) §	NR	19 (12–50)/28 (10–57)	110 (90–190)/140 (80–190)	100 (30–400)/ 140 (20–200)	2/2	3 (2–5)/ 3 (2–7)	Fever, blood transfusion, elongated drainage, Ileus controlled with nasogastric decompression
Jeon 2013	LPN	US	U	Retrospective cohort study	Sliding clips	NR	13/24	60.1 ± 13.8/ 55.3 ± 11.7	28.3 ± 5.5/27.4 ± 7.3	2.5 ± 0.8/2.0 ± 0.7	7.1 ± 1.7/ 6.6 ± 1.6 *	NR	24.5 ± 5.3/ 31.9 ± 8.9	248.5 ± 37.2/ 256.7 ± 39.2	319.2 ± 311.3/ 331.3 ± 221.6	2/2	3.8 ± 1.3/3.8 ± 1.2	Postoperative hemorrhage, urine leakage, others
Shang 2013	LPN	China	Bi	Retrospective cohort study	2 layers	30 days	34/30	49 (25–83)/ 47 (19–74)	25.6/25.4	4/3.8	8.7 ± 1.0/ 8.6 ± 1.2*	NR	18/24.8	73 (45–135)/79.5 (40–135)	20 (5–600)/20 (5–350)	4/4	NR	Urinary fistula, extraction-site hernias, atelectasis, delayed hemorrhage
Schauer 2014	OPN	Austria	U	Retrospective cohort study	NR	NR	15/35	59.1 ± 13.7/ 65.5 ± 10.5	NR	3.5 ± 1.6/3.6 ± 1.2	9.0 ± 2.1/ 8.1 ± 1.8§	NR	NR	NR	15.6 ± 5.6/14.4 ± 8.9	NR	NR	Urinoma, pyrexia
Wang 2014	LPN	China	Bi	Retrospective cohort study	Sliding clips	1–11 months	36/40	51.3 ± 10.1/ 50.8 ± 11.2	NR	3.1 ± 1.2/3.0 ± 1.4	NR	10.4 ± 3.2 /19.4 ± 6.7	15.2 ± 4.2/ 24.1 ± 5.6	78.5 ± 15.4/90.3 ± 18.1	60.5 ± 21.2/ 110.4 ± 21.1	0/2	5.9 ± 2.1/6.8 ± 2.3	Blood urine, urine leak

BMI Body massive index, *US* the United States, *RAPN* Robot-assisted partial nephrectomy, *LPN* Laparoscopic partial nephrectomy, *OPN* Open partial nephrectomy, *U* Unidirectional barbed suture, *Bi* Bidirectional barbed suture, *B* Barbed suture group, *C* Control group, *NR* Not reported
*RENALScore
§PAUDA Score
¶Charlson Score

Table 2 Results of meta-analysis comparing barbed and control suture group

Outcomes of interest	Results of the combined studies						Study heterogeneity	
	Studies no.	Barbed group patients no.	Control group patient no.	SMD/MD/OR	95% CI	*P* value	I^2	P value
Warm ischemia time	5	124	159	−6.55	−8.86 to −4.24	< 0.00001	50%	0.09
Warm ischemia time*	4	93	128	−7.85	−9.48 to-6.22	< 0.00001	0%	0.56
Operative time	4	93	128	−11.29	−17.87 to −4.71	0.0008	17%	0.30
Estimated blood loss	5	108	163	0.50	−1.41 to 0.42,	0.29	91%	< 0.00001
Estimated blood loss*	4	72	123	−0.07	−0.36 to 0.23	0.66	0%	0.81
Perioperative blood transfusion	6	160	191	0.56	0.26 to 1.24	0.15	0%	0.58
Hospital stay	4	93	128	−0.21	−0.58 to 0.15	0.26	0%	0.49
Postoperative complications	8	190	241	0.44	0.24 to 0.80	0.007	0%	0.92

CI Confidence Interval, *SMD* Standardized Mean Deviation, *MD* Mean Deviation
*Sensitive analysis

WIT in laparoscopic partial nephrectomy significantly decreased. (MD = – 7.85, 95% CI -9.48 to-6.22, $P < 0.00001$, Additional file 1: Figure S1).

Operative time

Four studies of the laparoscopic partial nephrectomy reported data of operative time [18, 19, 22, 25] (Fig. 2b). The pooling of raw data presented a statistically significant association between the suture types (barbed sutures vs. conventional sutures) and operative time based on 221 cases (MD = – 11.29, $P = 0.0008$, 95% CI -17.87 to – 4.71) with low heterogeneity ($I^2 = 17\%$).

Estimated blood loss

Five studies reported outcomes of estimated blood loss [18, 19, 22, 24, 25] (hemoglobin level or volume of blood loss). (Figure 2c) The pooling outcomes of the 271 cases did not present significantly benefits of barbed suture over conventional suture (SMD = – 0.50, 95% CI -1.41 to 0.42, $P = 0.29$). This finding was, however, highly limited due to a very high level of heterogeneity with random effect model ($I^2 = 91\%$).

Since Wang's study [25] account for the bidirectional barbed suture (Quill SRS), while others applied unidirectional barbed suture (V-Loc™ 180), we therefore excluded this study for a sensitivity analysis. And the newly pooled results (195 cases) showed the same result while with low heterogeneity. (SMD = – 0.07, 95% CI -0.36 to 0.23, $P = 0.66$, $I^2 = 0\%$, Additional file 1: Figure S2).

Perioperative blood transfusion

Six studies reported data of perioperative blood transfusion based on 351 participants. [19–23, 25] (Fig. 2d). Pooling of these cohort studies did not suggest a statistically significant association between the suture types and perioperative blood transfusion (OR = 0.56, 95% CI 0.26 to 1.24, $P = 0.15$, $I^2 = 0\%$). Moreover, subgroup analysis presented similar results, regardless of unidirectional or bidirectional barbed suture. (Additional file 1: Figure S3).

Hospital stay

Four studies, with 221 patients recruited, reported about hospital stay [18, 19, 22, 25] (Fig. 2e). Pooling of those outcomes did not present a statistically significant association between the application of barbed suture and hospital duration. (MD = – 0.21, 95% CI -0.58 to 0.15, $P = 0.26$, $I^2 = 0\%$).

Postoperative complications

Eight cohort studies reported raw event data postoperative complications [18–25] and the postoperative complications were evaluated based on the modified Clavien classification(Fig. 2f, Table 1) Pooling data of all the 431 cases showed that significantly fewer postoperative complications were found in patients with barbed suture versus conventional suture. (OR = 0.44, $P = 0.007$, 95% CI 0.24 to 0.80, $I^2 = 0\%$). Then the subgroup analyses (Additional file 1: Figure S4) by barbed suture types showed: compared with unidirectional barbed suture (V-Loc™), the use of barbed suture statistically decreases the postoperative complications. (OR = 0.48, 95% CI 0.24 to 0.94, $P = 0.03$, $I^2 = 0\%$); as for bidirectional barbed suture (Quill SRS), pooled data did not show significant differences between both groups (OR = 0.35, 95% CI 0.10 to 1.18, $P = 0.09$, $I^2 = 0\%$).

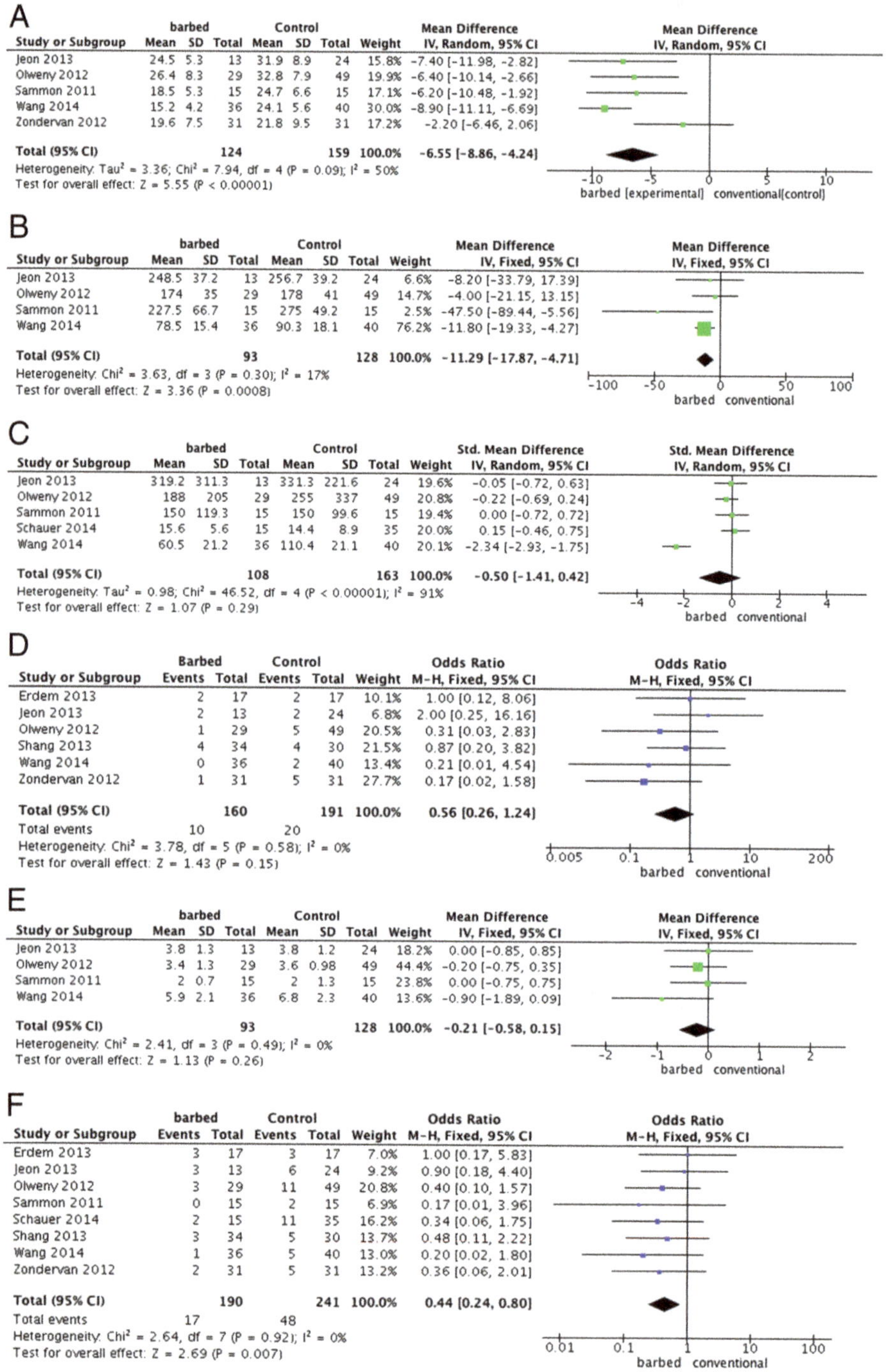

Fig. 2 Pooled estimate of outcomes: (**a**) A forest plot of warm ischemia time with or without barbed suture; (**b**) A forest plot of operative time with or without barbed suture; (**c**) A forest plot of estimated blood loss with or without barbed suture; (**d**) A forest plot of perioperative blood transfusion with or without barbed suture; (**e**) A forest plot of hospital stay with or without barbed suture; (**f**) A forest plot of postoperative complications with or without barbed suture

Changes in renal function

As the reflection of renal function, sCr and/or eGFR were reported by four studies [20, 21, 23, 24] (Table 3). Measurement tools differed among four studies and only median and range data were reported. Though not readily for pooling, all did not suggest that significant changes between two suture groups in terms of both renal function indicators.

Table 3 Changes in renal function before and after PN (sCr & eGFR)

Author/ year	Surgery	Cohort	N	Increase in sCr umol/L median [range]	P	Decline in eGFR ml/min/1.73 m^2 median [range]	P	Measurement tools
Zondervan 2012	OPN & LPN	Barbed	31	10.0(−70.7to114.0)	0.970	0.0(−4.3to14.2)	0.735	Creatinine was measured in the pre and postoperative period. Pre and postoperative estimated GFR were calculated using the CKD Epidemiology Collaboration (CKD-Epi) glomerular filtration equation
		Control	31	8.8(−26.5to123.8)		0.0(−4.6to18.6)		
Erdem 2013	LPN	Barbed	17	0(−0.3to2.3)	0.190	0(−23.0to39.0)	0.176	Functional renal preservation was assessed through the comparison of pre-operative and early postoperative eGFR, which was calculated using the Chronic Kidney Disease Epidemiology Collaboration formula. The early postoperative eGFR was based on an sCr measurement obtained after the peak sCr within the first 3 days of surgery.
		Control	17	0.1(−0.1to0.6)		9.0(−12to62)		
Shang* 2013	LPN	Barbed	34	2.59(−4.0 to 159.2)	0.797	7.7(−35.9to41.1)	0.065	RENAL nephrometry score system
		Control	30	2.65(−21.0 to 70.7)		8.9(−30.6to37.0)		
Schauer 2014	OPN	Barbed	15	20.1(−13.9to 51.9)	0.33	21.2(−18.0to38.0)	0.38	Postoperative changes in renal function parameters, serum creatinine levels, and eGFRs after surgery and before discharge.
		Control	35	10.3(−18.7to 61.5)		10.5(−26.1to42.5)		

PN partial nephrectomy, *LPN* laparoscopic partial nephrectomy, *OPN* open partial nephrectomy, *eGFR* estimated glomerular filtration rate, *sCr* serum creatinine
*The time point for renal function tests after surgery in this study was one month later after discharge from hospital, while the tests in other studies was right before the discharge from hospital

Discussion

In this systematic review, we have included all the controlled studies to test the effects of barbed suture on PN. The pooling of all the cohort studies showed significant decreases in WIT, operative time, and postoperative complications in barbed suture group; the quality of included cohort studies was high to moderate. The subgroup analysis suggested that unidirectional barbed suture significantly minimized the postoperative complications, which seems to be safer than the traditional suture.

As the most important factor after partial nephrectomy, the pooled outcome of WIT witnessed an overall significant reduction in barbed suture groups, especially laparoscopic partial nephrectomies. This means barbed suture can effectively reduce the WIT during laparoscopic partial nephrectomies so as to improve the postoperative renal function.

SCr and eGFR were the most commonly used tools to evaluate renal function after PN [1], but the change of these two indexes were only reported in four studies [20, 21, 23, 24]. Since all the raw data suggested no significant shift between both groups, many researchers believed that the results needed larger sample size [24] and longer follow up time to confirm, say at least 5-year follow up [21]. Besides, there are many ways to determine loss of renal function and evaluate the effects of surgery on renal function, such as renal scan and volumetric assessment of the kidney, which were not reported in the articles included [26, 27]. Moreover, as the concentrations of them are enormously influenced by age, gender, muscle mass and so on [1, 3], a more convincing way to evaluate renal function loss in the patients, such as renal scintigraphy, needs to be focused on for future studies. Furthermore, the statistical decrease of operative time in barbed group also indicated that barbed suture was effective in partial nephrectomy either by a robot-assisted, laparoscopic, or open technique [28].

With regard to blood issue, both outcomes of estimated blood loss and transfusion were comparable. After performing the sensitivity analysis on the outcomes of estimated blood loss, the heterogeneity dropped from 91 to 0% with the pooled outcomes of still no significant difference. Similarly, the subgroup analysis of blood transfusion by different barbed suture did not suggest any difference from the overall effect. However, Zondervan et al [20]. reported that no difference was owing to the fact that hemostatic agents applied during surgery were not considered, thus this may be a confounding factor that need take into account in the future.

Meanwhile, number of postoperative complications was significantly minimized in barbed suture groups. Besides, subgroup analysis indicated that unidirectional barbed suture turned out to be safer than the convention suture while bidirectional barbed suture did not. However, no human study concerned the safety and efficacy among different barbed sutures. Thus the feasibility and safety among different barbed sutures in vivo study need to take into consideration [29, 30].

The pooled outcome in this study provides a reliable evidence for the relationship between the barbed suture and some important surgical indicators for PN.

However, there are limitations of this study [1]. Even though two cohort studies adjusted their analyses via matching pairs, the pooled data may also be influenced by many factors, such as surgeons' preference or learning curves due to none of RCTs recruited [2]. Because not all the studies evaluated the tumor via RENAL, PAUDA or Charlson scores before surgeries, it is impossible to perform subgroup analyses based on those indexes and future studies should uniform the standards to evaluate renal tumors [3]. The literatures search was extensive, but the barbed suture only suggested for all T1 kidney tumors rather than some suitable T2-may be or T3 cases and still did not involve animal studies, letters to the editors, and conference publications; and [4] because only 8 studies were recruited, the risk of publication bias could not be evaluated by the Begg's funnel plots.

Nevertheless, our result renews a latest meta-analysis on barbed suture in PN. Based on what we know, this is to date the most comprehensive meta-analysis and systematic review exploring the relationship between barbed and traditional suture in PN.

Conclusions

The barbed suture may be a useful surgical innovation which can modify perioperative results for surgeons and patients. Significant decline of suture time, operative time and postoperative complications were found using barbed suture during PN. Unidirectional barbed suture seemed to be safer. Because of the limitations of quality, especially that matched renal tumor complexity is not utilized, this state-of-the-art need to be proved by evidences with higher quality, and randomized-controlled studies with longer follow up and larger sample sizes will be needed to prove the findings of the present studies.

Additional file

Additional file 1: Figure S1. A forest plot of sensitivity analysis of warm ischemia time with or without barbed suture. **Figure S2.** A forest plot of sensitivity analysis of Estimate blood loss with or without barbed suture. **Figure S3.** A forest plot of subgroup analysis of perioperative blood transfusion with or without barbed suture. **Figure S4.** A forest plot of subgroup analysis of postoperative complications with or without barbed suture. **Table S1.** Quality assessment of studies in the meta-analysis based on Newcastle-Ottawa Scale (NOS). (DOCX 92 kb)

Acknowledgements

Supported by Grant No. 81403276 from the National Natural Science Foundation of China and Grant No. JH20140066 from the Technology Support Program of Science and Technology Department of Sichuan Province.

Authors' contributions

YL, BL: Project development, data analysis and management, manuscript writing and editing. SL: Data collection, data analysis and management. LD: Data analysis and management, management manuscript writing and editing. JH, KW, HL: project development, manuscript writing and editing. All authors read and approved the final manuscript.

Author details

[1]Department of Urology, Institute of Urology (Laboratory of Reconstructive Urology), West China Hospital, Sichuan University, Chengdu, Sichuan, People's Republic of China. [2]West China School of Medicine, Sichuan University, Guoxuexiang 37, Chengdu 610041, Sichuan, China. [3]West China Hospital, Sichuan University, Guoxuexiang 37, Chengdu 610041, Sichuan, China.

References

1. Volpe A, Blute ML, Ficarra V, Gill IS, Kutikov A, Porpiglia F, et al. Renal ischemia and function after partial nephrectomy: a collaborative review of the literature. Eur Urol. 2015;68(1):61–74.
2. Porpiglia F, Bertolo R, Amparore D, Fiori C. Nephron-sparing suture of renal parenchyma after partial nephrectomy: which technique to go for? Some best practices. Eur Urol Focus. In press.
3. Lane BR, Babineau DC, Poggio ED, Weight CJ, Larson BT, Gill IS, et al. Factors predicting renal functional outcome after partial nephrectomy. J Urol. 2008; 180(6):2363–8 discussion 8-9.
4. Becker F, Van Poppel H, Hakenberg OW, Stief C, Gill I, Guazzoni G, et al. Assessing the impact of ischaemia time during partial nephrectomy. Eur Urol. 2009;56(4):625–34.
5. Gao ZL, Gu GL, Wu JT, Wang L. Comparison of the transperitoneal and a semi-open retroperitoneal approach for right-sided laparoscopic donor nephrectomy. Ann Transplant. 2011;16(4):40–6.
6. Benway BM, Wang AJ, Cabello JM, Bhayani SB. Robotic partial nephrectomy with sliding-clip renorrhaphy: technique and outcomes. Eur Urol. 2009;55(3): 592–9.
7. Gettman MT, Blute ML, Chow GK, Neururer R, Bartsch G, Peschel R. Robotic-assisted laparoscopic partial nephrectomy: technique and initial clinical experience with DaVinci robotic system. Urology. 2004;64(5):914–8.
8. Seideman C, Park S, Best SL, Cadeddu JA, Olweny EO. Self-retaining barbed suture for parenchymal repair during minimally invasive partial nephrectomy. J Endourol. 2011;25(8):1245–7 discussion 7-8.
9. Ruff GL. The history of barbed sutures. Aesthet Surg J. 2013;33(3 Suppl):12s–6s.
10. Warner JP, Gutowski KA. Abdominoplasty with progressive tension closure using a barbed suture technique. Aesthet Surg J. 2009;29(3):221–5.
11. Bai Y, Pu C, Yuan H, Tang Y, Wang X, Li J, et al. Assessing the impact of barbed suture on Vesicourethral anastomosis during minimally invasive radical prostatectomy: a systematic review and meta-analysis. Urology. 2015; 85(6):1368–75.
12. Li H, Liu C, Zhang H, Xu W, Liu J, Chen Y, et al. The use of unidirectional barbed suture for Urethrovesical anastomosis during robot-assisted radical prostatectomy: a systematic review and meta-analysis of efficacy and safety. PLoS One. 2015;10(7):e0131167.
13. Lin YF, Lai SK, Liu QY, Liao BH, Huang J, Du L, et al. Efficacy and safety of barbed suture in minimally invasive radical prostatectomy: a systematic review and meta-analysis. Kaohsiung J Med Sci. 2017;33(3):107–15.
14. Weld KJ, Ames CD, Hruby G, Humphrey PA, Landman J. Evaluation of a novel knotless self-anchoring suture material for urinary tract reconstruction. Urology. 2006;67(6):1133–7.
15. Rashid RM, Sartori M, White LE, Villa MT, Yoo SS, Alam M. Breaking strength of barbed polypropylene sutures: rater-blinded, controlled comparison with nonbarbed sutures of various calibers. Arch Dermatol. 2007;143(7):869–72.
16. Dindo D, Demartines N, Clavien PA. Classification of surgical complications: a new proposal with evaluation in a cohort of 6336 patients and results of a survey. Ann Surg. 2004;240(2):205–13.
17. Wells GA, Shea B, Peterson JEA, Welch V, Losos M, Tugwell P. The Newcastle-Ottawa scale (NOS) for assessing the quality of nonrandomised studies in meta-analyses; 2000.
18. Sammon J, Petros F, Sukumar S, Bhandari A, Kaul S, Menon M, et al. Barbed suture for renorrhaphy during robot-assisted partial nephrectomy. J Endourol. 2011;25(3):529–33.
19. Olweny EO, Park SK, Seideman CA, Best SL, Cadeddu JA. Self-retaining barbed suture for parenchymal repair during laparoscopic partial nephrectomy; initial clinical experience. BJU Int. 2012;109(6):906–9.

20. Zondervan PJ, Gozen AS, Opondo D, Rassweiler JJ, de la Rosette JJ, Laguna MP. Partial nephrectomy: is there an advantage of the self-retaining barbed suture in the perioperative period? A matched case-control comparison. World J Urol. 2012;30(5):659–64.
21. Erdem S, Tefik T, Mammadov A, Ural F, Oktar T, Issever H, et al. The use of self-retaining barbed suture for inner layer renorrhaphy significantly reduces warm ischemia time in laparoscopic partial nephrectomy: outcomes of a matched-pair analysis. J Endourol. 2013;27(4):452–8.
22. Jeon SH, Jung S, Son HS, Kimm SY, Chung BI. The unidirectional barbed suture for renorrhaphy during laparoscopic partial nephrectomy: Stanford experience. J Laparoendosc Adv Surg Tech A. 2013;23(6):521–5.
23. Shang JW, Ma X, Zhang X, Li HZ, Shi TP. Comparison of two different renorrhaphy techniques in retroperitoneal laparoscopic partial nephrectomy for complex tumor. Chin Med J. 2013;126(24):4629–32.
24. Schauer I, Theimer O, Klatte T, Waldert M, Klingler HC, Margreiter M. Use of self-retaining barbed sutures decreases cold ischemia time in open nephron-sparing surgery. Wien Klin Wochenschr. 2014;126(11–12):329–34.
25. Wang K, Zhang YL, Lin CH, Liu DF, Men CP, Wang JM, et al. Application of self-retaining bidirectional barbed absorbable suture in retroperito- neoscopic partial nephrectomy. Int Braz J Urol. 2014;40(2):220–4.
26. Porpiglia F, Bertolo R, Fiori C. Words of wisdom: re: residual parenchymal volume, not warm ischemia time, predicts ultimate renal functional outcomes in patients undergoing partial nephrectomy. Eur Urol. 2016;69(1):176–7.
27. Bertolo RG, Zargar H, Autorino R, Fiori C, Kaouk JH, Russo P, et al. Estimated glomerular filtration rate, renal scan and volumetric assessment of the kidney before and after partial nephrectomy: a review of the current literature. Minerva Urol Nefrol. 2017;69(6):539–47.
28. Campbell SC, Novick AC, Belldegrun A, Blute ML, Chow GK, Derweesh IH, et al. Guideline for management of the clinical T1 renal mass. J Urol. 2009; 182(4):1271–9.
29. Jordan MC, Holscher-Doht S, Jakubietz MG, Jakubietz RG, Meffert RH, Schmidt K. Suture material for flexor tendon repair: 3-0 V-Loc versus 3-0 Stratafix in a biomechanical comparison ex vivo. J Orthop Surg Res. 2014;9:72.
30. Iavazzo C, Mamais I, Gkegkes ID. The role of knotless barbed suture in gynecologic surgery: systematic review and meta-analysis. Surg Innov. 2014:528–39.

8

Robotic-assisted partial nephrectomy with sequential clamping of segmental renal arteries for multiple ipsilateral renal tumors: Initial outcomes

Jie Yang†, Jia-dong Xia†, Jian-xin Xue†, Ning-hong Song, Chao Liang, Di Xi, Ya-min Wang and Zeng-jun Wang*

Abstract

Background: To assess the technical feasibility and outcomes of robotic-assisted partial nephrectomy (RPN) with sequential segmental renal artery (SRA) clamping for multiple ipsilateral renal tumors (MIRTs).

Methods: From April 2016 to February 2018, consecutive eleven cases successfully underwent RPN with sequential SRA clamping under the guidance of dual-source computed tomography (DSCT).

Results: Ten cases had two lesions and two cases had three at the ipsilateral kidneys. The mean size and the mean R.E.N.A.L score for the dominant lesion of single case were 3.3 cm and 5.7, respectively. Twenty-two lesions (84.6%) had one target SRA and four (15.4%) had two target SRAs. Satisfactory ischemic areas were achieved by sequentially clamping two (81.8%) or three (18.2%) target SRAs with mean clamping time of 18.8 (15.0–27.0) min for single lesion, and the mean of total clamping time for single case was 37.5 (32.0–52.0) min. Only the complications of grade 1–2 were found and no positive surgical margin was discovered. The mean follow-up time was 5.4 months and no local recurrence or metastasis was found. The mean postoperative eGFR was 71.2 ml/minute/1.73m^2 that was only an insignificant reduction (9.3%) compared with the preoperative baseline.

Conclusion: This novel nephron-sparing technique, RPN with sequential SRA clamping, represents a good alternative for selected patients with MIRTs. With the guidance of DSCT and skilled robotic experience, this technique is feasible and can maximize renal function preservation. Large-scale multicenter clinical studies are still needed to further prove these initial outcomes.

Keywords: Multiple ipsilateral renal tumors, Robotic-assisted partial nephrectomy, Segmental renal artery, Dual-source computed tomography, Sequential clamping, Estimated glomerular filtration rate

Background

Multiple ipsilateral renal tumors (MIRTs) are characterized as at least two tumor foci in the same kidney, separated by normal tissue [1, 2]. The exact incidence of MIRTs was currently unreported. According to the available related data, we conservatively estimated the incidence between 4.5 and 7.9% [3]. Radical nephrectomy (RN) has been regarded as the standard treatment in previous studies. Unfortunately, patients with MIRTs would be highly predisposed to form contralateral renal tumors at the morbidity of about 5% [4, 5], thus RN is definitely not the optimal treatment for MIRTs.

Since 2003, a series of reports have suggested that nephron-sparing surgery (NSS) can provide a reliable oncologic cure and better postoperative function outcomes compared with RN in selected MIRT patients [5–7]. Meanwhile, robot-assisted partial nephrectomy (RPN) was reported in 2004 along with the growing confidence in robotic-assisted laparoscopic technique [8, 9]. Then Rogers et al. firstly reported RPN with main renal artery (MRA) clamping for the treatment of MIRTs in 2008 [10]. However, the excision of multiple lesions

* Correspondence: zengjunwang2002@sina.com
†Jie Yang, Jia-dong Xia and Jian-xin Xue contributed equally to this work.
Department of Urology, First Affiliated Hospital of Nanjing Medical University, Nanjing 210029, Jiangsu, China

inevitably requires more MRA clamping time, which will aggravate the ischemic/ reperfusion injury of normal spared nephron [11–13].

In order to further optimize the surgery treatment of MIRTs, we originally propose a novel clamping procedure of lesion-feeding arteries in RPN, the sequential clamping of precise segmental renal arteries (SRAs) [14]. Under the guidance of dual-source computed tomography (DSCT) [11–14], the technique has been successfully applied in the procedure of laparoscopic partial nephrectomy (LPN) for the treatment of MIRT in our center since 2010 and reported in 2017 [15]. But precise hilar microdissection required by sequential SRA clamping and one-time resection/renorrhaphy for multiple renal tumors are two major challenges of the technique in laparoscopic procedure. Robot-assisted platform can greatly help to overcome these challenges because of its two technical advantages. The first is its clearer 3D- field of vision with greater magnification than ordinary laparoscopic surgery, which can facilitate the identification of small branches of the renal arteries [10]. The other one is its more precise operating angle that can realize the quick resection and renorrhaphy of multiple lesions [9]. The aim of this study is to describe the application of sequential SRA clamping technique in the procedure of RPN and assess the technical feasibility for the treatment of MIRTs. Herein, we present our initial experience and short-term outcomes of this technique in a series of twelve patients.

Methods

Inclusion criteria

From April 2016 to February 2018, consecutive twelve MIRT cases, preoperatively diagnosed as renal cell carcinoma (RCC) or renal angiomyolipomas (AMLs) by computed tomography (CT) (Additional file 1: Figure S1), underwent RPN with sequential SRA clamping in our center. Under the guidance of preoperative DSCT, all cases had at least two SRAs feeding different lesions (Additional file 1: Figure S1C). All cases had normal contralateral renal function, evaluated by Gate's method before operation [16]. No case had bilateral or hilar lesions or metastatic foci, and no case had unacceptable anesthetic/operative risk based on the primary operator's judgment.

Surgical methods

All RPNs with sequential SRA clamping were performed by an experienced surgeon (Z.W.) independently through a transperitoneal approach [17, 18]. The standard SRA clamping technique was described in our previous studies on LPN [11–15]. Before operation, an additional DSCT was taken out to establish three-dimensional (3D) dynamic renal vascular models for every case (Fig. 1a). Thus, the anatomic relationship of SRAs with lesions was obtained and the feeding SRAs of every lesion could be precisely identified before operation (Fig. 1a).

Patients under general anesthesia were placed in the modified flank position at 60 degrees (Additional file 2: Figure S2A). The placement of five ports in the abdomen region (Additional file 2: Figure S2B) and subsequently docking with the DaVinci robot arms (Intuitive Surgical, Sunnyvale, CA, USA) were same as previously reported by other centers [17, 18]. When the MRA was identified at the renal hilum, further dissection was performed to isolate target SRAs for precisely clamping with neurosurgical bulldogs [11–15] (Fig. 1b). Following an easy-to-difficult procedure to expose each tumor (Fig. 2a, c), we first handled the renal tumor with a lower R.E.N.A.L score. With precisely clamping of the feeding SRA, a satisfying local ischemic area around the low-score lesion was achieved, and then we excised the tumor closely around its capsule with a margin of 1–2 mm normal parenchyma (Fig. 2a, b). If the ischemic area could not encompass the whole lesion after single branch was clamped, multiple SRAs would be done. When the excision was completed, renorrhaphy was performed to achieve haemostasis and the closure of incised calices using 2–0/3–0 barbed sutures (QUILL SRS, PA, USA) and hem-o-lok clips (Sanlian Xinghai Medical Innovation Co. Ltd., Jiangsu, China) before the feeding SRA was unclamped [17, 18]. It was also necessary to clamp additional SRAs when there was arterial bleeding from lesion beds. If there was excessive bleeding in the surgical field of vision, or clamping multiple SRAs could not obtain satisfactory ischemic area, conversion to MRA clamping or open procedure was required. Then, another high-score lesion with its feeding SRA was dealt with following the above procedure (Fig. 2c, d) (Additional file 3: Video S1).

Perioperative evaluations

We reviewed and recorded demographics, lesion characteristics, laboratory results, operative outcomes, and pathology reports. Serum creatinine (Scr) and estimated glomerular filtration rate (eGFR) at baseline and on the postoperative 30th day were applied to assess the function outcomes. All patients underwent a preoperative radiologic evaluation with contrast-enhanced CT to delineate the renal lesions and its size, as well as invasion depth. In addition, to delineate the renal vascular segmentation and indicate the target artery, CT angiography (CTA) with 3D reconstruction model was imaged before operation.

Data analysis

Complications were recorded according to the modified Clavien-Dindo classification [19]. eGFR was calculated

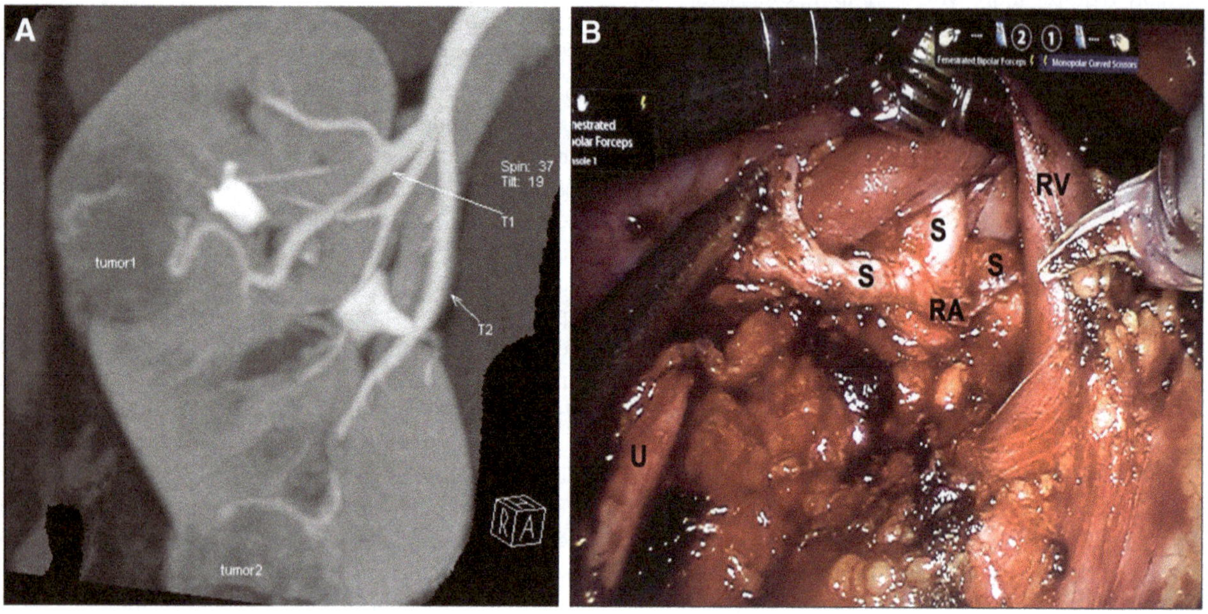

Fig. 1 The preoperative picture (**a**) of dual-source computed tomography (DSCT) angiography precisely predicts the two segmental renal arteries (SRAs) (T1 and T2) feeding two different lesions (tumor1 and tumor2) in the right kidney respectively, as confirmed by the hilar anatomy during robot-assisted partial nephrectomy (RPN) (**b**). T = target SRA

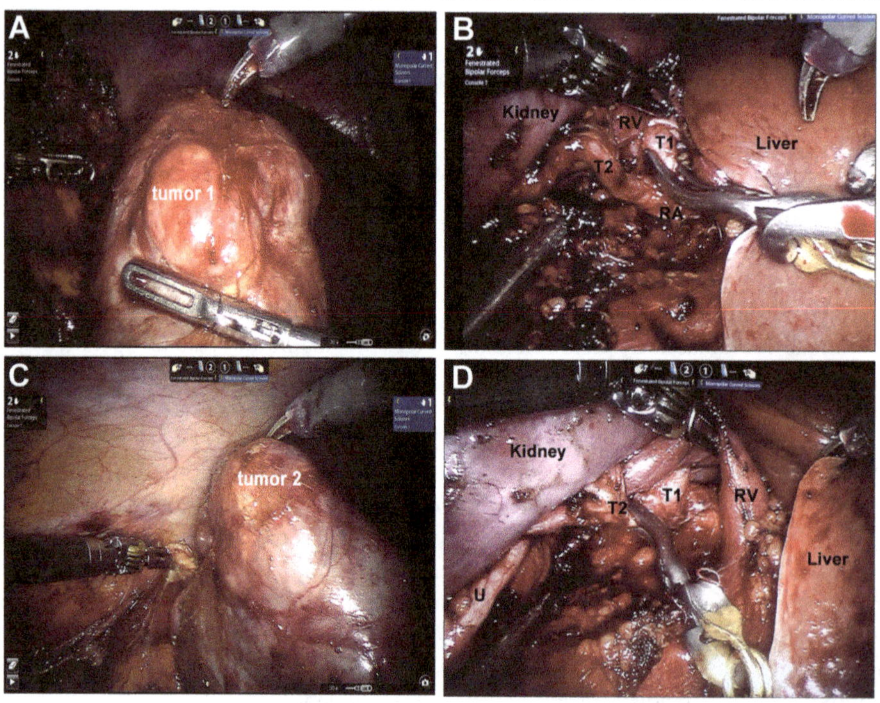

Fig. 2 Sequentially clamping the target segmental renal artery (SRA) 1 (**b**) and 2 (**d**) respectively for the ipsilateral high-score (**a**) and low-score (**c**) tumors in the right kidney. T = target SRA; U = ureter; RA = renal artery; RV = renal vein

using the Modification of Diet in Renal Disease equation: GFR in $mL/min/1.73\,m^2 = 186 \times Scr^{-1.154} \times age^{-0.203} \times$ (0.742 if female) [20]. The highest one of R.E.N.A.L nephrometry scores was considered for each patient [21]. Descriptive continuous variables were expressed with mean ± standard deviation. Descriptive categorical variable were summarized using frequencies and percentages. All statistical calculations were performed with the SPSS Statistics software v.19 (IBM, Armonk, NC, USA).

Results

Patient and lesion characteristics

The demographic and preoperative characteristics of twelve patients are summarized in Additional file 4: Table S1. The mean age was 62.7 years, and mean preoperative Scr and eGFR were 92.8 (range: 74.1–122.3) μmol/l and 78.5 (range: 54.8–113.0) ml/minute/1.73m^2, respectively. Ten cases had two lesions and two cases had three at the ipsilateral kidneys. Nine cases were diagnosed with RCCs of stage cT1a-cT1b and three were with AMLs by preoperative CT scanning. The mean size for single lesion was 2.7 cm, and the mean size and the mean R.E.N.A.L score for the dominant lesion of single case was 3.3 cm and 5.7, respectively. Two cases (16.7%) had a posterior lesion, six cases (50.0%) had at least a mesophytic lesion and one (8.3%) had an endophytic lesion. According to the 3D-reconstruction models of preoperative DSCT, twenty-two lesions (84.6%) had one target SRA and four (15.4%) had two target SRAs.

Operative outcomes

RPNs were completed in all twelve cases without conversion to open procedure or total nephrectomy. Eleven of twelve cases were completed successfully with sequential SRA clamping, and one patient converted to MRA clamping after three target SRAs were clamped but without satisfactory bleeding control. The operative outcomes of the eleven cases are summarized in Table 1. The mean operative time was 91.7 (range: 72.0–155.0) min with mean estimated blood loss (EBL) of 150.0 (range: 50.0–350.0) ml, and no patient underwent any

Table 1 Operative outcomes

Variables	n (%) or Mean (range)
Cases with successfully sequential SRA clamping, *n*	11 (91.7)
Operative time, *min*	91.7 (72.0–155.0)
Total clamping time for single case, *min*	37.5 (32.0–52.0)
Clamping time for single lesion, *min*	18.8 (15.0–27.0)
Clamped SRAs for single case, *n*	
2	9 (81.8)
3	2 (18.2)
Distribution of target SRAs, *n*	
Anterior	7 (63.6)
Combined (anterior and posterior)	4 (36.4)
Total renorrhaphy time for single case, *min*	20.8 (16.0–27.0)
Estimated blood loss, *ml*	150.0 (50.0–350.0)
Postoperative drainage volume, *ml*	125.0 (70.0–350.0)
Postoperative hospital stay, *day*	4.9 (4.0–7.0)
Complications, *n*	
Functional prolonged ileus (grade 1)	2 (18.2)
Low-grade fever (grade 1)	1 (9.1)
Gross hematuria (grade 2)	1 (9.1)
Pathological findings, *n*	
Clear cell carcinoma	7 (63.6)
Papillary cell carcinoma	1 (9.1)
AML	3 (27.3)
Postoperative Scr[a], *μmol/l*	103.6 (77.9–124.2)
Postoperative eGFR[a], *ml/minute/1.73m^2*	71.2 (52.7–106.4)

Abbreviation: *SRA* segmental renal artery, *AML* angiomyolipoma, *Scr* Serum creatinine, *eGFR* estimated glomerular filtration rate
[a]Values were tested or calculated on the postoperative 30th day

intraoperative or postoperative blood transfusion. Under the guidance of preoperative DSCT, satisfactory ischemic areas were achieved by sequentially clamping two (81.8%) or three (18.2%) target SRAs with mean clamping time of 18.8 (range: 15.0–27.0) min for single lesion, and the mean of total clamping time for single case was 37.5 (range: 32.0–52.0) min. (Table 1).

The mean volume of postoperative drainage was 125.0 (range: 70.0–350.0) ml, and the mean hospital stay after operation was 4.9 (4.0–7.0) days. Only the complications of grade 1–2 were found in the cohort without any one of grade 3–5, and one case had gross hematuria and recovered with only drug treatment. Pathological diagnoses were consistent with preoperative imaging diagnoses in all case and no positive surgical margin was discovered (Table 1). Only one tumor had invasion of the perinephric fat (stage pT3a), and all other tumors were stage pT1a- pT1b in eight cases with RCCs.

The mean follow-up time was 5.4 (range: 2.0–8.0) months and no further embolization or surgical procedure was required. All patients had a normal value of Scr (range: 77.9–124.2 μmol/l) on the postoperative 30th day, and the mean postoperative eGFR was 71.2 ml/minute/1.73m^2 that was only an insignificant reduction (9.3%) compared with the preoperative baseline (Table 1). No local recurrence or metastasis was found during the follow-up.

Discussion

The goal of managing MIRTs is to prevent renal tumors dissemination and maximize nephron sparing and postoperative function outcomes. With the development of robot-assisted platform and minimally invasive surgery techniques, the one-time resection of MIRTs with nephron sparing is becoming possible. Warm ischemia (WI) injury plays a principal role that influences the postoperative function outcomes in NSS, and the time of WI should be less than 20 min [15, 22]. Currently, many novel techniques have emerged to decrease WI injury, which are laudable endeavors [11–15, 23–26]. One of main methods is to convert total parenchymal ischemia to local ischemia [11–15]. In 2010, our center first successfully applied LPN with SRA clamping for the treatment of RCCs that has been proved safe and feasible [15]. The technique can minimize the scope of intraoperative WI injury and provide better postoperative function outcomes [12]. Logically, WI time during partial nephrectomy (PN) for MIRTs would be the accumulation of multiple single-lesion processing time if the MRA clamping is applied. Thus the WI time of spared nephrons is less likely to be controlled within 20 min, which will inevitably damage the postoperative function outcomes.

Fortunately, we found a considerable proportion of MIRT patients had at least two SRAs feeding different lesions by preoperative high-quality 3D-DSCT angiography. According to the anatomic characteristic between SRAs and multiple lesions, we originally applied the sequential clamping technique of target SRAs in RPN to avoid the WI time of any spared nephrons more than 20 min. In our cohort, although the mean of total clamping time for single case was 37.5 min, the mean clamping time for single lesion is only 18.8 min that successfully prevents spared nephrons from severe WI injury. All the patients had a normal value of Scr on the postoperative 30th day and the mean postoperative eGFR only had an insignificant reduction compared with the preoperative baseline. (Table 1).

Relying on the advantages of precision, flexibility and stability, the robotic-assisted laparoscopic system facilitates surgeons to perform many complex procedures, like precise hilar microdissection and one-time resection/renorrhaphy for multiple renal lesions. Compared with our previous report on LPN procedure in 2017 [15], RPN with sequential SRA clamping shows more advantages. In despite of the larger tumor size (mean 2.7 vs. 2.5 cm) and higher R.E.N.A.L score (mean 5.7 vs. 4.4) in RPN cohort than in LPN, RPN cohort manifests the better operative outcomes, such as less blood loss (mean 150 vs. 190 ml), shorter operation time (mean 91.7 vs 125 min) and clamping time for single lesion (mean 18.8 vs. 23 min). Therefore, it is foreseeable that the technique of sequential SRA clamping should be more powerful in RPN than in LPN for treating MIRTs.

To our knowledge, this is the initial report of the sequential SRA clamping technique in the procedure of RPN. There have been several reports that described the performance of RPN for MIRTs with MRA clamping or no clamping [24, 27–29]. However, MRA clamping of more than 20 min may cause severe renal ischemia/ reperfusion injury and function damage [27, 28]. At the other extreme, no clamping of renal hilum may lead to more blood loss, greater risk of open procedure or total nephrectomy, and longer surgery time than hilar control [24, 29]. Compared to the above two techniques, SRA clamping only blocks the blood flow of the selected renal segment located by lesions and preserves the supply to other segments. Furtherly, sequential clamping of multiple SRAs can effectively limit the WI time of each involved segment within the recommended 20 min for the one-time resection of MIRTs. Thus this technique minimizes WI injury to the whole kidney by the alternate conversion of ischemic regions, as is evidenced by the insignificant decrease of the postoperative eGFR in our cohort. Moreover, this technique provides better visualization than no clamping, and may help resect less normal parenchyma and avoid positive margins. In our cohort, the mean EBL was 150.0 ml without any intraoperative or postoperative blood transfusion. Only the complications of grade 1–2 were found and no positive surgical margin was discovered.

In this study, we describe our initial experience with sequential SRA clamping in RPN for MIRT treatment. A limitation of this technique is the target SRAs should be isolated precisely. However, SRAs could be dissected in only half of cases, which indicates this technique may not be feasible in certain instances such as cases with dense perirenal fat or short segmental arteries [30]. Moreover, during the NSS study, we did find some MIRT cases unsuitable for sequential SRA clamping before surgery or in operation. For instance, preoperative DSCT revealed only unique SRA feeding multiple lesions or clamping multiple SRAs could not obtain satisfactory ischemic area. Now we have been collecting such cases to compare with those successfully undergoing sequential SRA clamping, and the results from the comparison will be reported in our next article.

Although the advantages of this technique were discovered in this report, some shortcomings should be taken into consideration. First of all, the report only was a retrospective description of single center with a small sample size of twelve cases, for which some complication rates could not be evaluated. Second, we didn't compare the technique with other approaches to PN, so some more reliable and robust results couldn't be achieved. Our report only indicates the technique may facilitate a minimally invasive approach to NSS in patients with MIRTs. Third, the mean follow-up time was only 5.4 months. The long-term recurrence rate couldn't be evaluated due to the lack of a long-term follow-up. Thus large-scale multicenter clinical studies are still needed to further prove the advantages of RPN with sequential SRA clamping in MIRT treatment.

Conclusion

This novel nephron-sparing technique, RPN with sequential SRA clamping, represents a good alternative for selected patients with MIRTs. With the guidance of DSCT and skilled robotic experience, this technique can facilitate the challenges of minimally invasive approaches to NSS for MIRT patients, who expect a long-term survival while maintaining adequate renal function. The technique is feasible, can be performed in security and maximize renal function preservation. Hence, more cases, longer follow-up, and comparisons with other approaches to PN are needed to confirm these initial outcomes.

Additional files

Additional file 1: Figure S1. The pictures of preoperative computed tomography (CT) scanning and three-dimensional reconstruction (C) show a 2.4*2.7 cm tumor (A) and a 2.1*2.3 cm tumor (B) co-locating in the right kidney of a 57-year-old woman. (TIF 6027 kb)

Additional file 2: Figure S2. The schematic drawing (A) and operative photograph (B) of patient positioning and port placement for right robot-assisted partial nephrectomy. IC = iliac crest, CM – costal margin; Ro = robotic port; As = assistant port; Cam = camera port. (TIF 4531 kb)

Additional file 3: Video 1. Robotic-Assisted partial nephrectomy with sequential clamping of segmental renal arteries for two ipsilateral renal tumors in the right kidney. (WMV 121213 kb)

Additional file 4: Table S1. Demographics and imaging features of tumors. (DOCX 20 kb)

Acknowledgements
Not applicable.

Authors' contributions
ZJW and NHS conceived and designed the study; YMW and DX as corresponding researchers collected clinical information and interviewed patients; CL and JDX organized and input the data; YMW checked and verified data input by CL and JDX; ZJW performed the operations; JY and JXX performed statistical analyses; JY and JDX drafted the manuscript; JY and JXX revised the manuscript. All authors have read and approved the final version.

References

1. Ljungberg B, Campbell SC, Choi HY, et al. The epidemiology of renal cell carcinoma. Eur Urol. 2011;60(4):615–21.
2. Lang H, Lindner V, Martin M, et al. Prognostic value of multifocality on progression and survival in localized renal cell carcinoma. Eur Urol. 2004; 45(6):749–53.
3. Tsivian M, Moreira DM, Caso JR, et al. Predicting occult multifocality of renal cell carcinoma. Eur Urol. 2010;58(1):118–26.
4. Klatte T, Patard JJ, Wunderlich H, et al. Metachronous bilateral renal cell carcinoma: risk assessment, prognosis and relevance of the primary-free interval. J Urol. 2007;177(6):2081–6.
5. Blute M, Thibault GP, Leibovich BC, et al. Multiple ipsilateral renal tumors discovered at planned nephron sparing surgery: Importance of tumor histology and risk of metachronous recurrence. J Urol. 2003;170(3):760–3.
6. Krambeck AE, Iwaszko M, Leibovich BC, et al. Long-term outcome of multiple ipsilateral renal tumours found at the time of planned nephron-sparing surgery. BJU Int. 2008;101:1375–9.
7. Minervini A, Serni S, Giubilei G, et al. Multiple ipsilateral renal tumors: retrospective analysis of surgical and onco-logical results of tumor enucleation vs radical nephrectomy. Eur J Surg Oncol. 2009;35:521–6.
8. Ljungberg B, Cowan NC, Hanbury DC, et al. EAU guidelines on renal cell carcinoma: the 2010 update. Eur Urol. 2010;58:398–406.
9. Gettman MT, Blute ML, Chow GK, et al. Robotic-assisted laparoscopic partial nephrectomy: technique and initial clinical experience with DaVinci robotic system. Urology. 2004;64(5):914–8.
10. Rogers CG, Singh A, Blatt AM, et al. Robotic partial nephrectomy for complex renal tumors: surgical technique. Eur Urol. 2008;53(3):514–21.
11. Shao P, Tang L, Li P, et al. Application of a vasculature model and standardization of the renal hilar approach in laparoscopic partial nephrectomy for precise segmental artery clamping. Eur Urol. 2013;63(6): 1072–81.
12. Li P, Qin C, Cao Q, et al. A retrospective analysis of laparoscopic partial nephrectomy with segmental renal artery clamping and factors that predict postoperative renal function. BJU Int. 2016;118(4):610–7.
13. Qian J, Li P, Qin C, et al. Laparoscopic partial nephrectomy with precise segmental renal artery clamping for clinical T1b tumors. J Endourol. 2015; 29(12):1386–91.
14. Shao P, Tang L, Li P, et al. Precise segmental renal artery clamping under the guidance of dual-source computed tomography angiography during laparoscopic partial nephrectomy. Eur Urol. 2012;62(6):1001–8.
15. Zhu J, Jiang F, Li P, Shao P, Liang C, Xu A, Miao C, Qin C, Wang Z, Yin C. Application and analysis of retroperitoneal laparoscopic partial nephrectomy with sequential segmental renal artery clamping for patients with multiple renal tumor: initial experience. BMC Urol. 2017;17(1):82.

16. Gates GF. Split renal function testing using Tc-99m DTPA. A rapid technique for determining differential glomerular filtration. Clin Nucl Med. 1983;8:400–7.
17. Kara O, Akca O, Zargar H, et al. Robotic partial nephrectomy in the treatment of renal Angiomyolipoma. J Endourol. 2016;30(3):275–9.
18. Andrade HS, Zargar H, Caputo PA, et al. Five-year oncologic outcomes after Transperitoneal robotic partial nephrectomy for renal cell carcinoma. Eur Urol. 2016;69(6):1149–54.
19. Dindo D, Demartines N, Clavien PA. Classification of surgical complications: a new proposal with evaluation in a cohort of 6336 patients and results of a survey. Ann Surg. 2004;240:205.
20. Levey AS, Coresh J, Greene T, et al. Using standardized serum creatinine values in the modification of diet in renal disease study equation for estimating glomerular filtration rate. Ann Intern Med. 2006;145(4):247–54.
21. Kutikov A, Uzzo RG. The R.E.N.A.L. nephrometry score: a comprehensive standardized system for quantitating renal tumor size, location and depth. J Urol. 2009;182(3):844–53.
22. Porpiglia F, Fiori C, Bertolo R, et al. Long-term functional evaluation of the treated kidney in a prospective series of patients who underwent laparoscopic partial nephrectomy for small renal tumors. Eur Urol. 2012;62: 130–5.
23. Gill IS, Patil MB, Abreu AL, et al. Zero ischemia anatomical partial nephrectomy: a novel approach. J Urol. 2012;187(3):807–14.
24. Rizkala ER, Khalifeh A, Autorino R, et al. Zero ischemia robotic partial nephrectomy: sequential preplaced suture renorrhaphy technique. Urology. 2013;82(1):100–4.
25. LPN D, Caputo PA, Krishnan J, et al. Robot-assisted partial nephrectomy with intracorporeal renal hypothermia using ice slush: step-by-step technique and matched comparison with warm ischaemia. BJU Int. 2016;117(3):531–6.
26. Rogers C, Sukumar S, Gill IS. Robotic partial nephrectomy: the real benefit. Curr Opin Urol. 2011;21(1):60–4.
27. Boris R, Proano M, Linehan WM, et al. Initial experience with robot assisted partial nephrectomy for multiple renal masses. J Urol. 2009;182(4):1280–6.
28. Laydner H, Autorino R, Spana G, et al. Robot-assisted partial nephrectomy for sporadic ipsilateral multifocal renal tumours. BJU Int. 2012;109(2):274–80.
29. Guillonneau B, Bermudez H, Gholami S, et al. Laparoscopic partial nephrectomy for renal tumor:single center experience comparing clamping and no clamping techniques of the renal vasculature. J Urol. 2003;169:483–6.
30. Klatte T, Ficarra V, Gratzke C, et al. A literature review of renal surgical anatomy and surgical strategies for partial nephrectomy. Eur Urol. 2015; 68(6):980–92.

9

Comparison of the long-term follow-up and perioperative outcomes of partial nephrectomy and radical nephrectomy for 4 cm to 7 cm renal cell carcinoma

Yu-Li Jiang[1,2*], Cheng-Xia Peng[1,2], Heng-Zi Wang[1,2] and Lu-Jie Qian[1,2]

Abstract

Background: The efficacy of partial nephrectomy (PN) for T1b renal cell carcinoma (RCC) is controversial. The oncological outcomes, the change in postoperative renal function and the perioperative complications are unclear.

Methods: We searched PUBMED, EMBASE and the Cochrane Central Register for studies from March 1998 to March 2018 for studies comparing PN to radical nephrectomy (RN) for the treatment of T1b RCC. After data extraction and quality assessment, we used RevMan 5.2 to pool the data. Then, we used Stata 12.0 to perform sensitivity analyses and meta-regression. We used the GRADE profiler to evaluate the evidence according to the GRADE approach.

Results: A total of 16 studies involving 33,117 patients were included in our meta-analysis. No significant difference was found in the 5-year overall survival (OS), 10-year OS, 5-year recurrence free survival (RFS) and 10-year RFS. The 5-year cancer-special survival (CSS) and 10-year CSS were better in RN compared to PN, respectively, at RR = 1.02, $P < 0.05$ and RR = 1.04, $P < 0.05$. PN was better than RN in the preservation of renal function (WMD = -9.15, 95% CI: − 10.30 to − 7.99, $P < 0.05$). The confidence level grading of the evidence was moderate for 5-year OS, 10-year OS, 5-year CSS, 10-year CSS, 5-year RFS, 10-year RFS, tumor recurrence, decline in eGFR, and postoperative complications.

Conclusions: PN may provide comparable outcomes in terms of RFS & OS, and better renal function preservation although CSS was worse.

Keywords: Renal cell carcinoma, Partial nephrectomy, Radical nephrectomy, Overall survival, Cancer special survival, Recurrence-free survival

Background

Renal cell carcinoma, also called renal adenocarcinoma, comprises 85% of malignant renal cell carcinomas (RCCs), accounts for 2–3% of all cancer diagnoses and is a common urology cancer [1]. The increased chance of detection of small renal masses has attracted urology surgeons to focus on making and revising operation methods and treatments for T1b renal cell carcinoma. The incidence of diagnosis of RCC has increased steadily by 2.5% (the most common histological variant of RCC is clear-cell carcinoma).

In the last several decades, radical nephrectomy (RN), has been the standard treatment for RCC. Since 1980, Nov et al. reported that partial nephrectomy has been adopted for some selective renal cell carcinoma patients [2]. PN has been accepted as a standard surgical approach, especially in the last decade, for the treatment of patients with a renal mass < 4 cm, with equivalent oncological outcomes and better renal preservation than RN [3]. Initially, PN was performed solely in patients with imperative indications, but it is also being adopted for patients with

* Correspondence: renren108@126.com
[1]Department of Urology, The Affiliated Hospital of Hang Zhou Normal University, Hangzhou 310015, China
[2]School of Medicine, Hang Zhou Normal University, Hangzhou 310016, China

relative indications. Even though both EAU guidelines and AUA guidelines recommend the use of PN as a standard treatment, evidence supporting this recommendation is insufficient [4, 5]. The present study showed that the oncological long-term outcomes between patients treated with PN and RN were similar, but patients treated with RN had a higher mortality rate than those treated with PN [6–9]. However, there are few studies addressing the surgical indications for the treatment of T1b renal tumors.

The advantages of PN for the treatment of T1b renal tumor are still controversial. Several studies have reported that PN could have a similar effect on the control of cancer as RN. Kim et al. performed a meta-analysis to compare the outcomes of PN and RN in cases of localized renal tumors. They reported that PN had a greater advantage over RN [10]. However, the studies involved patients with T1a renal tumor masses. The study reported cancer-specific mortality and all-cause mortality. In addition, Mir et al. conducted a meta-analysis comparing PN and RN and combined cases with T1b and T2 renal tumor masses. Therefore, we performed a meta-analysis comparing PN and RN for the treatment of patients with T1b RCC.

The aim of this meta-analysis was to compare long-term oncological outcomes in patients with 4 to 7 cm RCC treated with PN and RN.

Methods

This meta-analysis was performed in accordance with the Preferred Reporting Items for Systemic Reviews and Meta-analysis (PRISMA) statement. We searched PUBMED, EMBASE and the Cochrane Central Register for studies which published in English dating from March 1998 to March 2018. The search terms were renal tumors, kidney cancer, renal cancer, T1b, 4–7 cm, nephron-sparing-surgery or PN, radical nephrectomy, PN and RN, NSS and RN. We also used the combined Boolean operators "AND" or "OR" Title/Abstract. The two investigators (YLJ and HZW) reviewed the results in the case of discrepancies. The inclusion criteria were as follows: (1) comparative PN or NSS and RN for the treatment of 4–7 cm renal tumors and (2) evaluation of at least one oncological result such as RFS, CSS, and OS.

The exclusion criteria were as follows: (1) case reports, reviews, and articles without applicable data; (2) studies that included both T1b and T2 or renal tumors larger than 7 cm; and (3) studies that were not comparative in nature.

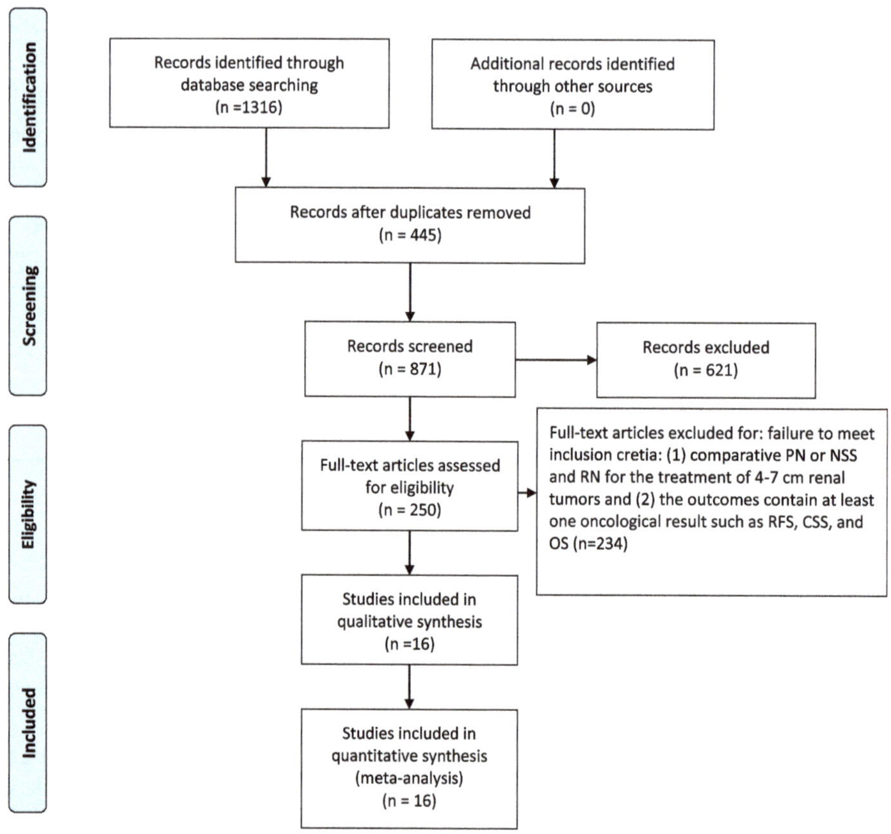

Fig. 1 Flow diagram of the process for the selection of relevant studies

The process of identifying relevant studies is summarized in Fig. 1.

Statistical analysis

We used Review Manager Version 5.2 software (The Cochrane Collaboration, Oxford, UK) and Stata 12.0 to perform the analysis of the included data. We used the GRADE approach to evaluate the quality of the evidence. We used Cochran's Q to evaluate the heterogeneity; if the value of Q < 50% or $P > 0.01$, we believed little heterogeneity was present. However, if Q > 50%, $P < 0.01$, evident heterogeneity existed. For quantitative data, we used weight mean difference (WMD) or standard mean difference (SMD) to calculate continuous data. We used OR and 95% confidence interval (CI) to evaluate binary data. We used LnRR instead of RR and SE to normalize the distribution of the data. We used Stata 12.0 to perform funnel plots to evaluate the publication bias among the studies (Additional file 1: S1 File).

Evidence grading

We used the GRADE profiler to create the evidence grading. Assessment of the underlying quality of the evidence, major statistical results, and grading of the evidence for each outcome made the body of the evidence. The evidence was graded as high, moderate,

Table 1 Basic Characteristics of the Included Studies

Study	Study type	Group	Sample Size	Age(y)	Sex F/M	Pathologic tumor size (cm)	Follow-up month(s)
Kim2012	retrospective	PN	18	47.3	5/13	5.0	78.2
		RN	52	57.3	16/36	5.5	66.5
Badalato2011	retrospective	PN	1047	58.4	677/370	4.86	120
		RN	10,209	60.7	4166/6043	5.27	120
Jang2016	retrospective	PN	100	55.3	29/71	4.9	48.1
		RN	100	55.7	29/71	4.9	42.6
Iizuka2012	retrospective	PN	67	57.6	16/51	4.9	31.3
		RN	195	58.1	76/119	5.3	93.0
Roos2011	retrospective	PN	73	60.4	7/66	5.0	55.2
		RN	100	61.1	62/38	5.5	78
Roos2012	retrospective	PN	85	NA	55/56	NA	120
		RN	118	NA	59/87	NA	120
Crepel2010	retrospective	PN	275	60.5	100/175	NA	40.7
		RN	1100	60.5	433/667	NA	46.7
Milonas2013	retrospective	PN	34	62.2	9/15	4.67	168
		RN	317	63.4	153/164	5.25	168
Thompson2009	retrospective	PN	286	NA	90/196	NA	57.6
		RN	873	NA	335/538	NA	57.6
Pignot2014	retrospective	PN	123	57.6	43/80	5.2	39.5
		RN	185	61.6	58/127	5.5	46.9
Antoneli2012	retrospective	PN	198	58.2	64/134	5.0	120
		RN	1426	62.4	524/902	5.7	120
Meskawi2013	retrospective	PN	1526	60.3	493/1033	5.14	60
		RN	6104	60.6	1966/4138	5.15	120
Weight2010	retrospective	PN	212	49	73/139	4.8	49
		RN	298	41	122/176	5.6	41
Simmoons2009	retrospective	PN	35	63.5	9/26	4.6	NA
		RN	75	63.4	36/39	5.3	NA
Robert2006	retrospective	PN	33	68.9	7/26	5.2	34.0
		RN	66	66.9	22/44	5.2	48.5
Patard2004	retrospective	PN	64	NA	NA	5.3	120
		RN	576	NA	NA	5.6	120

NA Not Available

lower, low or very low quality. The criteria for the evaluation of the evidence included the assessment of risk bias as determined from the results of the Cochran Risk of Bias Tool.

Results

A total of 1316 studies were obtained from the selected databases. The PRISMA flow diagram of the search process is summarized in Fig. 1. We removed 445 duplicates. From the selected databases, we obtained 144 reports. After screening the titles and abstracts, 89 full texts were excluded for failure to meet inclusion cretia. After detailed processing, 29 reports were excluded for failure to meet inclusion cretia. Finally, sixteen studies were included in our meta-analysis [11–26]. Table 1 summarizes the baseline characteristics and assessments.

Quality assessment of the included studies

We used the New-Ottawa Scale (NOS) to assess the included nonrandomized studies. We used a 9-point system to evaluate the NOS scores. The study score of 7–9 or above was considered high quality, a score of 4–6 was considered medium quality, and a score of 0–4 or below was considered low quality. Two reviewers (YLJ and CXP) evaluate the quality of the included studies. Table 2 shows the risk of bias of the selected studies.

5-year OS and 10-year OS

Eight studies reported the 5-year OS outcome. There was no significant difference in the 5-year OS between the PN and RN groups ($n = 13{,}016$, 1571 patients were in the PN group, 11,445 patients were in the RN group, 95% CI 1.0–1.05; $p = 0.05$, $I^2 = 84\%$, fixed-effect model, Fig. 2). Six studies reported the 10-year OS in our meta-analysis. No significant statistical difference between the PN and the RN group was noted ($n = 2678$, LnRR: 1.17, 95% CI: 0.91 to 1.10, $I^2 = 85\%$, fixed-effects model, Fig. 3)

.

5-year CSS and 10-year CSS

Nine studies included a 5-year CSS. There was a statistically significant difference between the PN and the RN group ($n = 19{,}406$, 2195 patients were in the PN group, 17,211 patients were in the RN group, LnRR: 1.02, 95% CI 1.01–1.03, $p = 0.001$, $I^2 = 68\%$, fixed-effective model, Fig. 4). Seven studies included a 10-year CSS. There was a statistically significant difference between the PN and the RN group ($n = 20{,}401$, 2302 patients were in the PN group, 18,099 patients were in the RN group, LnRR: 1.04, 95% CI 1.03–1.06, $p < 0.05$, $I^2 = 57\%$, fixed-effective model, Fig. 5).

5- and 10-year RFS

Six studies reported the 5-year RFS. No significant difference was found between the PN and the RN group ($n = 2349$ patients, 495 patients were included in the PN

Table 2 Newcastle-Ottawa Scale for risk of bias assessment of the included studies

Study	Design	Selection				Comparability	Outcome			Total
		Representativeness of exposed cohort	Selective of nonexposed Cohort	Ascertainment of exposure	Outcome not present at start		Assessment of outcome	Adequate follow-up length	Adequacy of follow-up	
Kim	R	*	*	*	*	**		*	*	8
Badalato	R	*		*	*	**		*	*	7
Jang	R	*	*	*	*	*	*	*	*	8
Iizuka	R	*		*	*	**	*	*	*	8
Roos2011	R	*		*	*	**	*	*	*	8
Roos2012	R	*		*	*		*	*	*	8
Crepel	R	*	*	*	*	**	*	*	*	9
Milonas	R	*		*	*	*	*	*	*	7
Thompson	R	*		*	*	**	*	*	*	8
Pignot	R	*		*	*	**	*	*	*	8
Antoneli	R	*		*	*	**	*	*	*	8
Meskawi	R	*		*	*	**		*	*	7
Weight	R	*	*	*	*	**	*	*	*	9
Simmoons	R	*		*	*	**	*	*	*	8
Robert	R	*	*	*	*	**	*	*	*	9
Patard	R	*		*	*	**		*	*	8

R Retrospective study

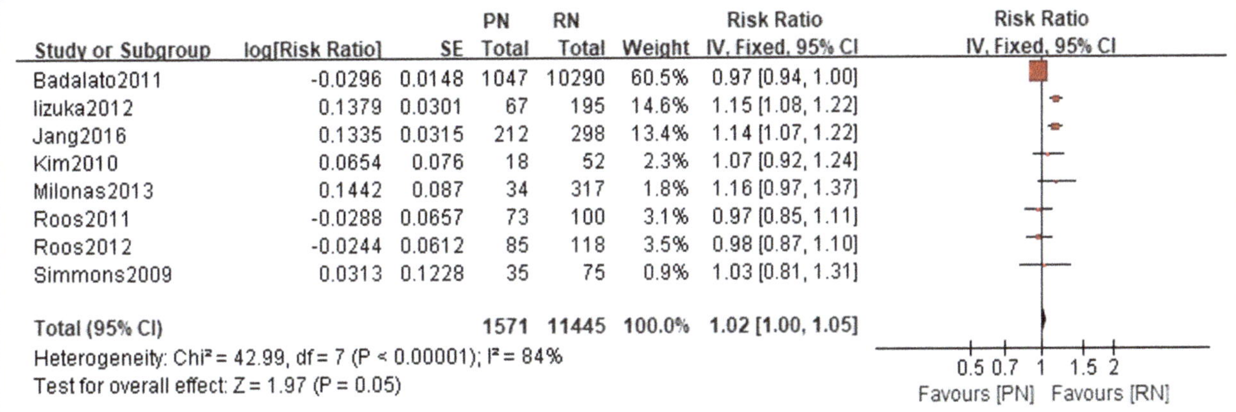

Fig. 2 Forest plot for 5-year OS between the PN and RN for T1b tumors

group, and 1854 patients were included in the RN group, LnRR: 0.99, 95% CI: 0.98 to 1.01, $\chi^2 = 7.22$, df = 5, $p = 0.20$, $I^2 = 31\%$, fixed-effects model, Fig. 6). Two studies reported the 10-year RFS. No significant difference was found between the PN and the RN group ($n = 373$ patients, 173 patients were included in the PN group. and 200 patients were included in the RN group, LnRR: 1.00, 95% CI: 0.91 to 1.10, $\chi^2 = 6.77$, df = 1, $p = 0.97$, $I^2 = 85\%$, fixed-effects model, Fig. 7).

Tumor recurrence

Eight studies included in our meta-analysis assessed tumor recurrence. The patients in the PN group had a lower rate of tumor recurrence compared to the RN group ($n = 2052$ patients, 531 patients were in the PN group, 1521 patients were in the RN group, OR: 0.68, 95% CI: 0.40 to 0.98, $\chi 2 = 6.07$, df = 7, $p = 0.04$, $I^2 = 0$, fixed-effects model, Fig. 8).

Postoperative complications

Three studies reported postoperative complications. There was no statistically significant difference between the PN and the RN group ($n = 798$ patients, 235 patients were in the PN group, 563 patients were in the RN group, LnRR = 1.45, 95% CI: 0.95 to 2,21, $I^2 = 0$, $\chi^2 = 0.01$, df = 2, $P = 0.99$, fixed-effect model, Fig. 9).

Declined eGFR

Four studies reported declined eGFR. There was a significant difference in declined eGFR between the PN and the RN group ($n = 1090$, 433 patients were in the PN group, 657 patients were in the RN group, WMD; − 9.15, 95% CI: − 10.30 to − 7.99, $\chi^2 = 36.27$, df = 3, $P < 0.05$, $I^2 = 0.92$, fixed-effects model, Fig. 10)

.

Sensitivity analysis

We sequentially omitted a single study one by one to determine which studies contributed the most to the heterogeneity of the results. In the 5-year and 10-year OS outcomes, we found that the studies performed by Badalato (2011) and Thompson (2009) greatly changed the overall outcome. In the declined eGFR outcome, the study performed by Weight (2009). probably changed the outcome greatly. In the 5-year CSS outcome, no study changed the outcome significantly. (Additional file 2: S2 File).

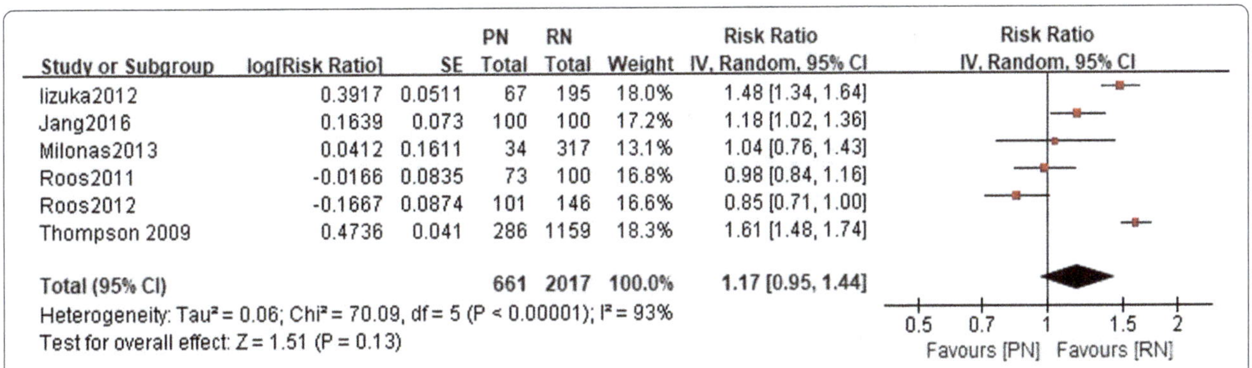

Fig. 3 Forest plot for 10-year OS between the PN and RN for T1b tumors

Study or Subgroup	log[Risk Ratio]	SE	PN Total	RN Total	Weight	Risk Ratio IV, Fixed, 95% CI
Antonelli 2012	-0.0292	0.025	198	1426	4.3%	0.97 [0.92, 1.02]
Kim2010	0.0023	0.0667	18	52	0.6%	1.00 [0.88, 1.14]
Meskawi2014	0.0169	0.0059	1526	14807	77.5%	1.02 [1.01, 1.03]
Milonas2013	0.1839	0.0405	34	317	1.6%	1.20 [1.11, 1.30]
Robert 2006	-0.0155	0.0344	33	66	2.3%	0.98 [0.92, 1.05]
Roos2011	-0.0259	0.0332	73	100	2.4%	0.97 [0.91, 1.04]
Roos2012	-0.0244	0.0612	101	146	0.7%	0.98 [0.87, 1.10]
Simmons2009	0.0704	0.1276	43	29	0.2%	1.07 [0.84, 1.38]
Weight2010	0.0378	0.0162	169	268	10.3%	1.04 [1.01, 1.07]
Total (95% CI)			**2195**	**17211**	**100.0%**	**1.02 [1.01, 1.03]**

Heterogeneity: $Chi^2 = 25.27$, $df = 8$ ($P = 0.001$); $I^2 = 68\%$
Test for overall effect: $Z = 3.41$ ($P = 0.0006$)

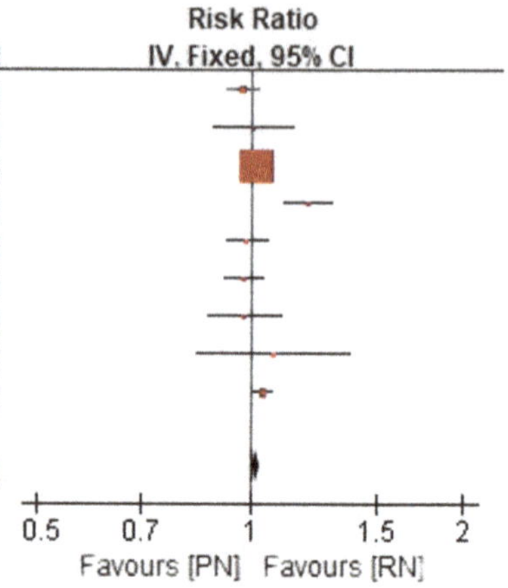

Fig. 4 Forest plot for 5-year CSS between the PN and RN for T1b tumors

Grading assessment

Additional file 3: Figure S3 shows a summary of evidence grading. The evidence was graded as moderate for 5-year OS, 10-year OS, 5-year CSS, 10-year CSS, 5-year RFS, 10-year RFS, tumor recurrence, declined eGFR, and postoperative complications. (Additional file 3: S3 File).

Discussion

The present systematic review and meta-analysis was performed to compare the long-term follow-up outcomes and perioperative outcomes of partial nephrectomy and radical nephrectomy for the treatment of T1b renal cell carcinomas. The present study was the first meta-analysis to compare long-term oncological outcomes. In addition, the present study provides us with moderate evidence determined by using the GRADE approach to evaluate the effectiveness of PN versus RN for the treatment of T1b renal tumors.

Our meta-analysis demonstrated that patients with T1b RCC presented comparable basic characteristics. Our study compared the long-term follow-up outcomes among patients receiving PN versus RN. These patients shared comparable common baseline characteristics. In our study, 5-year CSS, 5-year RFS and 5-year OS rates were not significantly different for patients undergoing PN versus RN. The indications for PN are exclusively for 4–7 cm RCC. In the present study, no significant differences in 5-year and 10-year OS were found between the PN and the RN groups for the treatment of T1b renal tumors. Zhang et al. found that OS was independent of the type of surgical procedure in the propensity score matching [27].

Our present study demonstrated that the 5-year and 10-year OS were not impacted by PN or RN. In addition, Weight et al. found that patients with T1b RCC had a better OS in the PN group compared to the RN group. Antonelli et al. and Thompson et al. also reported similar outcomes [11, 18]. However, Zhang et al. reported that the PN group had a better OS according to both Cox-regression and Kaplan-Meier analysis ($P < 0.01$). Several studies also reported that PN or RN do not influence the OS. These studies used propensity score matching to eliminate any potential confounding factors. Tumor size, tumor grading and age may influence the

Study or Subgroup	log[Risk Ratio]	SE	PN Total	RN Total	Weight	Risk Ratio IV, Fixed, 95% CI
Antonelli 2012	0.0325	0.0259	198	1426	6.3%	1.03 [0.98, 1.09]
Jang2016	0.0176	0.045	100	458	2.1%	1.02 [0.93, 1.11]
Meskawi2014	0.0477	0.0071	1526	14807	83.3%	1.05 [1.03, 1.06]
Milonas2013	0.0394	0.0928	34	317	0.5%	1.04 [0.87, 1.25]
Roos2011	-0.0495	0.0445	73	100	2.1%	0.95 [0.87, 1.04]
Roos2012	-0.0467	0.0409	85	118	2.5%	0.95 [0.88, 1.03]
Thompson 2009	0.1126	0.0357	286	873	3.3%	1.12 [1.04, 1.20]
Total (95% CI)			**2302**	**18099**	**100.0%**	**1.04 [1.03, 1.06]**

Heterogeneity: $Chi^2 = 13.84$, $df = 6$ ($P = 0.03$); $I^2 = 57\%$
Test for overall effect: $Z = 6.76$ ($P < 0.00001$)

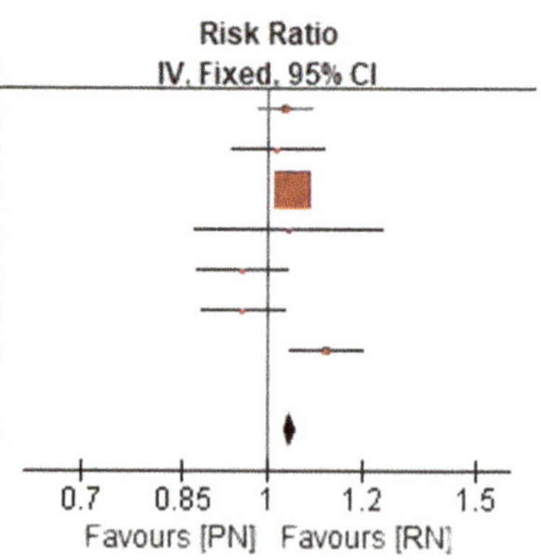

Fig. 5 Forest plot for 10-year CSS between the PN and RN for T1b tumors

Study or Subgroup	log[Risk Ratio]	SE	PN Total	RN Total	Weight	Risk Ratio IV, Fixed, 95% CI
Antonelli 2012	-0.0052	0.0074	198	1426	85.2%	0.99 [0.98, 1.01]
Jang2016	0	0.0571	100	100	1.4%	1.00 [0.89, 1.12]
Kim2010	0.2052	0.0951	18	52	0.5%	1.23 [1.02, 1.48]
Roos2011	-0.0799	0.0574	73	100	1.4%	0.92 [0.82, 1.03]
Roos2012	-0.0186	0.0225	71	101	9.2%	0.98 [0.94, 1.03]
Simmons2009	-0.0318	0.0458	35	75	2.2%	0.97 [0.89, 1.06]
Total (95% CI)			**495**	**1854**	**100.0%**	**0.99 [0.98, 1.01]**

Heterogeneity: Chi² = 7.22, df = 5 (P = 0.20); I² = 31%
Test for overall effect: Z = 1.01 (P = 0.31)

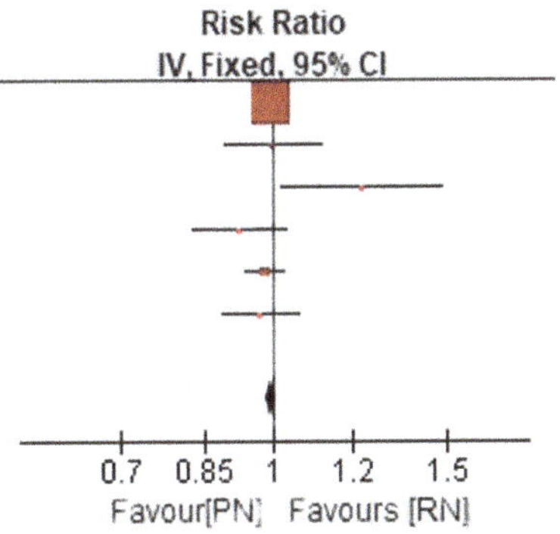

Fig. 6 Forest plot for 5-year RFS between the PN and RN for T1b tumors

OS of the two groups. After propensity score matching, no significant difference was found in the baseline covariates, which lowered the effects of potential confounders in the regression models. In addition, it was found that the OS of T1b RCC following treatment was similar between the PN and the RN groups in cases where patients with underlying conditions were treated with PN. Roos et al. found that the difference in OS was related to selection bias. Additionally, they found that tumor size was an independent factor affecting the OS of patients treated with RN instead of PN. Roos et al. reported that tumor size was related to a reduced OS for patients with RN and not PN. They also demonstrated that the feasibility of PN was dependent upon tumor location [24]. The selection bias present in the included studies with regards to the tumor pathology (clear-cell carcinoma vs non-clear cell carcinoma) may account for the higher heterogeneity of the 10-year OS outcome.

Our study showed that patients receiving RN for the treatment of a T1b renal tumor had a longer 5-year and 10-year CSS compared to those receiving PN. Similarly, Leibovich et al. reported that patients receiving PN had a higher 5-year CSS [8]. However, several articles reported no significant difference in the 5-year CSS rate in patients with T1b RCC treated with PN versus RN [17, 23, 25]. Tumor location, tumor size and selection bias may account for this difference. It is believed that selection bias may have influenced these results. Additionally, these differences may also be due to the cancer subtype and TNM stage. Crepel et al. reported the CSS rate and suggested that PN should have equal consideration [12]. However, Lee et al. found no significant difference between the two types of treatment using Cox analysis. These differences did not persist after adjusting for some preoperative covariates. In their study, the patients were usually younger and had smaller tumors in the PN group than in the RN group. They showed that age, tumor size and T stage may be potential predicting factors to evaluate the CSS [14]. In our study, the patients in the PN presented a smaller tumor size than those in the RN group. This factor may have contributed to the results.

Several studies showed that the CSS was better in the PN than in the RN group. Weight et al. and Thompson et al. found that patients receiving RN had almost a two-fold greater mortality than those receiving PN [18]. Milonas et al. found that the estimated 12-year CSS was lower than RN, thus indicating that disease relapse was lower than that in patients receiving RN [18]. Antonelli et al. found that the CSS decreased in the case of patients receiving PN for Fuhrman grade IV RCC (clear cell carcinoma) [11].

Weight et al. reported,a total of 510 patients, that the lack of histological subtyping and tumor size did not have a significant effect on the outcome [19].

Tumor recurrence in patients with T1b renal tumors who received PN was lower than those who underwent RN. Similarly, Milonas et al. and Mitchell et al. reported

Study or Subgroup	log[Risk Ratio]	SE	PN Total	RN Total	Weight	Risk Ratio IV, Fixed, 95% CI
Jang2016	0.1924	0.0875	100	100	30.1%	1.21 [1.02, 1.44]
Roos2011	-0.0799	0.0574	73	100	69.9%	0.92 [0.82, 1.03]
Total (95% CI)			**173**	**200**	**100.0%**	**1.00 [0.91, 1.10]**

Heterogeneity: Chi² = 6.77, df = 1 (P = 0.009); I² = 85%
Test for overall effect: Z = 0.04 (P = 0.97)

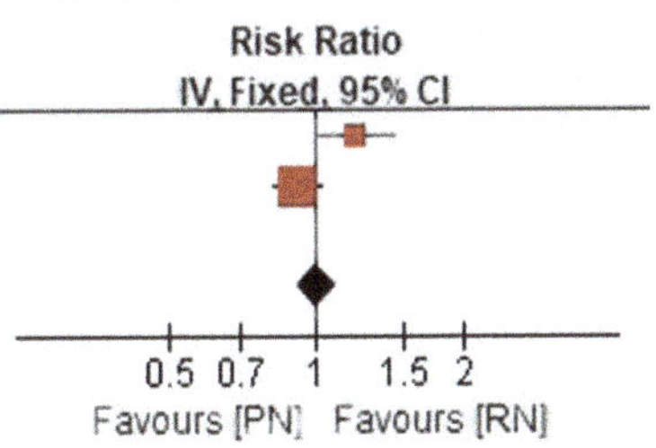

Fig. 7 Forest plot for 10-year RFS between the PN and RN for T1b tumors

Study or Subgroup	PN Events	PN Total	RN Events	RN Total	Weight	Odds Ratio M-H, Fixed, 95% CI
Antonelli 2012	4	52	37	277	15.3%	0.54 [0.18, 1.59]
Iizuka2012	7	67	28	195	18.2%	0.70 [0.29, 1.68]
Jang2016	6	100	12	100	16.0%	0.47 [0.17, 1.30]
Kim2010	2	18	18	52	11.7%	0.24 [0.05, 1.14]
Patard 2004	3	85	39	576	13.7%	0.50 [0.15, 1.67]
Roos2011	8	73	11	100	11.7%	1.00 [0.38, 2.61]
Roos2012	9	101	11	146	11.6%	1.20 [0.48, 3.01]
Simmons2009	2	35	2	75	1.7%	2.21 [0.30, 16.39]
Total (95% CI)		**531**		**1521**	**100.0%**	**0.68 [0.46, 0.98]**
Total events	41		158			

Heterogeneity: Chi² = 6.07, df = 7 (P = 0.53); I² = 0%
Test for overall effect: Z = 2.04 (P = 0.04)

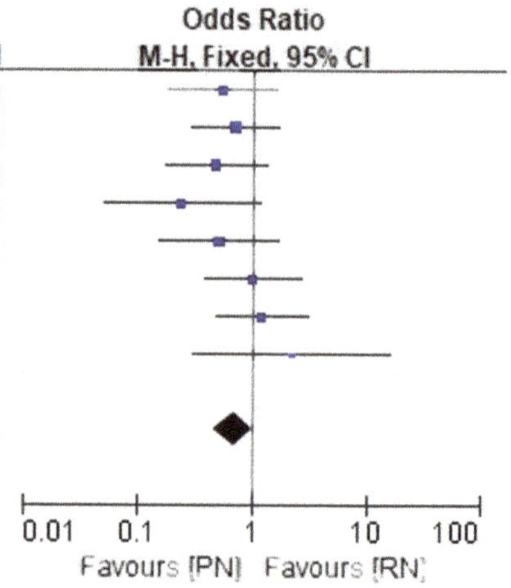

Fig. 8 Forest plot for Tumor recurrence between the PN and RN for T1b tumors

that PN was associated with a higher risk of tumor relapse compared to RN [16, 18]. A recent study performed by Roos et al. reported that patients with papillary renal carcinoma had a higher tumor recurrence rate than those with clear cell carcinoma [26]. In addition, Robert also found that there was no significant difference in recurrence-free survival and cancer-specific survival in patients with T1b RCC treated by PN versus RN [16]. However, Patard et al. found that RN was associated with a lower rate of local and systemic recurrence compared to PN [17]. This was different from the results shown in our study. Furthermore, they found that altering the type of surgical intervention (PN or RN) did not result in a higher incidence of tumor recurrence. In addition, Leibov et al. reported that no significant difference was found in CSS and distant metastasis rates between PN and RN. They also found that tumor stage was not related to tumor recurrence [8]. This may be associated with the histology of the renal tumor and the clinical stage or the pathology stage. Additionally, these studies had a shorter follow-up period. Furthermore, the surgical expertise of the urologist may have also contributed to the selection bias. Additionally, Patard et al. found that the two surgical approaches may impact tumor recurrence. Tumor recurrence may be linked to the histological tumor subtype and grade. The relationship between tumor recurrence and positive margins is unclear. In addition, it is unclear whether the selection of PN or RN is relevant to pathology of the tumor. Lastly, the clinical stage of an RCC is different from the pathological stage [17].

In our study, for patients with larger T1b renal tumors, patients in PN were comparable with RN for 5-year RFS and 10-year RFS. Robert et al. also found that the tumor diameter was an independent factor related to RFS. They found that the histological subtype, stage, grade, and surgical technique were not significant predictors of recurrence-free survival [16].

This was compared with our study. Lu et al. found that tumor enucleation was associated with a lower morbidity and mortality compared to PN [28].

Several studies also reported that preservation of renal function could lower the risk of cardiovascular complications and increase the OS, indicating that PN has the advantage of preserving renal function [13, 19, 22, 25, 29]. Lane et al. also found that patients with preexisting CKD

Study or Subgroup	PN Events	PN Total	RN Events	RN Total	Weight	Odds Ratio M-H, Fixed, 95% CI
Jang2016	15	100	11	100	26.5%	1.43 [0.62, 3.28]
Milonas2013	3	34	21	317	10.5%	1.36 [0.38, 4.83]
Roos2011	40	101	45	146	63.0%	1.47 [0.87, 2.50]
Total (95% CI)		**235**		**563**	**100.0%**	**1.45 [0.95, 2.21]**
Total events	58		77			

Heterogeneity: Chi² = 0.01, df = 2 (P = 0.99); I² = 0%
Test for overall effect: Z = 1.72 (P = 0.09)

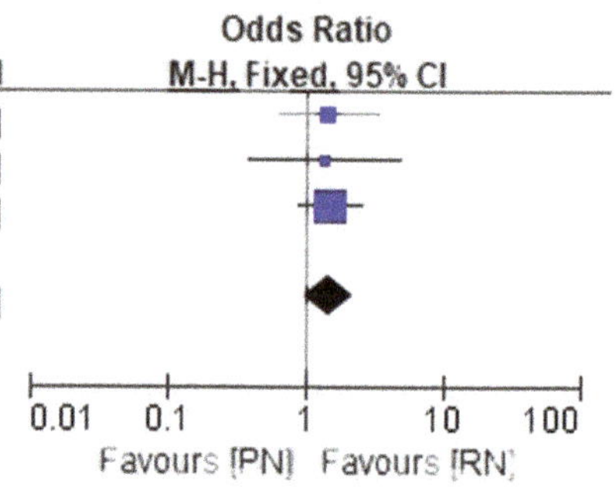

Fig. 9 Forest plot for postoperative complications between the PN and RN for T1b tumors

Study or Subgroup	PN Mean	PN SD	PN Total	RN Mean	RN SD	RN Total	Weight	Mean Difference IV, Fixed, 95% CI
Kim2010	12	9.1	18	18.1	12.5	52	4.6%	-6.10 [-11.51, -0.69]
Kopp 2015	12.5	3.5	80	20.2	7.3	122	58.8%	-7.70 [-9.21, -6.19]
Pignot 2014	16.7	13.3	123	21.4	17.5	185	11.2%	-4.70 [-8.15, -1.25]
Weight2010	12	13	212	27	13	298	25.4%	-15.00 [-17.29, -12.71]
Total (95% CI)			**433**			**657**	**100.0%**	**-9.15 [-10.30, -7.99]**

Heterogeneity: $Chi^2 = 36.27$, $df = 3$ ($P < 0.00001$); $I^2 = 92\%$
Test for overall effect: $Z = 15.53$ ($P < 0.00001$)

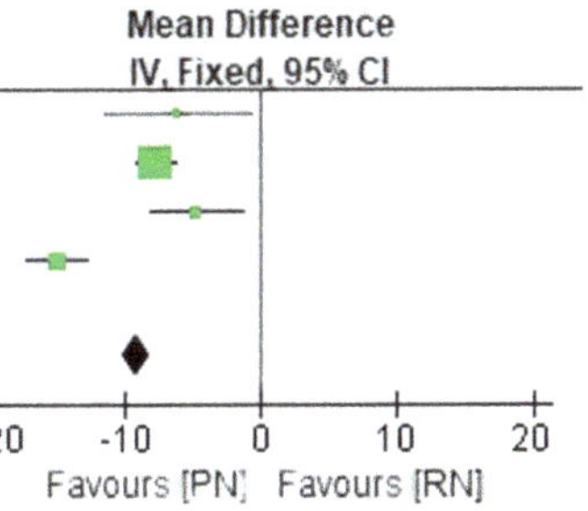

Fig. 10 Forest plot for Declined eGFR between the PN and RN for T1b tumors

were at a higher risk of death by increasing the incidence of patients developing chronic renal insufficiency. Therefore, it was unclear whether PN or RN were factors impacting CKD via different routes [30]. Roos et al. also determined via multivariate analysis that tumor size was not an independent predictor and was not associated with CKD [26]. Badalato et al. found that, due to the preservation of renal function, patients receiving PN had a higher health-related quality of life [23]. Simmons also proposed that the main factor restricting the selection of surgical methods was tumor location rather than tumor diameter [25]. In addition, the indications for PN should be broadened to reduce the chance of the development of postoperative CKD. Additionally, Pignot et al. reported that tumor size, receiving PN and age are all factors that could impact renal function loss [22].

In our study, the rate of postoperative complications was comparable between PN group and RN group. Several articles also reported a similar result [11, 14, 15]. However, Mir MC et al. performed a meta-analysis demonstarting that the PN had a higher likelihood of postoperative complications than RN (RR 1.74). They included both clinical T1b and T2 tumors [31]. Van Poppel H et al. reported a similarly results founding that higher urinary fistula and reoperation rate in PN [32]. In addition, Meskawi et al. reported that, after a learning phase, PN would become feasible in urology [15].

Furthermore, uncommon RCCs, for example, papillary RCC, may present metastasis to distant locations. Therefore, for papillary RCC larger than between 4 cm and 7 cm, RN should be selected. The urologist should decide on which surgical approach to take to treat T1b RCC based on tumor location, histology of the tumor, mean Fuhrman grade, and tumor diameter. In addition, the PN group may have a higher mortality rate. Using multivariate analysis, Weight et al. reported that patients receiving RN had a higher risk of death than those receiving PN.

Our study has several limitations. First, the included studies were non-RCTs, which may reduce the quality of the evidence used. Second, our meta-analysis used LnRR instead of LnHR to demonstrate the OS, CSS and RFS. Third, the studies included in suffered from bias, especially selective bias (surgeons use PN or RN according to their personal preference), thus introducing heterogeneity. Additionally, the studies included in this study used different surgical techniques, such as LPN, OPN, a fact which may have increased the overall bias. Furthermore, the tumor histology could, to an extent, have affected the postoperative follow-up outcomes. However, after sensitivity analyses and meta-regression, no explicit causes of heterogeneity have been detected. Further studies should determine whether tumor location, tumor diameter or tumor grading are determining factors in the selection of PN or RN.

Conclusions

Our meta-analysis showed that PN may provide comparable outcomes in terms of RFS & OS, and better renal function preservation. In addition, RN ensures a better CSS compared to PN. PN had an equal incident of postoperative complications compared to RN.

Additional files

Additional file 1: Figure S1. (a)-1(d). Funnel plots of the study. (a) 5-year css (b)5-year os (c)10-year os(d) Declined eGFR. (ZIP 82 kb)

Additional file 2: Figure S2. (a)-2(d) Sensitive analysis of the (a) 5-year css (b)5-year os (c)10-year os(d) Declined eGFR. (ZIP 95 kb)

Additional file 3: Figure S3. Summary of evidence grading. (PNG 81 kb)

Abbreviations

CSS: Cancer-special survival; NOS: New-Ottawa Scale; NSS: Nephron-sparing-surgery; OS: Overall survival; PN: Partial nephrectomy; PRISMA: Preferred Reporting Items for Systemic Reviews and Meta-analysis; RCC: Renal cell carcinoma; RFS: Recurrence-free survival; RN: Radical nephrectomy; SMD: Standard mean difference; WMD: Weight mean difference

Acknowledgements

Not applicable.

Authors' contributions

YLJ and CXP designed the study. YLJ wrote the manuscript. YLJ and CXP analyzed the data. LJQ and HZW searched the articles. All authors read and approved the final manuscript.

References

1. Jemal A, Bray F, Center MM, Ferlay J, Ward E, Forman D. Global cancer statistics. CA Cancer J Clin. 2011;61:69–90.
2. Novick AC, Streem S, Montie JE, Pontes JE, Siegel S, Montague DK, et al. Conservative surgery for renal cell carcinoma: a single-center experience with 100 patients. J Urol. 1989;141:835–9.
3. Lee CT, Katz J, Shi W, Thaler HT, Reuter VE, Russo P. Surgical management of renal tumors 4 cm. Or less in a contemporary cohort. J Urol. 2000;163:730–6.
4. Ljungberg B, Bensalah K, Canfield S, Dabestani S, Hofmann F, Hora M, et al. EAU guidelines on renal cell carcinoma: 2014 update. Eur Urol. 2015;67:913–24.
5. Campbell SC, Novick AC, Belldegrun A, Blute ML, Chow GK, Derweesh IH, et al. Guideline for management of the clinical T1 renal mass. J Urol. 2009;182:1271–9.
6. Huang WC, Levey AS, Serio AM, Snyder M, Vickers AJ, Raj GV, et al. Chronic kidney disease after nephrectomy in patients with renal cortical tumours: a retrospective cohort study. Lancet Oncol. 2006;7:735–40.
7. Bensalah K, Crepel M, Patard JJ. Tumor size and nephron-sparing surgery: does it still matter? Eur Urol. 2008;53:691–3.
8. Leibovich BC, Blute M, Cheville JC, Lohse CM, Weaver AL, Zincke H. Nephron sparing surgery for appropriately selected renal cell carcinoma between 4 and 7 cm results in outcome similar to radical nephrectomy. J Urol. 2004;171:1066–70.
9. Hadjipavlou M, Khan F, Fowler S, Joyce A, Keeley FX, Sriprasad S. Partial vs radical nephrectomy for T1 renal tumours: an analysis from the British Association of Urological Surgeons Nephrectomy Audit. BJU Int. 2016;117:62–71.
10. Kim SP, Thompson RH, Boorjian SA, Weight CJ, Han LC, Murad MH, et al. Comparative effectiveness for survival and renal function of partial and radical nephrectomy for localized renal tumors: a systematic review and meta-analysis. J Urol. 2012;188:51–7.
11. Antonelli A, Ficarra V, Bertini R, Carini M, Carmignani G, Corti S, et al. Elective partial nephrectomy is equivalent to radical nephrectomy in patients with clinical T1 renal cell carcinoma: results of a retrospective, comparative, multi-institutional study. BJU Int. 2012;109:1013–8.
12. Crepel M, Jeldres C, Perrotte P, Capitanio U, Isbarn H, Shariat SF, et al. Nephron-sparing surgery is equally effective to radical nephrectomy for T1BN0M0 renal cell carcinoma: a population-based assessment. Urology. 2010;75:271–5.
13. Jang HA, Kim JW, Byun SS, Hong SH, Kim YJ, Park YH, et al. Oncologic and functional outcomes after partial nephrectomy versus radical nephrectomy in T1b renal cell carcinoma: a multicenter, matched case-control study in Korean patients. Cancer Res Treat. 2016;48:612–20.
14. Lee H, Oh JJ, Byun SS, Jeong CW, Kwak C, Jeong BC, et al. Can partial nephrectomy provide equal oncological efficiency and safety compared with radical nephrectomy in patients with renal cell carcinoma (>/=4cm)? A propensity score-matched study. Urol Oncol. 2017;35:379–85.
15. Meskawi M, Becker A, Bianchi M, Trinh QD, Roghmann F, Tian Z, et al. Partial and radical nephrectomy provide comparable long-term cancer control for T1b renal cell carcinoma. Int J Urol. 2014;21:122–8.
16. Mitchell RE, Gilbert SM, Murphy AM, Olsson CA, Benson MC, McKiernan JM. Partial nephrectomy and radical nephrectomy offer similar cancer outcomes in renal cortical tumors 4 cm or larger. Urology. 2006;67:260–4.
17. Patard JJ, Shvarts O, Lam JS, Pantuck AJ, Kim HL, Ficarra V, et al. Safety and efficacy of partial nephrectomy for all T1 tumors based on an international multicenter experience. J Urol. 2004;171:2181–5 quiz 435.
18. Thompson RH, Siddiqui S, Lohse CM, Leibovich BC, Russo P, Blute ML. Partial versus radical nephrectomy for 4 to 7 cm renal cortical tumors. J Urol. 2009;182:2601–6.
19. Weight CJ, Larson BT, Gao T, Campbell SC, Lane BR, Kaouk JH, et al. Elective partial nephrectomy in patients with clinical T1b renal tumors is associated with improved overall survival. Urology. 2010;76:631–7.
20. Iizuka J, Kondo T, Hashimoto Y, Kobayashi H, Ikezawa E, Takagi T, et al. Similar functional outcomes after partial nephrectomy for clinical T1b and T1a renal cell carcinoma. Int J Urol. 2012;19:980–6.
21. Brewer K, O'Malley RL, Hayn M, Safwat MW, Kim H, Underwood W 3rd, et al. Perioperative and renal function outcomes of minimally invasive partial nephrectomy for T1b and T2a kidney tumors. J Endourol. 2012;26:244–8.
22. Pignot G, Bigot P, Bernhard JC, Bouliere F, Bessede T, Bensalah K, et al. Nephron-sparing surgery is superior to radical nephrectomy in preserving renal function benefit even when expanding indications beyond the traditional 4-cm cutoff. Urol Oncol. 2014;32:1024–30.
23. Badalato GM, Kates M, Wisnivesky JP, Choudhury AR, McKiernan JM. Survival after partial and radical nephrectomy for the treatment of stage T1bN0M0 renal cell carcinoma (RCC) in the USA: a propensity scoring approach. BJU Int. 2012;109:1457–62.
24. Roos FC, Brenner W, Muller M, Schubert C, Jager WJ, Thuroff JW, et al. Oncologic long-term outcome of elective nephron-sparing surgery versus radical nephrectomy in patients with renal cell carcinoma stage pT1b or greater in a matched-pair cohort. Urology. 2011;77:803–8.
25. Simmons MN, Weight CJ, Gill IS. Laparoscopic radical versus partial nephrectomy for tumors >4 cm: intermediate-term oncologic and functional outcomes. Urology. 2009;73:1077–82.
26. Roos FC, Brenner W, Thomas C, Jager W, Thuroff JW, Hampel C, et al. Functional analysis of elective nephron-sparing surgery vs radical nephrectomy for renal tumors larger than 4 cm. Urology. 2012;79:607–13.
27. Zhang M, Zhao Z, Duan X, Deng T, Cai C, Wu W, et al. Partial versus radical nephrectomy for T1b-2N0M0 renal tumors: a propensity score matching study based on the SEER database. PLoS One. 2018;13:e0193530.
28. Lu Q, Ji C, Zhao X, Fu Y, Guo S, Liu G, et al. Histopathologic analysis of tumor bed and peritumoral pseudocapsule after in vitro tumor enucleation on radical nephrectomy specimen for clinical T1b renal cell carcinoma. Urol Oncol. 2017;35:603.e15–20.
29. Scosyrev E, Messing EM, Sylvester R, Campbell S, Van Poppel H. Renal function after nephron-sparing surgery versus radical nephrectomy: results from EORTC randomized trial 30904. Eur Urol. 2014;65:372–7.
30. Lane BR, Campbell SC, Demirjian S, Fergany AF. Surgically induced chronic kidney disease may be associated with a lower risk of progression and mortality than medical chronic kidney disease. J Urol. 2013;189:1649–55.
31. Mir MC, Derweesh I, Porpiglia F, Zargar H, Mottrie A, Autorino R. Partial nephrectomy versus radical nephrectomy for clinical T1b and T2 renal tumors: a systematic review and meta-analysis of comparative studies. Eur Urol. 2017;71:606–17.
32. Van Poppel H, Da Pozzo L, Albrecht W, Matveev V, Bono A, Borkowski A, et al. A prospective randomized EORTC intergroup phase 3 study comparing the complications of elective nephron-sparing surgery and radical nephrectomy for low-stage renal cell carcinoma. Eur Urol. 2007;51:1606–15.

10

Metachronous renal cell carcinoma with metastasis to the urinary bladder and distant organs, 28 years after radical nephrectomy

Mustufa Babar[1], Saad Hamdani[1], Corinne Liu[2], Jogarao Vedula[3] and David S. Schnapp[1*]

Abstract

Background: Metachronous renal cell carcinoma after radical nephrectomy is extremely rare. Renal cell carcinoma commonly metastasizes to distant organs. However, metastasis to the urinary bladder is very uncommon.

Case presentation: Herein, we report a case of metachronous renal cell carcinoma with metastasis to the urinary bladder, left acetabulum, left rib, lungs, thyroid, right renal vein and inferior vena cava. The patient had undergone a left-sided radical nephrectomy 28 years ago. The pathological diagnosis of a fragment of the bladder tumor was consistent with Fuhrman grade 2 clear cell renal cell carcinoma.

Conclusions: Although metachronous renal cell carcinoma after radical nephrectomy is rare, active surveillance should be still considered. Renal cell carcinoma has shown to unusually metastasize to the urinary bladder, a rarely reported organ of metastasis. Treatment options, such as immunotherapy, are available to patients with such metastasis and long-term survivorship can be achieved.

Keywords: Renal cell carcinoma, Bladder metastasis, Nephrectomy

Background

As the third most common urological cancer and with newly reported cases arising each year due to increased usage of imaging procedures, renal cell carcinoma (RCC) proves to be a relevant adult malignancy [1]. Although extremely rare, RCC has the ability to undergo metachronous metastasis many years after radical nephrectomy. Furthermore, RCC frequently metastasizes to distant organs. However, metastasis to the urinary bladder is extremely rare with less than 40 reported cases in literature [2]. We present a case of metachronous RCC with metastasis to the bladder, as well as distant organs, 28 years after radical nephrectomy.

Case presentation

A 79-year-old man, who had a left-sided radical nephrectomy 28 years ago as a result of renal cell carcinoma, is presented with urinary retention for six months. Renal ultrasound revealed the right kidney to be 13.6 cm, normal echogenicity without hydronephrosis, and a mildly distended bladder. Urodynamic testing indicated obstruction.

The patient returned one month later with gross hematuria. Computed tomography (CT) scan of the abdomen and pelvis revealed an intraluminal 3.7*3.2 cm mass on the right side of the urinary bladder (Fig. 1a) and a 1.7 cm lytic lesion in the left acetabulum, which was suspicious for metastatic disease (Fig. 1b). Furthermore, the right kidney demonstrated subcentimeter hypodense lesions. Magnetic resonance imaging (MRI) of the visceral pelvis showed an enhancing 2.5 cm lesion in the left superior acetabular region with disruption of the medial cortex that was consistent with metastatic disease.

A transurethral resection of the bladder removed a 4.2*3.5*0.6 cm single fragment of aggregate soft, tan-brown colored bladder tissue. The pathological diagnosis

* Correspondence: dr.david.schnapp@dssurology.com
[1]DSS Urology, Queens Village, New York, USA
Full list of author information is available at the end of the article

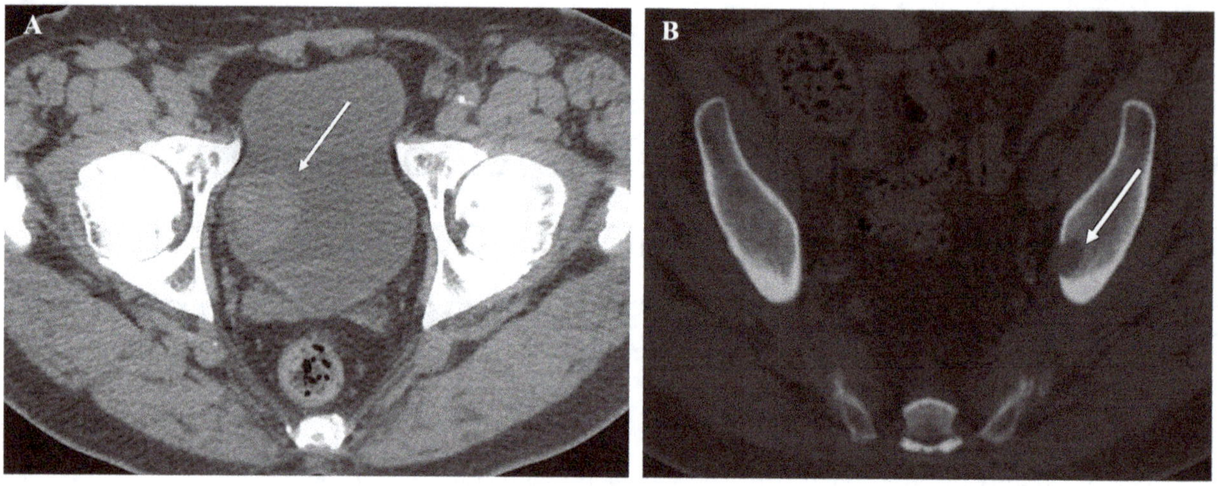

Fig. 1 **a** Non-contrast CT abdomen and pelvis demonstrates a hyperattenuating intraluminal bladder mass (white arrow). **b** Non-contrast CT abdomen and pelvis reveal a lytic lesion with cortical destruction and extraosseous soft tissue extension in the left ilium (white arrow), consistent with osseous metastasis

of a fragment of the partially necrotic bladder tumor was consistent with Fuhrman grade 2 clear cell renal cell carcinoma (Fig. 2). Bone scan showed negative findings. However, positron emission tomography computed tomography scan with fluorodeoxyglucose (PET-CT FDG) of the skull base to thighs revealed scattered hypermetabolic lytic osseous lesions in the left acetabulum, a lytic lesion in the 1st left rib, a hypermetabolic 4.4 cm right para-aortic retroperitoneal lesion, numerous subcentimeter scattered lungs nodules, and a 17 mm right thyroid nodule. Furthermore, an MRI of the abdomen revealed multiple hypoenhancing masses in the right kidney which were suspicious for renal neoplasm associated with metastatic disease (Fig. 3a). The MRI also showed a tumor thrombus in the right renal vein and inferior vena cava (Fig. 3b), and pulmonary nodules (Fig. 3c).

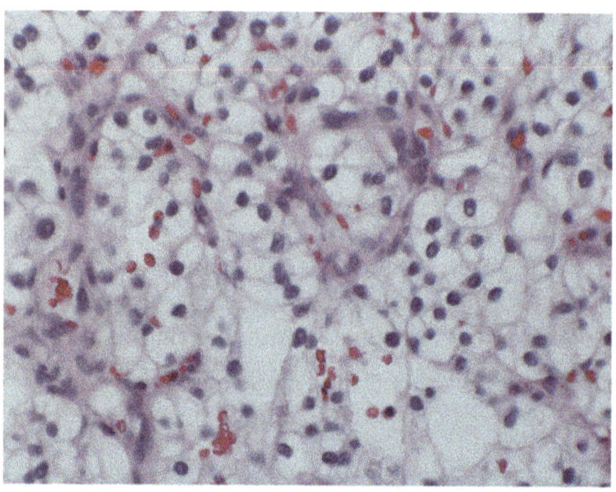

Fig. 2 Fuhrman grade 2 renal cell carcinoma metastatic to the urinary bladder. Hematoxylin-eosin stain, reduced from 40x

At first, the patient decided not to undergo any systemic treatment plan as he desired to pursue the situation through a holistic approach. A few weeks later, however, the patient agreed to start chemotherapy. He was given sunitinib 12.5 mg which was later increased to 25 mg. However, he was unable to tolerate the increased sunitinib dosage due to gross hematuria. Consequently, the patient was given nivolumab through a Port-a-Cath and has remained in stable condition for over two years.

Discussion and conclusions

Metachronous RCC after radical nephrectomy is extremely rare and reported to occur at 1.2% [3]. Although metachronous RCC occurrence is typically 5 years post nephrectomy [4], rare cases show metachronous RCC occurrence after 24 years [5]. Metachronous RCC requires patients to receive active surveillance as an independent viable option based on personal and financial grounds [4]. Several surveillance protocols, such as routine imaging, physical examination, and laboratory testing, have been suggested as surveillance options barring aggressiveness and staging of the tumor [6]. Furthermore, it is recommended to remain under surveillance 5–10 years post nephrectomy [4]. However, our case suggests that surveillance for life may be necessary.

RCC can metastasize to many distant organs, with lungs, bones, liver and distant lymph nodes being the most common. These common sites of metastasis can be monitored and effectively treated with resection [4]. However, RCC metastasis to the bladder is extremely rare, accounting for less than 2 % of all bladder tumors [7]. Consequently, bladder metastasis is more challenging

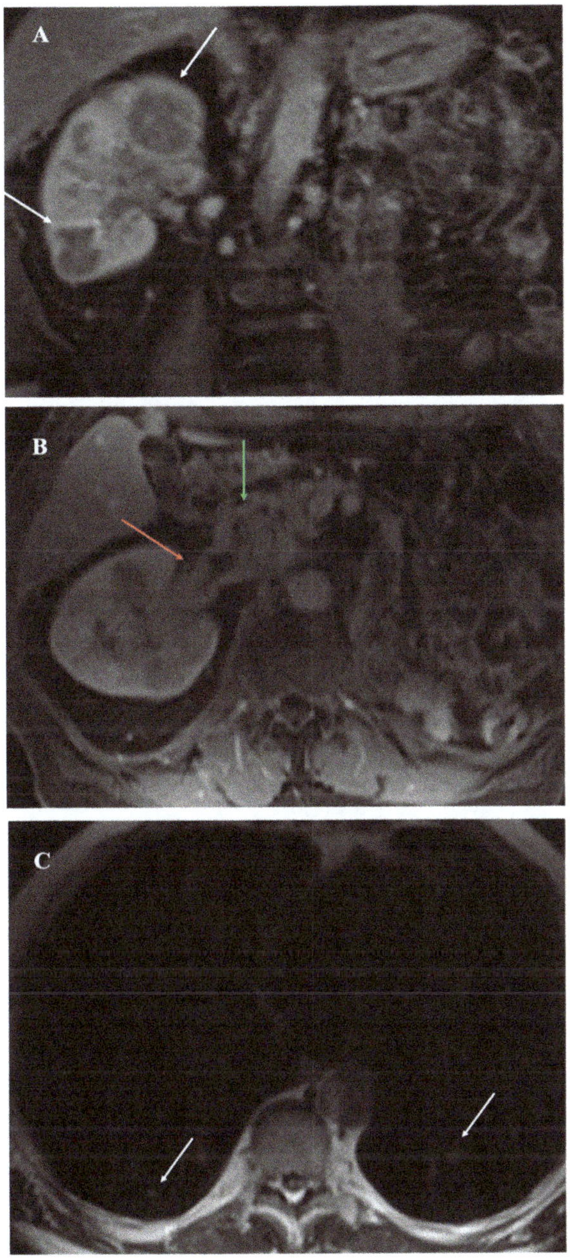

Fig. 3 **a** Gadolinium enhanced T1 weighted coronal image of the abdomen demonstrates multiple hypoenhancing masses throughout the right kidney (white arrows). **b** Gadolinium enhanced T1 weighted axial image of the abdomen demonstrates right renal vein (red arrow) and inferior vena cava invasion (green arrow) by tumor. **c** Axial T2 weighted image demonstrates several scattered pulmonary nodules (white arrows)

to treat due to its irregularity. Bladder metastasis frequently presents itself with gross hematuria. Although most patients with RCC metastasis to the bladder die within the first year of diagnosis, long-term survivorship of more than six years have been reported [8, 9]. The mechanism of RCC metastasis to the bladder remains a subject of discussion but several theories have been proposed.

One theory suggests retrograde venous embolism from renal venous drainage through a tumor thrombus [8–10]. More specifically, Abeshouse states that a tumor thrombus found in the left renal vein, as opposed to the right renal vein, is responsible for RCC metastasis to pelvic organs since the left renal vein is the central network of venous circulation to adjacent organs [9, 10]. In our case, the patient had a tumor thrombus in the right renal vein as well as a prior left-sided radical nephrectomy. As a result, for our case, the mechanism of retrograde venous embolism through the left renal vein is unlikely to be responsible for the bladder metastasis observed.

Another theory of RCC metastasis to the bladder suggests metastasis to occur through the lymphatic system, which involves the penetration and embolization of tumor cells through vascular lymphatic vessels [8]. However, lymphatic invasion and an interconnected vascular network between the kidneys and the bladder is not observed [9]. Therefore, RCC metastasis to the bladder through the lymphatic system is an unlikely route.

Raviv et al. used the term "drop metastases" to describe a fascinating theory of RCC metastasis to the bladder by direct seed implantation of cancer cells through the urinary tract [8, 9]. This route of metastasis is proposed due to the presence of tumor cells in the urine of patients with RCC metastasis to the bladder [8]. However, the likelihood of metastasis to the urinary tract was found to be low in these patients which makes this route questionable [9]. In addition, because our patient had systemic metastasis to distant organs, "drop metastases" may not be the suggestable metastatic route in our case.

Another theory of tumor metastasis, known as hematogenous metastasis, involves tumor cells penetrating blood vessels and invading different organs through the general circulation [11]. Since our patient had multiple sites of metastasis, including the bladder, bones, lungs, thyroid, and veins, our case suggests hematogenous metastasis to be responsible for RCC metastasis to the bladder and distant organs. The tumor thrombus observed in the patient's right renal vein may have spread into his inferior vena cava before extending to the heart and lungs and eventually diffusing to other parts of the body through the systemic circulation [12]. However, since there are many interconnections between these theories of metastasis, several of these routes may be responsible for the unique metastasis observed.

Treatment for RCC metastasis is offered on a case by case basis. For bladder lesions as a result of RCC metastasis, transurethral resection or partial cystectomy is recommended [8]. For metastasis to other organs, systemic treatment options, such as chemotherapy and radiation therapy, should be offered. A chemotherapy option that is found to be effective in managing metastatic and metachronous RCC uses target treatment agents such as sunitinib and sorafenib. These agents provide a novel approach in managing RCC by targeting vascular endothelial and platelet-derived growth factors [11]. Furthermore, immunotherapy, involving nivolumab or IL-2 cytokines, is also found to be effective in managing RCC.

Metachronous RCC after radical nephrectomy is probable, although rare, making active surveillance an important option. In addition, RCC has shown to unusually metastasize to the urinary bladder, a rarely reported organ of metastasis. Although there is no general accepted theory, several theories have been proposed to account for the unique route of metastasis to the bladder. Treatment options are available to patients with such metastasis and long-term survivorship can be achieved. Our patient is alive for more than two years after metachronous RCC with metastasis to the bladder, and other organs, under immunotherapy involving nivolumab.

Abbreviations

CT: Computed tomography; MRI: Magnetic resonance imaging; PET-CT FDG: Positron emission tomography computed tomography scan with fluorodeoxyglucose; RCC: Renal cell carcinoma

Acknowledgements

Not applicable.

Authors' contributions

MB and SH made substantial contributions in drafting the manuscript. DSS substantially revised the manuscript for structure and intellectual accuracy. CL provided radiology images and appropriate image descriptions. JV prepared the histology image. All authors have approved the final version of the publication. All authors have agreed both to be personally accountable for the author's own contributions and to ensure that questions related to the accuracy or integrity of any part of the work, even ones in which the author was not personally involved, are appropriately investigated, resolved, and the resolution documented in the literature.

Author details

[1]DSS Urology, Queens Village, New York, USA. [2]Department of Radiology, Memorial Sloan Kettering Cancer Center, New York, USA. [3]Department of Pathology, NYU Winthrop Hospital, Mineola, New York, USA.

References

1. Chow W-H, Devesa SS, Warren JL, et al. Rising incidence of renal cell Cancer in the United States. JAMA. 1999;281:1628.
2. Zhang M, Wah C, Epstein JI. Metastatic renal cell carcinoma to the urinary bladder: a report of 11 cases. Am J Surg Pathol. 2014;38:1516.
3. Bani-Hani AH, Leibovich BC, Lohse CM, et al. Associations with contralateral recurrence following nephrectomy for renal cell carcinoma using a cohort of 2,352 patients. J Urol. 2005;173:391.
4. Abara E, Chivulescu I, Clerk N, et al. Recurrent renal cell cancer: 10 years or more after nephrectomy. Can Urol Assoc J. 2010;4:E45.
5. Donaldson JC, Slease RB, DuFour DR, et al. Metastatic renal cell carcinoma 24 years after nephrectomy. JAMA. 1976;236:950.
6. Chin AI, Lam JS, Figlin RA, et al. Surveillance strategies for renal cell carcinoma patients following nephrectomy. Rev Urol. 2006;8:1.
7. Roberts DI. Secondary neoplasms of the Genito-urinary tract. Br J Urol. 1978;50:68.
8. Shiraishi K, Mohri J, Inoue R, et al. Metastatic renal cell carcinoma to the bladder 12 years after radical nephrectomy. Int J Urol. 2003;10:453.
9. Raviv S, Eggener SE, Williams DH et al: Long-Term Survival after "Drop Metastases" of Renal Cell Carcinoma to the Bladder. Urology 2002;60:697xiii.
10. Abeshouse BS. Metastasis to ureters and urinary bladder from renal carcinoma: report of two cases. J Int Coll Surg. 1956;25:117.
11. Doo SW, Kim WB, Kim BK, et al. Metastasis of renal cell carcinoma to the bladder. Korean J Urol. 2013;54:69.
12. Brufau BP, Cerqueda CS, Villalba LB, et al. Metastatic renal cell carcinoma: radiologic findings and assessment of response to targeted antiangiogenic therapy by using multidetector CT. RadioGraphics. 2003;33:1691.

11

Significant impact of three-dimensional volumetry of perinephric fat on the console time during robot-assisted partial nephrectomy

Daisuke Motoyama*, Yuto Matsushita, Hiromitsu Watanabe, Keita Tamura, Toshiki Ito, Takayuki Sugiyama, Atsushi Otsuka and Hideaki Miyake

Abstract

Background: To assess the impact of volumetry of perinephric fat (PNF) on the perioperative outcomes of robot-assisted partial nephrectomy (RAPN).

Methods: Between 2016 and 2019, a single surgeon performed RAPN for 128 patients with clinical T1a-b renal tumors at our institution, and the 70 most recent patients were included in this study to minimize the effects of surgical experience. PNF was defined as a fatty area around the kidney within the anatomical structures, including the lateroconal fascia, fusion fascia, psoas muscle, lumbar quadrate muscle and diaphragm, and its volume was calculated based on reconstructed three-dimensional computed tomography images using the SYNAPSE VINCENT system.

Results: In this series, the trifecta and MIC (margin, ischemia and complications) score system outcomes were achieved in 69 (98.6%) and 64 patients (91.4%), respectively. The median PNF volume in the 70 patients was 166.05 cm^3, which was significantly correlated with both the body mass index (BMI) and Mayo adhesive probability (MAP) score (correlation coefficient = 0.68 and 0.74, respectively). There was no significant difference in the R.E.N.A.L. nephrometry score, PNF volume or console time during RAPN among 5 groups consisting of 14 consecutive patients. Of several factors examined, the console time was significantly affected by the sex, MAP score and PNF volume, and only the PNF volume was independently associated with the console time.

Conclusion: Even if performed by an experienced robotic surgeon beyond the initial learning curve, the PNF volume may influence the console time during RAPN.

Keywords: Three-dimensional volumetry, Perinephric fat, Robot-assisted partial nephrectomy, Mayo adhesive probability score

Background

Partial nephrectomy (PN) is currently regarded as the standard of care for patients with localized small renal masses because it has been demonstrated to provide equivalent cancer control with the added benefit of preserving renal function when compared with radical nephrectomy [1]. In recent years, robotic technology has been applied to the field of PN, with significant advancements in surgical techniques and instruments. Robot-assisted PN (RAPN) has become prevalent due to marked improvements of perioperative outcomes [2–4], with a shorter learning curve than laparoscopic PN [5, 6]. However, it is well known that the surgical complexity of RAPN varies depending on a wide variety of factors [7]. Thus, it is not uncommon to encounter cases in which it is difficult to perform RAPN even by experienced robotic surgeons.

Currently, there are several image-based morphometry scoring systems that enable the quantification of relevant anatomical findings to help predict the potential complexity of PN, such as the R.E.N.A.L. nephrometry score, PADUA prediction score and centrality index (C-index)

* Correspondence: urom1124@yahoo.co.jp
Department of Urology, Hamamatsu University School of Medicine, 1-20-1 Handayama, Higashi-Ku, Hamamatsu 431-3192, Japan

[8–10]; however, patient-specific factors are not considered by these systems. Of numerous non-tumor-specific factors, those associated with perinephric fat (PNF) are reported to affect the complexity of PN [11–14]. One such factor is the presence of adherent perinephric fat (APF), which makes it difficult to mobilize the kidney and isolate the renal tumor [11]. Recently, Davidiuk et al. advocated the Mayo adhesive probability (MAP) score in order to accurately predict the presence of APF [15], and its usefulness was confirmed in several previous studies [16, 17]. However, this score is somewhat subjective regarding the definitions of both APF and the score itself, and is not intended to directly predict the surgical difficulty of PN.

Considering these findings, we focused on the PNF volume, which may influence the complexity of RAPN, and conducted 3-dimensional (3D) volumetry for PNF on a total of 70 patients undergoing RAPN performed by a single experienced robotic surgeon in order to assess the impact of PNF volume on their perioperative outcomes.

Methods

Patients

The research ethics committee of our institution approved the design of this study (approval number, E15–115), and the need to obtain informed consent for involvement in this study from all of the included patients was waived because of its retrospective design. Between April 2016 and April 2019, RAPN was performed for a total of 128 consecutive patients with localized clinical T1a-b renal tumors by a single experienced robotic surgeon using the da Vinci Xi (Intuitive Surgical Inc., Sunnyvale, California, USA) at our institution. Of these 128, the 70 most recent patients who underwent RAPN under a uniform surgical procedure were included in order to minimize the effects of surgical experience.

Evaluation

All 70 patients were preoperatively examined by contrast-enhanced computed tomography (CT) with a 64-detector row scanner, Aquilion (Toshiba Medical System, Tokyo, Japan) under the following conditions: tube voltage of 120 KV, tube currents depending on the CT-AEC, rotation time of 0.5 s/VOT, pitch factor of 0.828 and slice thickness of 0.5 or 0.6 mm. All data for the 70 patients concerning clinicopathological characteristics and perioperative findings were obtained from their medical records, and we defined the console time in this study as the time from roll-in to roll-out for the patient-cart of the robotic system. For each patient, the MAP score and R.E.N.A.L. nephrometry score were assessed according to the preoperative features on contrast-enhanced CT, as previously described [8, 15], and the severity of postoperative complications that occurred during hospitalization was evaluated using the Clavien-Dindo system [18]. Three to 5 days after RAPN, contrast-enhanced CT was routinely performed in order to precisely observe the postoperative status of the resected kidney, particularly the presence of renal pseudoaneurysm [19]. In this series, the achievement of trifecta, a widely employed key surrogate for successful PN, including RAPN, was defined as the simultaneous fulfillment of the three following factors: negative surgical margins, ischemia time ≤ 25 min and no postoperative complications corresponding to grade 3 or 4 using the Clavien-Dindo system [4]. The margin, ischemia and complications (MIC) score was also analyzed as an alternative strict surrogate based on the definition of ischemia time ≤ 20 min, in addition to negative surgical margins and no Clavien-Dindo grade 3 or 4 complications [20].

Surgical procedure

A single trained surgeon (H.M.) performed RAPN for all 70 patients included in this study employing a 3-arm da Vinci Xi robotic system. Before RAPN, 3D images were reconstructed from the digital imaging and communications in medicine (DICOM) data of the contrast-enhanced CT images for each patient using the SYNAPSE VINCENT system (FUJIFILM, Inc., Tokyo, Japan), which were directly visualized on the screen of the surgeon's console with the TilePro multi-input display functions during RAPN [21]. At our institution, the trans-peritoneal approach is often selected, except for patients with dorsal hilar tumors or a history of intra-peritoneal surgery. One to three additional trocars, including the AirSeal iFS (CONMED Japan KK, Tokyo, Japan), were placed to be used by assistant surgeons. To evaluate the tumor distribution and plan the excision margins, an ARIETTA 70 probe (Hitachi, Inc., Tokyo, Japan) was used for ultrasound examinations. After clamping the main renal arteries with the Bulldog on the affected side, the tumor was excised using cold scissors maintaining a secure margin of approximately 5 mm, and an inner running suture using 3–0 V-Loc (COVIDIEN Japan, Inc., Tokyo, Japan) was placed to repair the collecting system and large vessels. Following early unclamping of renal arteries, additional inner suturing and/or soft coagulation (VIO300D; ERBE Elektromedizin GmbH, Tübingen, Germany) was then carried out to stop the bleeding from interlobar or segmental arteries, followed by renorrhaphy using 2–0 V-Loc [22].

Three-dimensional Volumetry

For the volumetry of PNF, the region of interest (ROI) for PNF on the affected side was defined as the fatty area within the anatomical structures, including the laterоconal fascia, fusion fascia, psoas muscle, lumbar quadrate muscle and diaphragm. Based on the ROI, 3D images for PNF were reconstructed from the DICOM data of non-contrast-enhanced CT, and the volume of PNF was quantitatively calculated using the SYNAPSE VINCENT system (Fig. 1) [23].

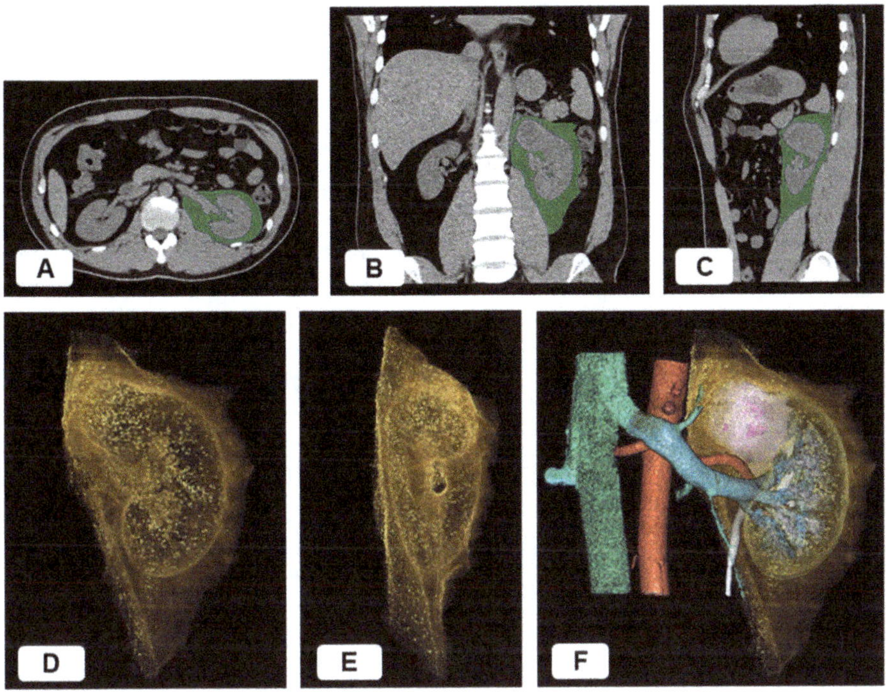

Fig. 1 **a**, **b**, **c**: Preoperative non-contrast-enhanced computed tomography images for a patient with a localized renal mass located at the upper pole of the left kidney. The green area shows the region of interest corresponding to the perinephric fat defined as the fatty area within the anatomical structures, including the laterocolonal fascia, fusion fascia, psoas muscle, lumbar quadrate muscle and diaphragm. **a**, Axial section. **b**, Coronal section. **c**, Sagittal section. **d**, **e**, **f**: The three-dimensional (3D) images for the perinephric fat reconstructed from the digital imaging and communications in medicine data according to the region of interest. The volume of this 3D structure was then calculated quantitatively. **d**, Anterior 3D view. The shape of the kidney and its upper tumor are stereoscopically excluded from the 3D structure. **e**, Inside 3D view. The lumens of renal hilar vessels are empty. **f**, Overlaid anterior 3D view showing the perinephric fat and other anatomical structures, including the kidney, artery, vein, ureter and tumor

Statistical analysis

All statistical analyses were performed using R ver. 3.1.1 software (R Development Core Team, https://www.r-project.org/index.html), and *p*-values less than 0.05 were considered significant. Spearman's rank correlation analysis was used to assess the association between the PNF volume and other parameters. Differences in the R.E.N.A.L. nephrometry score, PNF volume and console time during RAPN among the 5 groups consisting of 14 consecutive patients were assessed by the Kruskal-Wallis chi-squared test. Logistic regression analyses were conducted to examine the association between several parameters and the console time. Several variables with significant differences in the univariate analysis were selected and reanalyzed as the factors in the multivariate analysis.

Results

The baseline clinical characteristics and perioperative outcomes of the 70 patients included in this study are summarized in Table 1. In this series, the median body mass index (BMI), MAP score and PNF volume on the affected side were 23.90 kg/m^2 (ranged from 17.0 to 31.8 kg/m^2), 0 (ranged from 0 to 4) and 166.05 cm^3 (ranged from 22.1 to 1399.3 cm^3), respectively, and the trifecta and MIC score system outcomes were achieved in 69 (98.6%) and 64 patients (91.4%), respectively.

Scatter plots of the PNF volume according to the BMI and MAP score are presented in Fig. 2. The PNF volume was significantly correlated with both the BMI and MAP score in the 70 patients included in this study; however, the correlation coefficient was 0.68 between the PNF volume and BMI, whereas that between the PNF volume and MAP score was 0.74. The comparison of the R.E.N.A.L. nephrometry score, PNF volume and console time during RAPN among the 5 groups is also shown in Fig. 2. No significant difference was noted in the R.E.N.A.L. nephrometry score, PNF volume or console time among these 5 groups.

The outcomes of logistic regression analyses assessing the impacts of several parameters, including the PNF volume, on the console time as an index reflecting the complexity of RAPN are presented in Table 2. Univariate analysis identified the sex, MAP score and PNF volume as significant predictors of the console time. However, of these significant parameters, only the PNF was independently associated with the console time during RAPN by multivariate analysis.

Table 1 Patient characteristics and perioperative outcomes ($n = 70$)

Sex (%)	
Male	41 (58.6)
Female	29 (41.4)
Age (years), median (range)	63 (18–85)
Body mass index (kg/m^2), median (range)	23.90 (17.0–31.8)
Mayo adhesive probability score, median (range)	0 (0–4)
Perinephric fat volume (cm^3), median (range)	166.05 (22.1–1399.3)
Diabetes mellitus (%)	17 (24.3)
Hypertension (%)	29 (41.4)
Preoperative chronic kidney disease (%)	12 (17.1)
Tumor side (%)	
Right	38 (54.3)
Left	32 (45.7)
Hilar tumor (%)	15 (21.4)
Tumor size (mm), median (range)	23 (5–57)
R.E.N.A.L. nephrometry score, median (range)	7 (4–10)
Surgical approach (%)	
Transperitoneal	53 (75.7)
Retroperitoneal	17 (24.3)
Operative time (min), median (range)	167.5 (103–248)
Console time (min), median (range)	98.0 (60–194)
Estimated blood loss (ml), median (range)	50 (0–620)
Warm ischemia time (min), median (range)	12 (6–21)
Histological subtype (%)	
Clear cell renal cell carcinoma	46 (65.7)
Other malignant tumor	12 (17.1)
Angiomyolipoma	7 (10.0)
Other benign tumor	5 (7.1)
Positive surgical margins (%)	1 (1.4)
Major complications (Clavien-Dindo 3 or 4) (%)	0 (0)
Achievement of trifecta outcomes (%)	69 (98.6)
Achievement of MIC score system outcomes (%)	64 (91.4)

MIC, margin, ischemia and complications

Discussion

Currently available classification systems to estimate the complexity of PN are based on only tumor-specific factors, such as size and location, without taking patient-specific factors into account [8–10]. There have been a number of studies demonstrating obesity, particularly increased visceral fat, to be a potential patient-specific factor associated with surgical difficulty and frequent postoperative complications in renal surgery, including PN [11–14]. To date, several parameters reflecting obesity, such as the BMI, PNF thickness and APF, have been evaluated as predictors of the complexity of PN [11–17]; however, which parameter has the most significant impact on the complexity of PN remains controversial. Furthermore, the complexity of PN may be considerably influenced by the introduction of the robotic technique to this surgical field [2–6]. Taken together, the significance of obesity should be reanalyzed using more objective parameters to predict the surgical difficulty of PN in the era of robotic surgery. In this study, we hypothesized that the exact PNF volume can serve as a better predictor for the complexity of RAPN; therefore, this study was conducted to characterize the effects of the PNF volume on the perioperative outcomes in a total of 70 consecutive patients with clinical T1 renal tumors who underwent RAPN performed by a single experienced robotic surgeon beyond the initial learning curve.

In this study, we measured the PNF volume based on reconstructed 3D images using the SYNAPSE VINCENT system, which is a widely employed method to measure the volumetry of a specific target that has been reported to be able to calculate the exact volume with high reproducibility and interobserver concordance [23, 24]. The median PNF volume in the 70 patients included in this series was 166.05 cm^3, but it ranged between 22.1 and 1399.3 cm^3, suggesting its diverse distribution. We found a significant association between the PNF volume and other related parameters, such as the BMI and MAP score; however, these correlations were not close. Accordingly, it may be difficult to use either the BMI or MAP score as an alternative to the PNF volume measured by the method in this study.

Considering the effects of surgical experience on perioperative outcomes of RAPN, this study included the latest 70 patients undergoing RAPN at our institution during the period of this study. Furthermore, we confirmed the absence of a significant difference in the R.E.N.A.L. nephrometry score and PNF volume among the 5 groups. Based on these findings, this series consisted of patients with comparatively homogeneous features, and no significant difference in the console time during RAPN was noted. Therefore, the data from this cohort of patients may be sufficient to assess the impact of the PNF volume on the perioperative outcomes.

In this series, as achievement of the trifecta and MIC score system outcomes in the 70 patients was favorable, the components consisting of these systems, including the surgical margin status, ischemia time and postoperative complications, were not used as surrogates of the difficulty of RAPN. Therefore, we regarded the console time during RAPN as an index reflecting the complexity of RAPN, and assessed the effects of several parameters, including the PNF volume, on the console time. Of these, only the PNF volume was independently associated with the console time during RAPN. Our findings suggest that measurement of the PNF volume, rather than the BMI or MAP score, can help predict the level of difficulty of RAPN.

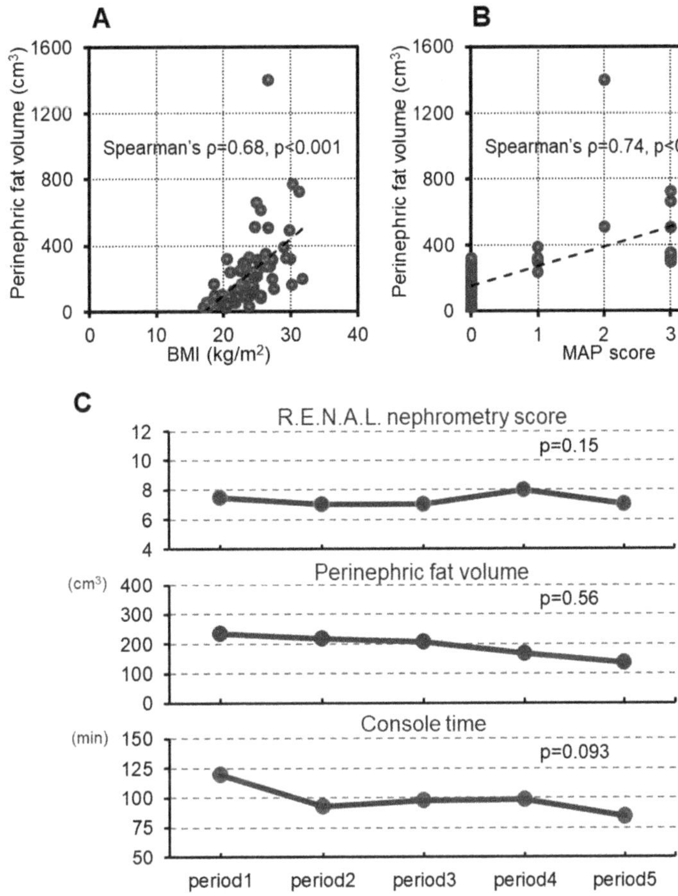

Fig. 2 a: Assessment of the association between the perinephric fat volume and body mass index (BMI) by Spearman's rank correlation analysis. **b:** Assessment of the association between the perinephric fat volume and Mayo adhesive probability (MAP) score by Spearman's rank correlation analysis. **c:** Comparison of the median R.E.N.A.L. nephrometry score, perinephric fat volume and console time among the 5 groups consisting of 14 consecutive patients from the 70 most recent patients who underwent robot-assisted partial nephrectomy at our institution. Periods 1, 2, 3, 4 and 5 consisted of cases 1–14, 15–28, 29–42, 43–56 and 57–70, respectively

Table 2 Univariate and multivariate analyses of several factors as predictors prolonging the console time during robot-assisted partial nephrectomy

	Univariate analysis[a]			Multivariate analysis [a]		
	OR	95% CI	*p*-value	OR	95% CI	*p*-value
Age (< 65 versus ≥65 years)	0.71	0.28–1.84	0.49	–	–	–
Sex (male versus female)	3.47	1.27–9.50	0.015	1.29	0.39–4.32	0.68
Body mass index (< 22.0 versus ≥22.0 kg/m^2)	0.52	0.18–1.53	0.23	–	–	–
Mayo adhesive probability score (0–2 versus 3–5)	0.07	0.01–0.57	0.013	0.18	0.02–1.67	0.13
Diabetes mellitus (positive versus negative)	3.32	0.93–13.85	0.052	–	–	–
R.E.N.A.L. nephrometry score (4–6 versus 7–12)	0.36	0.13–1.05	0.062	–	–	–
Hilar tumor (positive versus negative)	1.80	0.56–5.75	0.32	–	–	–
Surgical approach (transperitoneal versus retroperitoneal)	0.58	0.19–1.75	0.33	–	–	–
Surgical experience (less versus more than half)	2.00	0.77–5.18	0.15	–	–	–
Perinephric fat volume (< 166.05 versus ≥166.05 cm^3)[b]	0.14	0.05–0.40	< 0.001	0.23	0.07–0.77	0.017

OR odds ratio, *CI* confidence interval

[a]The median value for console time (98.0 min) for the included patients was used as the cutoff point in this analysis

[b]The median value for perinephric fat volume (166.05 cm^3) for the included patients was used as the cutoff point in this analysis

Variance inflation factors ranged from 1.10 to 1.25 in the present multivariate model

It is of interest to explore the etiology of why the console time during RAPN is independently affected by the PNF volume, irrespective of other factors, including the BMI or MAP score. BMI is a common factor to characterize the degree of obesity, but it reflects total body fat composition, and patients with the same BMI may have varying distributions of PNF. Indeed, several studies reported that the parameters associated with the distribution of intraabdominal fat are better predictors for PN outcomes than BMI [11, 25]. Furthermore, although it was originally developed to assess the probability of APF during PN [15], the MAP score, which is based on the posterior PNF thickness and stranding, was found to be significantly related to prolongation of the console time, particularly that of the dissection phase time, during RAPN [17]. However, the reproducibility of the MAP score was reported to be unsatisfactory [16], and the presence of APF itself may not be always affect the difficulty of PN [15]. Considering these findings, the volume of PNF, which markedly affects all surgical steps throughout the procedure of RAPN, is more likely to be associated with the complexity of RAPN than the BMI or MAP score.

There are several limitations in this study. First, as this was a retrospective study including a small number of patients, it will be necessary to confirm the findings presented in this study in a prospective study with a larger sample size. Second, RAPN for all 70 patients included in this series was performed by a single experienced robotic surgeon to minimize the effects of surgical experience on the study outcomes; therefore, the present findings cannot be applied to all cohorts of patients undergoing RAPN. Third, the procedure to exactly measure the PNF volume used in this study is slightly complicated; however, we believe that most urologists will be able to measure the PNF volume in approximately 10 min after a few procedures. Fourth, the volume of renal sinus fat, which usually has little impact on the RAPN procedure, was included in the measurement of the 3D volume because it is difficult to define the anatomical boundary line between perinephric and renal sinus fat. On the other hand, the definition of PNF in this series did not include the flank pad, although it may affect the complexity of RAPN, particularly when performed via the retroperitoneal approach. Last, although it is a standard value in our country, the BMI range in this series was lower than those in previous studies from the United States and Europe [15, 16]. Thus, it may be difficult to apply the present findings to cohorts with the significantly greater BMI.

Conclusion

This study included a total of 70 patients with clinical T1a-b renal tumors who were treated by RAPN performed by a single experienced robotic surgeon beyond the initial learning curve, and the significance of the PNF volume as a predictive factor for the complexity of RAPN was analyzed. Considering the favorable trifecta and MIC score system outcomes, this study regarded the console time during RAPN as a surrogate for the index reflecting the surgical difficulty of RAPN, and only the PNF volume was found to be independently associated with the console time, irrespective other significant parameters, including the MAP score. Collectively, our study suggests that measurement of the PNF volume can serve as a reliable predictor of the complexity of RAPN if performed by an experienced robotic surgeon beyond the initial learning curve. To further investigate the significance of the PNF volume during RAPN, it will be of interest to assess the impact of the PNF volume on other surrogate points reflecting the surgical complexity in more diverse cohorts.

Abbreviations

3D: 3-dimentional; APF: Adherent perinephric fat; BMI: Body mass index; C-index: Centrality index; CT: Computed tomography; DICOM: Digital imaging and communications in medicine; MAP score: Mayo adhesive probability score; MIC: Margin, ischemia and complications; PN: Partial nephrectomy; PNF: Perinephric fat; RAPN: Robot-assisted partial nephrectomy; ROI: Region of interest

Acknowledgements

Not applicable.

Authors' contributions

D.M. and H.M. designed the study, collected the clinical data, performed the statistical analysis, participated in the operation and drafted the manuscript. Y.M., H.W., K.T., T.I., T.S. and A.O. participated in the operation and revised the manuscript. All authors read and approved the final manuscript.

References

1. Gill IS, Aron M, Gervais DA, et al. Clinical practice. Small renal mass. N Engl J Med. 2010;362:624–34.
2. Xia L, Wang X, Xu T, et al. Systematic review and meta-analysis of comparative studies reporting perioperative outcomes of robot-assisted partial nephrectomy versus open partial nephrectomy. J Endourol. 2017;31: 893–909.
3. Chang KD, Abdel Raheem A, Kim KH, et al. Functional and oncological outcomes of open, laparoscopic and robot-assisted partial nephrectomy: a multicentre comparative matched-pair analyses with a median of 5 years' follow-up. BJU Int. 2018;122:618–26.
4. Motoyama D, Aki R, Matsushita Y, et al. Early single-center experience with robotic partial nephrectomy using the da Vinci xi: comparative assessment with conventional open partial nephrectomy. Current Urol. In Press.
5. Haseebuddin M, Benway BM, Cabello JM, et al. Robot-assisted partial nephrectomy: evaluation of learning curve for an experienced renal surgeon. J Endourol. 2010;24:57–61.
6. Motoyama D, Matsushita Y, Watanabe H, et al. Initial learning curve for robot-assisted partial nephrectomy performed by a single experienced robotics surgeon. Asian J Endosc Surg. 2019. https://doi.org/10.1111/ases.12683.
7. Patton MW, Salevitz DA, Tyson MD, et al. Robot-assisted partial nephrectomy for complex renal masses. J Robot Surg. 2016;10:27–31.
8. Kutikov A, Uzzo RG. The R.E.N.a.L. nephrometry score: a comprehensive standardized system for quantitating renal tumor size, location and depth. J Urol. 2009;182:844–53.
9. Simmons MN. Morphometric characterization of kidney tumors. Curr Opin Urol. 2011;21:99–103.
10. Simmons MN, Ching CB, Samplaski MK, et al. Kidney tumor location measurement using the C index method. J Urol. 2010;183:1708–13.

11. Gorin MA, Mullins JK, Pierorazio PM, et al. Increased intra-abdominal fat predicts perioperative complications following minimally invasive partial nephrectomy. Urology. 2013;81:1225–30.
12. Macleod LC, Hsi RS, Gore JL, et al. Perinephric fat thickness is an independent predictor of operative complexity during robot-assisted partial nephrectomy. J Endourol. 2014;28:587–91.
13. Raman JD, Reynolds C, Hannon M. An increasing proportion of perinephric to subcutaneous fat is associated with adverse perioperative outcomes of robotic partial nephrectomy. J Robot Surg. 2016;10:255–9.
14. Ioffe E, Hakimi AA, Oh SK, et al. Effect of visceral obesity on minimally invasive partial nephrectomy. Urology. 2013;82:612–8.
15. Davidiuk AJ, Parker AS, Thomas CS, et al. Mayo adhesive probability score: an accurate image-based scoring system to predict adherent perinephric fat in partial nephrectomy. Eur Urol. 2014;66:1165–71.
16. Martin L, Rouviere O, Bezza R, et al. Mayo adhesive probability score is an independent computed tomography scan predictor of adherent perinephric fat in open partial nephrectomy. Urology. 2017;103:124–8.
17. Ishiyama R, Kondo T, Takagi T, et al. Impact of the Mayo adhesive probability score on the complexity of robot-assisted partial nephrectomy. J Endourol. 2018;32:928–33.
18. Dindo D, Demartines N, Clavien PA. Classification of surgical complications: a new proposal with evaluation in a cohort of 6336 patients and results of a survey. Ann Surg. 2004;240:205–13.
19. Takagi T, Kondo T, Tajima T, et al. Enhanced computed tomography after partial nephrectomy in early postoperative period to detect asymptomatic renal artery pseudoaneurysm. Int J Urol. 2014;2:880–5.
20. Buffi N, Lista G, Larcher A, et al. Margin, ischemia, and complications (MIC) score in partial nephrectomy: a new system for evaluating achievement of optimal outcomes in nephron-sparing surgery. Eur Urol. 2012;62:617–8.
21. Furukawa J, Miyake H, Tanaka K, et al. Console-integrated real-time three-dimensional image overlay navigation for robot-assisted partial nephrectomy with selective arterial clamping: early single-Centre experience with 17 cases. Int J Med Robot. 2014;10:385–90.
22. Kondo T, Takagi T, Morita S, et al. Early unclamping might reduce the risk of renal artery pseudoaneurysm after robot-assisted laparoscopic partial nephrectomy. Int J Urol. 2015;22:1096–102.
23. Muto S, Kawano H, Isotani S, et al. Novel semi-automated kidney volume measurements in autosomal dominant polycystic kidney disease. Clin Exp Nephrol. 2018;22:583–90.
24. Leslie S, Gill IS, de Castro Abreu AL, et al. Renal tumor contact surface area: a novel parameter for predicting complexity and outcomes of partial nephrectomy. Eur Urol. 2014;66:884–93.
25. Naeem N, Petros F, Sukumar S, et al. Robot-assisted partial nephrectomy in obese patients. J Endourol. 2011;25:101–5.

12

Treatment of urinary calculi after Yang-Monti ileal ureter reconstruction

Zhenxing Wang[1,2], Zhaolin Sun[2*], Guangheng Luo[2*], Ye Tian[2] and Xiushu Yang[2]

Abstract

Background: The development of ureteral calculi after Yang-Monti ileal ureter reconstruction has not been reported. This study was performed to explore the safety and effectiveness of ureteroscopy combined with laser lithotripsy in the treatment of ipsilateral lower ureteral calculi and lower calyceal calculi after Yang-Monti ileal ureter reconstruction.

Case presentation: A 48-year-old man was admitted to our hospital with ipsilateral distal ureteral calculi and ipsilateral lower calyceal calculi. One year prior to this admission, the patient had undergone Yang-Monti ileal ureter reconstruction due to long-segment ureteral stenosis. After conservative treatment failed, we used a rigid ureteroscope with a holmium laser to break up the distal ureteral calculi, and successfully removed the renal calculi with a digital flexible ureteroscope and basket extractor.

Conclusion: The successful outcome of the present case suggests that ureteroscopy combined with laser lithotripsy is a valuable option for the management of urinary calculi following Yang-Monti ileal ureter reconstruction.

Keywords: Ureter, Ureteroscopy, Urinary calculi, Holmium, Lasers

Background

The development of ureteral calculi after Yang-Monti ileal ureter reconstruction has not been reported. The treatment of ureteral stones is technically challenging, especially for surgeons with minimal experience in such procedures. We used ureteroscopy combined with laser lithotripsy to successfully treat a patient with ipsilateral distal ureteral calculi and ipsilateral lower calyceal calculi after Yang-Monti ileal ureter reconstruction due to long-segment ureteral stenosis.

Case presentation

The patient was a 48-year-old man with a 4-year history of ureteral calculi and a 2-year history of ureteral stenosis for which he had undergone multiple surgeries. Ureteral calculi recurred many times, resulting in repeated ureteral stricture that was treated three times by ureteroscopic holmium laser lithotripsy, and twice by ureteroscopic balloon dilation. He had been admitted to our hospital for left ureteral stenosis in June 2015. Examination at that time revealed a 20-cm stenosis in the middle and lower segments of the ureter. Noncontrast computed tomography showed inflammation and adhesion around the kidney as a result of multiple ureteral surgeries, making the patient unsuitable for autologous kidney transplantation. Yang-Monti ileal ureter reconstruction was performed, and the 6-month postoperative examination revealed left ureteral patency (Fig. 1), stable renal function, normal electrolyte levels, and no obvious mucus-like flocculation in the urine.

Ten months after the Yang-Monti ileal ureter reconstruction, the patient developed left lumbar pain and discomfort. Noncontrast computed tomography showed that the left kidney had a slightly smaller volume than the right, and that the left renal pelvis and renal calices were slightly expanded and hydronephrotic. Two nodule-shaped high-density shadows were present in the lower renal calyx; the diameter of the larger shadow was 4 to 5 mm. A liquid-density shadow was seen in the ileal lumen of the left ureter, with a small nodule-shaped

* Correspondence: 763920818@qq.com; 13809440294@163.com
[2]Department of Urology, Guizhou Provincial People's Hospital, No. 83 East Zhongshan Road, Guiyang 550002, Guizhou, China
Full list of author information is available at the end of the article

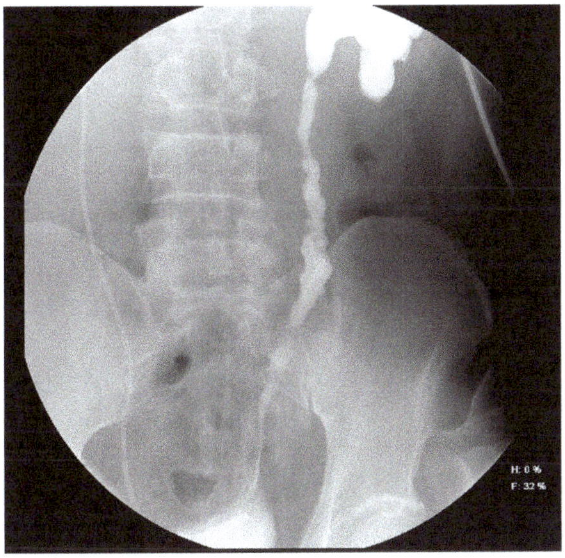

Fig. 1 Left ureteral patency at 6 months after Yang-Monti ileal ureter reconstruction

high-density shadow (3-mm diameter) at its end. Corticomedullary development was good. During excretion, accumulation of contrast agent could be seen in the left renal pelvis, renal calices, and ureter (Figs. 2, 3 and 4). The serum creatinine concentration was normal.

The patient was placed in the lithotomy position under general anesthesia. The ileal ureterovesical reimplantation opening was smoothly entered under direct vision using a 9.5-Fr semirigid ureteroscope (Richard Wolf Medical Instruments, Knittlingen, Germany). Ureteroscopic examination revealed that the calculi were attached to surgical sutures located from 1 cm from the inner end of the ileal ureter to the ureteral opening, and

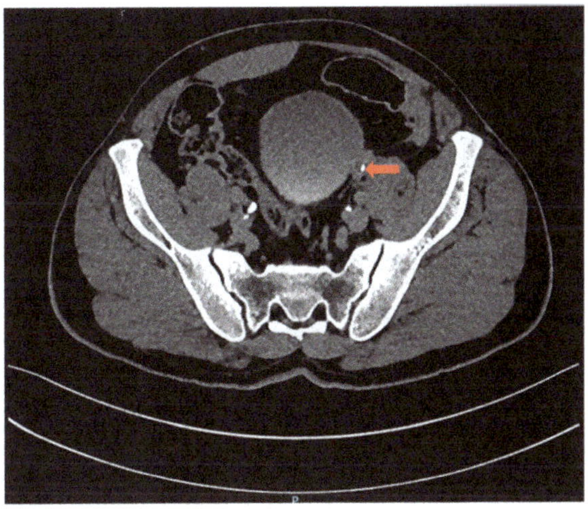

Fig. 3 A nodule-shaped high-density shadow in the ileal lumen of the left ureter (indicated by the arrow)

that the sutures were embedded under the ileal ureteral mucosa in a ring shape (Fig. 5). A basket extractor [NGage Nitinol Stone Extractor (NGE-017115), 1.7 Fr × 115 cm; Cook Medical, Bloomington, IN, USA] was used to hold the calculi and sutures, which were then broken up with a holmium laser (0.6 J, 30 Hz, 200-μm fiber; 60-W LISA Sphinx Holmium:Yttrium-Aluminium-Garnet Laser System, LISA Laser Products, Katlenburg-Lindau, Germany) and completely removed (Figs. 6, 7). Ureteroscopy revealed that the Yang-Monti ileal ureter had a thick and straight lumen, smooth mucosa, and no obvious folds or anastomoses between sections (Fig. 8). Using a Zebra guidewire (Boston Scientific, Marlborough, MA, USA) for guidance, a flexible ureteroscope working sheath (12/14 Fr × 115 cm, M006250226; Boston Scientific)

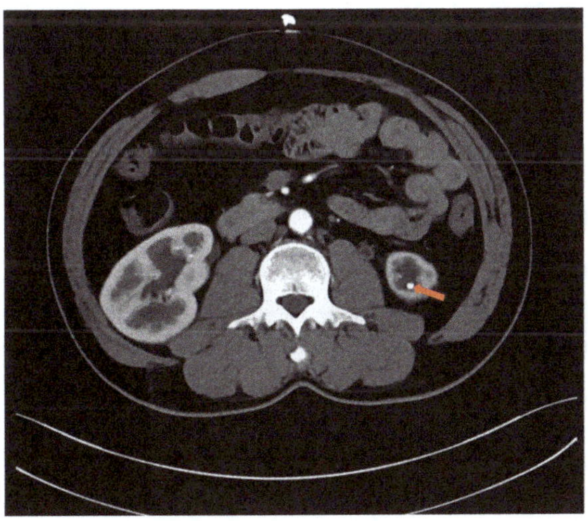

Fig. 2 Two nodule-shaped high-density shadows in the lower renal calyx (indicated by the arrows)

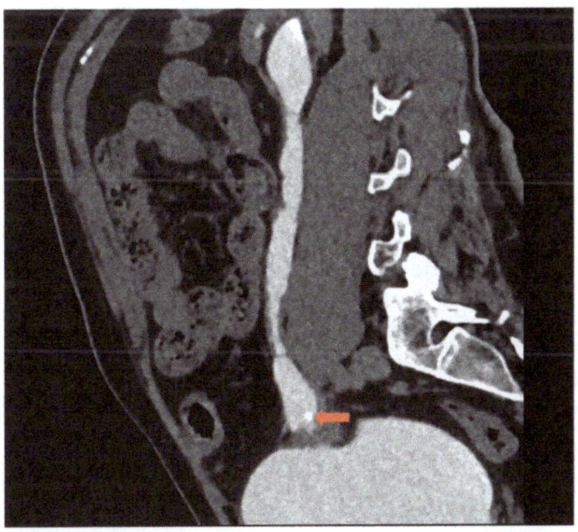

Fig. 4 A nodule-shaped high-density shadow in the ileal lumen of the left ureter (indicated by the arrow)

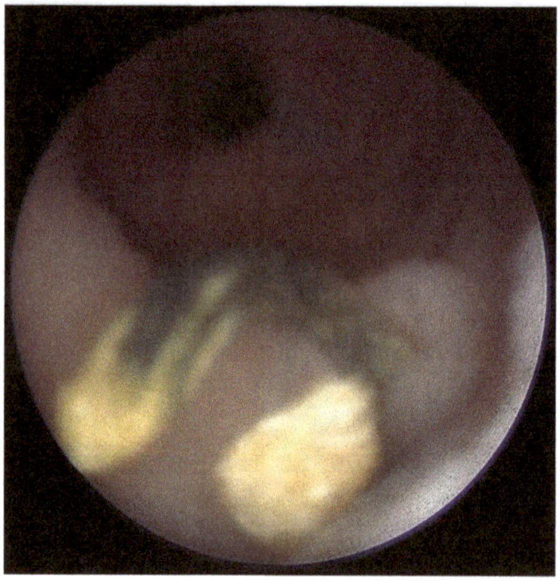

Fig. 5 The calculi were attached to surgical sutures, and the sutures were embedded under the ileal ureteral mucosa

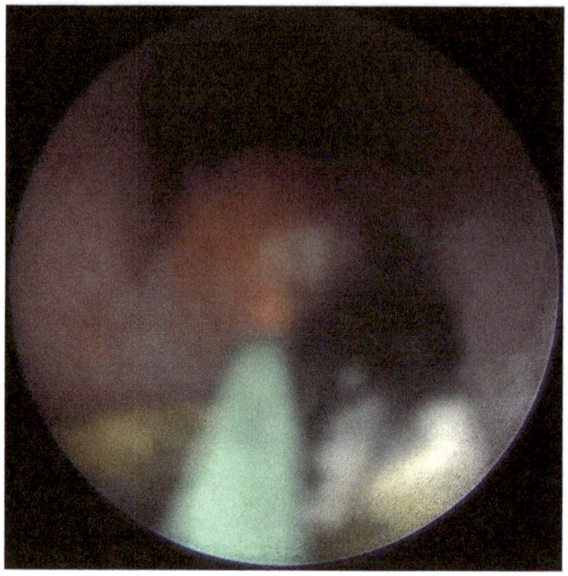

Fig. 7 The calculi and sutures were broken up with a holmium laser

was imbedded and inserted into the left renal pelvis under direct vision using a digital flexible ureteroscope (8.5 Fr, 11278VS; Karl Storz, Tuttlingen, Germany). Using a filling pump (26331020–1; Storz Medical, Tägerwilen, Switzerland) with an infusion pressure of 80 mmHg, the two lower calyceal calculi were identified, broken up, and removed. As a preoperative urine culture had revealed a urinary tract infection, antibiotics were administered postoperatively. Additionally, a 5-Fr ureteral catheter (Kangge Medical Instruments, Shanghai, China) and a urinary catheter were left indwelling, and were removed on postoperative day 3.

Discussion and conclusion

A previous study investigating minimally invasive treatment of ureteral calculi following ileal neobladder surgery reported that the cause of calculi development may be related to the presence of foreign bodies (e.g., ureteral stents and sutures) [1]. Furthermore, the generation of ileal ureteral calculi also has a very close relationship with intestinal mucous [2]; when the ileal anastomosis is

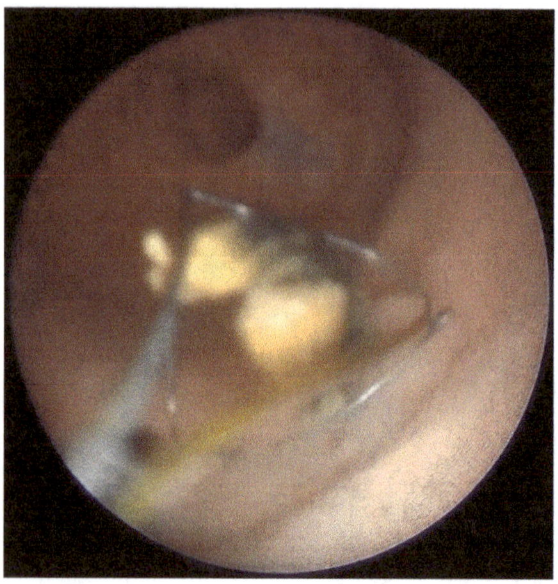

Fig. 6 A basket extractor was used to hold the calculi and sutures

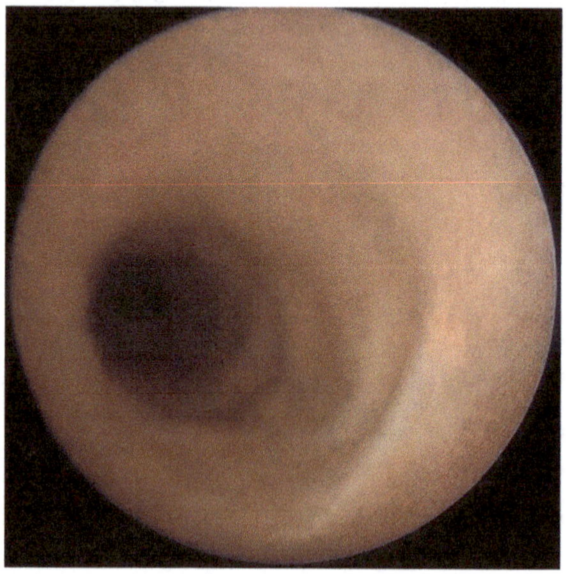

Fig. 8 The Yang-Monti ileal ureter had a thick and straight lumen and smooth mucosa

bulky, the intestinal mucous secreted in the ileal segment near the kidney during bowel movements is more likely to enter the kidney, accumulate in the renal pelvis within the calyx, and become a matrix or core of stone formation, along with urine salt deposition and stone formation [2]. If the ileal replacement ureter is too long and the postoperative replacement urine becomes stored in the ileum, this urine combines with the large amount of mucus secreted by the intestinal tract to form calculi, and ureteral calculi in the ureteral diversion may be formed by renal calculi falling through the urine drainage [3]. In the present case, the absorbable suture in the lower ileal ureteral segment from the previous ureteral reconstruction had not degraded or fallen off, and so served as a matrix or core for calculi formation; its long-term contact with urine resulted in urinary salt being continuously deposited to form calculi [4, 5]. The lower ileal ureteral calculi were successfully removed using a rigid ureteroscope combined with holmium laser lithotripsy to remove the sutures and attached calculi.

During the holmium laser removal of sutures, it is important to determine the shape and direction of the suture, cut the suture from its root near the ileal ureteral mucosa, and check the integrity of the suture to prevent leaving residual suture that will again enable calculi to form. Suture removal must be performed under direct vision. As the suture moves along with the movement of the perfusate, the suture must be fixed with a basket extractor to create adequate tension and thus prevent the suture from moving; this improves the success rate of suture removal, and reduces the risk of ileal ureteral injury.

A digital flexible ureteroscope was entered into the left renal collection system. As the calculi were small (maximum diameter of 5 mm) and oval-shaped with smooth surfaces, we were able to use a basket extractor to cover and remove the calculi. During removal, we discovered that the calculi had diameters that were larger than that of the working sheath for the flexible ureteroscope; hence, we covered each calculus and removed it together with the working sheath of the flexible ureteroscope. Using intraoperative ureteroscopic guidance, a 5-Fr double-J stent was placed upon completion of the surgery.

The key points gained from our experience are as follows. (1) The thinnest holmium laser fiber with the appropriate energy for cutting should be selected, so that the laser fiber can pass through the gap between the basket extractor and the ureteroscopic operation channel. It is best to conduct an in vitro analysis of suture materials, and then choose the best energy setting for cutting. The appropriate energy setting is that which can cut the suture while preventing damage to the ureter. (2) Good intraoperative control of the perfusion pressure must be maintained. Excessive pressure causes dilatation of the reconstructed ureteral lumen, increased pressure in the renal pelvis and renal calices, and an increased risk of postoperative infection. (3) The ileal ureter has a large lumen diameter. Even if the diameter of the intestinal canal is cut using the Yang-Monti method, the reconstructed ureteral lumen still has a large diameter, and thus the rigid ureteroscope, flexible ureteroscope, and working sheath of the flexible ureteroscope can be successfully retrograded to the renal pelvis. When the diameters of the calculi are smaller than the diameter of the ureteral lumen, a basket extractor can be used.

In summary, ureteroscopy combined with laser lithotripsy seems to be a valuable option for the management of urinary calculi following Yang-Monti ileal ureter reconstruction.

Declarations

No conflict of interest exits in the submission of this manuscript, and the manuscript has been approved by all authors for publication. The work described herein is original research that has not been published previously and is not under consideration for publication elsewhere, in whole or in part. All authors of the manuscript have read and agreed to its content and are accountable for all aspects of the accuracy and integrity of the manuscript in accordance with ICMJE criteria, and all agree to the terms of the BioMed Central License Agreement and Open Data Policy.

Authors' contributions

ZW wrote the first draft of the manuscript. ZS, GL, YT, and XY reviewed the manuscript and were involved in its critical revision before submission. All authors read and approved the final manuscript.

Author details

[1]Basic Medical College, Guizhou Medical University, Guiyang 550004, China.
[2]Department of Urology, Guizhou Provincial People's Hospital, No. 83 East Zhongshan Road, Guiyang 550002, Guizhou, China.

References

1. Hertzig LL, Iwaszko MR, Rangel LJ, Patterson DE, Gettman MT, Krambeck AE. Urolithiasis after ileal conduit urinary diversion: a comparison of minimally invasive therapies. J Urol. 2013;189(6):2152–7.
2. Linyu Z, Zhengzi Y, Tiankai S, et al. Long-term complications and prevention of ileal ureteral replacement[J]. Chinese J Surg. 1997;35(9):574.
3. Schott F, Becker B, Gross AJ, et al. Symptomatic distal ureteral stone in an Ileal ureter: treatment by combined supine Ureteroscopy and mini percutaneous Nephrolithotomy[J]. J Endourol Case Rep. 2017;3(1):90.
4. Mahdavi A, Mostafavi H. Hanging bladder calculi secondary to misplaced surgical suture[J]. Iran J Radiol. 2015;12(2):e11303.
5. Mcadams S, Sweet R, Anderson K. V6-09 technique for endoscopic removal of calcified permanent suture after PYELOPLASTY[J]. J Urol. 2015;193(4): e579–80.

13

Optimized management of urolithiasis by coloured stent-stone contrast using dual-energy computed tomography (DECT)

Giuseppe Magistro[1*], Patrick Bregenhorn[2], Bernhard Krauß[3], Dominik Nörenberg[3], Melvin D'Anastasi[3], Anno Graser[4], Philipp Weinhold[1], Frank Strittmatter[1], Christian G. Stief[1] and Michael Staehler[1]

Abstract

Background: We analysed in vitro the appearance of commonly used ureteral stents with dual-energy computed tomography (DECT) and we used these characteristics to optimize the differentiation between stents and adjacent stone.

Methods: We analysed in vitro a selection of 36 different stents from 7 manufacturers. They were placed in a self-build phantom model and measured using the SOMATOM® Force Dual Source CT-Scanner (Siemens, Forchheim, Germany). Each sample was scanned at various tube potentials of 80 and 150 peak kilovoltage (kVp), 90 and 150 kVp and 100 and 150 kVp. The syngo Post-Processing Suite software program (Siemens, Forchheim, Germany) was used for differentiation based on a 3–material decomposition algorithm (UA, calcium, urine) according to our standard stone protocol.

Results: Stents composed of polyurethane appeared blue and silicon-based stents were red on the image. The determined appearances were constant for various peak kilovoltage (kVp) values. The coloured stent-stone-contrast displayed on DECT improves monitoring, especially of small calculi adjacent to indwelling ureteral stents.

Conclusion: Both urinary calculi and ureteral stents can be accurately differentiated by a distinct appearance on DECT. For the management of urolithiasis patients can be monitored more easily and accurately using DECT if the stent shows a different colour than the adjacent stone.

Keywords: Urolithiasis, Stone disease, Dual-energy computed tomography, Stent-stone-contrast

Background

Urolithiasis is a common bothersome condition with a prevalence of 4–20% and an upward trend is reported in developed countries [1, 2]. Non-contrast enhanced computed tomography (NCCT) is the standard for diagnosing patients with acute flank pain [3]. Low-dose NCCT has emerged as the imaging technique of first choice in the acute setting. It provides both excellent sensitivity of 97% and specificity of 95% for the detection of urinary calculi [4]. NCCT determines accurately location, size, density and skin-to-stone distance, all of which are relevant determinants for treatment decision. With the introduction of technical innovations like dual-energy computed tomography (DECT) acquisition of additional information on chemical stone composition is now possible. The attenuation difference produced by two different x-ray energy spectra is utilized to differentiate uric-acid (UA) calculi from non-uric-acid (non-UA) stones. The post-processing software applied for analysis uses a 3-material decomposition algorithm, which characterizes a calculus as a mixture of UA, calcium and urine. Based on this algorithm, material-specific chromatic image-pixels with an attenuation ratio similar to UA are coloured red, those similar to non-UA stones appear blue. This classification is achieved with high accuracy, which is supported by a reported sensitivity of

* Correspondence: Giuseppe.Magistro@med.uni-muenchen.de
[1]Department of Urology, Ludwig-Maximilians-University of Munich, Marchioninistrasse 15, 81377 Munich, Germany
Full list of author information is available at the end of the article

up to 100% [5–12]. The fact can be decisive for optimal management as in case of UA stones pharmacological chemolitholysis is preferred to interventional approaches [3].

Of note, ureteral stents are also assigned a specific colour according to their material composition on DECT. The imaging of small stones adjacent to a ureteral stent is a common pitfall in the current diagnostic assessment. The option to display stent and stone in contrasting colour may help to optimize the detection. The colour-coded characteristics of calculi based on chemical composition are well documented, whereas for ureteral stents they do not. The determinants underlying the phenomenon of red and blue stents on DECT scans have not been elucidated yet. In the current work it was our main objective to characterize in vitro the appearance of different stents from various manufacturers using DECT.

Methods

In vitro setting

We purchased 36 commonly used stents from 7 manufacturers and analysed them on the third generation SOMATOM® Force Dual Source CT-Scanner (Siemens, Forchheim, Germany). We used a phantom model measuring 45 cm × 20 cm × 20 cm (height x width x depth) and filled it with water at body temperature (36 °C) (Fig. 1). The model itself and experimental settings had no influence on CT performance and analysis. Stents were fixed with clips, spanned throughout the phantom model and consecutive measurements were performed. Each sample was scanned at various tube potentials of 80 and 150 peak kilovoltage (kVp), 90 and 150 kVp and 100 and 150 kVp. We affixed a calculus of 2 mm in diameter of known chemical composition (calcium oxalate monohydrate; blue on DECT scan) to blue and red stents and repeated measurements.

CT protocol and post processing

The images were acquired on a SOMATOM® FORCE Siemens computed tomography (CT) scanner (Siemens, Forchheim, Germany) in dual-energy mode. The patients underwent imaging with 100/Sn150 kVp reflecting our current institutional dual-energy protocol. Continuous non-contrast images were obtained from the level of the diaphragm to the pubic symphysis. A slice thickness of 4 mm and interval of 4 mm were chosen to be consistent with our clinical practice. The images were reconstructed on a multimodality WorkPlace (Siemens) using CT syngo Post-Processing Suite software, version VA 50A (Siemens). Reconstructions used a 0.75-mm slice thickness and 0.7-mm interval, with a QR40 convolution kernel for optimal data analysis. DECT allows differentiating between uric acid (UA) and non-UA stones, which are colour-coded based on a post-processing algorithm. The syngo Post-Processing Suite software program utilizes a 3-material (UA, calcium, and urine) decomposition algorithm to assign colour (red or blue) based on the ratio of X-ray attenuations from the two tube potentials. Materials that more closely resemble the dual-energy characteristics (DEC) of UA stones are depicted in red and those that more closely resemble the DEC of non-UA stones are depicted in blue.

Results

Results are demonstrated in Fig. 2a. All polyurethane-based stents showed a blue appearance on DECT, whereas stents composed of silicone were red. The assigned colours were constant over various kVp values. The determined colour according to material composition of various stents from the same manufacturer was consistent throughout our measurements (Table 1). As shown in Fig. 2b, placing a pure calcium oxalate monohydrate stone (blue) of 2 mm in size next to a ureteral stent of blue colour makes it difficult to discern the fragment on both coronal and sagittal reformatted DECT

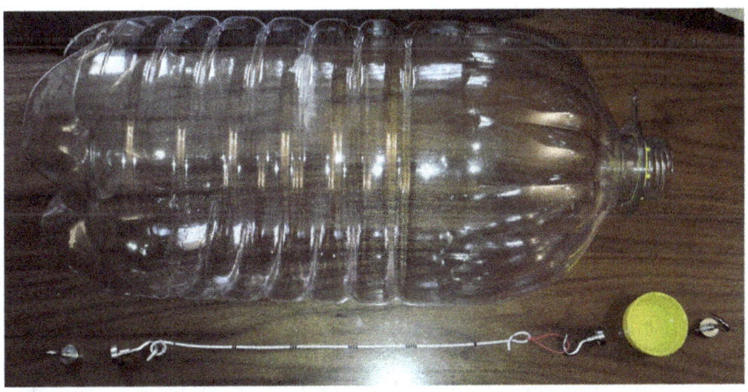

Fig. 1 A container was filled with water at body temperature (36 °C). Stents were fixed with clips at both ends and spanned throughout the phantom model for measurements

a

b

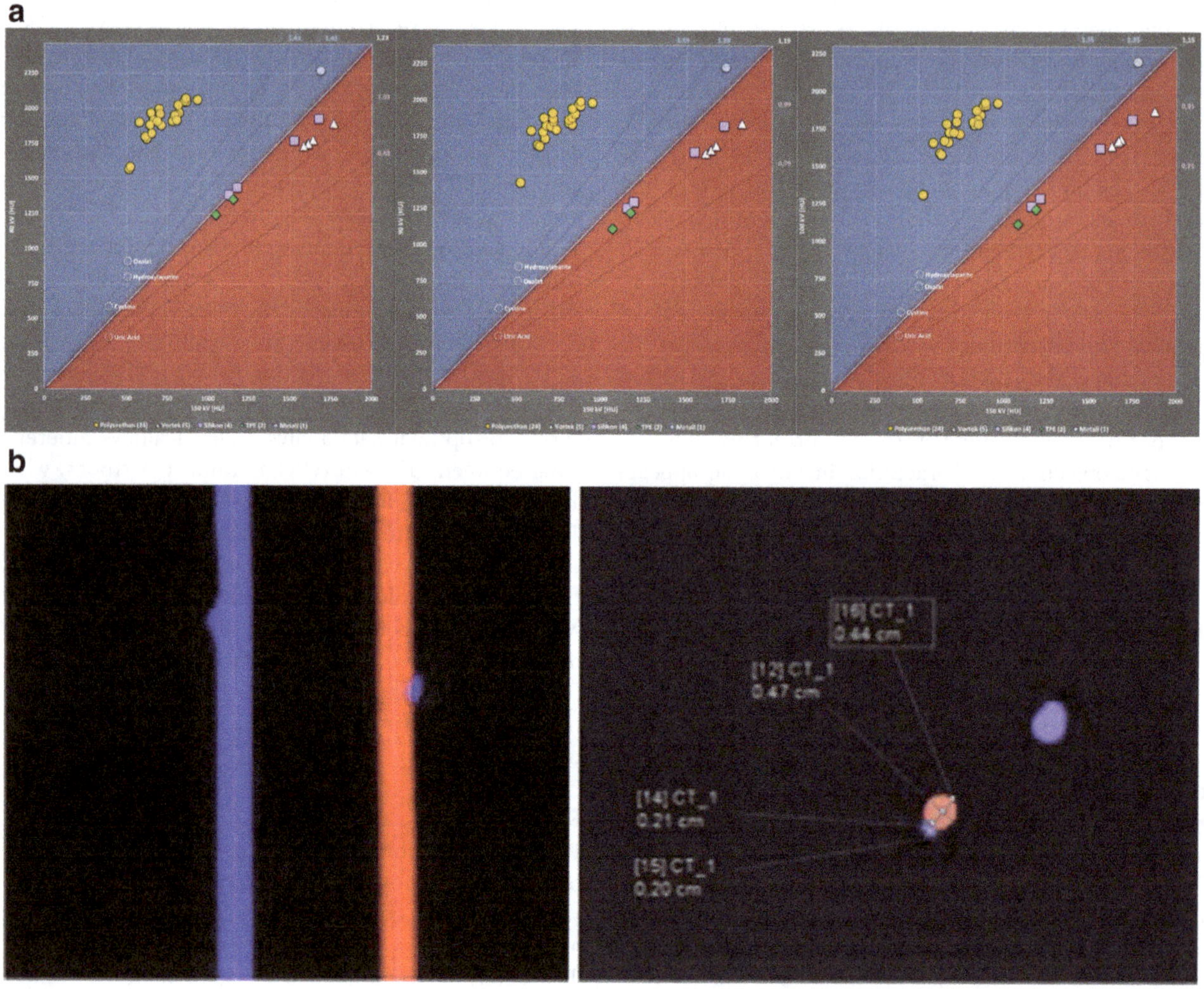

Fig. 2 a. Results acquired for various tube potentials (80/150 kVp; 90/150 kVp; 100/150 kVp). Respective Hounsfield units (HU) were measured and plotted. Stents above the cut-off of 1,15 appeared blue and samples below the cut-off appeared red. Reference values for known stone types are depicted as well. Polyurethane-based samples were blue, silicone-based stents were red. **b.** A pure calcium oxalate monohydrate stone of 2 mm (blue) was affixed to a blue and red stent on DECT. The enhanced stent-stone-contrast obtained for the red stent allows clear differentiation of the stone from the adjacent stent. For the blue stent a contour irregularity of the stent is indicative of stone presence, better displayed on coronal than sagittal images

images. Now, using a silicone-based stent, which appears red on DECT, the presence of the stone could be easily detected due to a clear stent-stone-contrast.

Discussion

Information on chemical stone composition optimizes management of urolithiasis in many ways. As mentioned above, DECT assures identification of UA stones with high accuracy, thus efficient chemolitholysis should be preferred rather than interventional treatment, if it is clinically appropriate and safe. However, the overall incidence of UA stones was estimated to be 11.7% for men and 7% for women [13]. Thus, the clinical impact on management is actually rather low. Furthermore, the unique ability to determine stone types may prevent inefficient treatment options. Extracorporeal shockwave lithotripsy (ESWL) achieves good results for renal stones ≤20 mm, but shockwave-resistant stones composed of calcium oxalate monohydrate or cystine are known negative predictors for success [14]. Both stone types can be identified with high diagnostic accuracy using DECT [15]. In these cases multiple ineffective procedures can be avoided in favour of a more effective treatment modality such as percutaneous nephrolithotomy (PNL).

A distinct appearance of ureteral stents on DECT has been observed, but a systematic analysis of this phenomenon is lacking [16]. In the current study we investigated in vitro a random selection of 36 various samples from 7 manufacturers and we were able to match appearance (blue or red) to material composition

Table 1 A random selection of 36 various stents was purchased from 7 manufacturers. Material composition and reference numbers for each model are displayed. Stents are classified according to their appearance as red or blue on DECT

Manufacturer	RED	BLUE
Uromed		Hydropur (polyurethane, 4640–28) Hydropur (polyurethane, 4687–28) Heparius (polyurethane, 4377–28) Heparius (polyurethane, 4387–28)
Urotech		Yellow-Star (polyurethane, TU-360628) Yellow-Star (polyurethane, EP-360628) Green-Star (polyurethane, EG-480628) White-Star (polyurethane, ES-370628) White-Star (polyurethane, ES-570730)
Cook	C-Flex Towers (TPE, 037732) Universa Soft (TPE, USH-722-T1) Black Silicone (silicone, 133,624)	Universa UFH (polyurethane, UFH-772-T1) Resonance (metal, RMS-060022-R)
Rüsch		Superglide DD (polyurethane, 334,841) Superglide integral (polyurethane, 334,248) Integral Stent Set (polyurethane, 334,201) DD-Ureterstent (polyurethane, 334,801)
Optimed		Optisoft (polyurethane, 3004–2400) Optipur (polyurethane, 3034–2400) Optisplint (polyurethane, 3064–2400) Carbosoft (polyurethane, 3090–2400)
Coloplast/ Porges	Vortek Tumor Stent (Vortek, BCCG75) Vortek (Vortek, ACB576) Vortek Hydrogel (Vortek, BCFA75) Vortek Hydrogel (Vortek, BNFA75) Vortek Mono-J (Vortek, ACA207) Silicone (silicone, AJ4275) Silicone (silicone, AJ4A75) Silikon Pyelostent (silicone, AJ4Y85) Silikon Stenostent (silicone, AJ4W85)	PU-R (polyurethane, AC4D75) PU-R (polyurethane, AC4B75) PU S (polyurethane, AC4274) Biosoft Duo (polyurethane, BNAA75)
IMP		Tumorstent (polyurethane, S137996070300)

of a stent. In our setting polyurethane based stents were always blue on DECT, stents composed of silicone appeared always red. We further demonstrated that an enhanced stent-stone-contrast by selecting a stent in a different colour than the adjacent stone facilitates safe and easy detection, even for 2 mm calculi. This enhanced stent-stone-contrast allows clear differentiation in both coronal and sagittal images. Without colour coding, as in NCCT, only a contour irregularity may be suggestive of an adjacent stone, which becomes speculative when calculi decrease in size. This diagnostic obstacle may be overcome using color-coding based on a post-processing algorithm as applied in DECT. We demonstrated that a pure calcium oxalate monohydrate stone (blue) of 2 mm could be clearly differentiated from a silicon-based stent (red). Next to a blue stent, the presence of the stone was indicative by a poorly defined irregularity, which was more prominent on the coronal scan. The analysis of other 2 mm stones with different composition but a distinct colour on DECT scans, could always be detected accurately when the stent appeared in contrasting colour.

This feature may be of value in various clinical scenarios for the management of urolithiasis. The advantage of DECT technology aids urologists in stent selection according to stone appearance and assures accurate monitoring of stone patients. It has to be acknowledged, that stenting is indicated only in case of obstructive pyelonephritis, anuria and analgesia not achieved medically. The impact of our findings still needs to be evaluated for the clinical management.

The early results of DECT imaging for the management of urolithiasis are promising, however, due to the infancy of this technology relevant issues still need to be addressed. Certain pitfalls have been reported including reduced specificity for small calculi < 3 mm and patients with large body habitus [17]. With the development of third-generation scanners and modification of protocol settings and post-processing the capacity and potential of the technology is still advancing [18].

Certain limitations of this study need to be acknowledged. First of all, although we present the analysis of the largest stent collection to date with convincing consistency, we cannot exclude that stents from different manufacturers may display a diverse phenotype. Certain coatings might have a profound impact on appearance on DECT. Second, we present mainly in vitro data. Prospective, clinical trails are necessary to confirm our first results in stone patients and to evaluate the true benefit for management.

Conclusions

Polyurethane-based stents are blue and stents composed of silicone appear red using DECT imaging. The enhanced stent-stone-contrast using DECT imaging is an additional feature that may be helpful for stent selection. Whenever available, it can contribute to an easy and accurate monitoring of stone patients. The coloured stent-stone-contrast displayed on DECT improves detection, especially of small calculi < 3 mm next to indwelling ureteral stents. Wherever DECT is available, urologists are encouraged to screen for blue and red stents in their institution and to choose ureteral stents according to stone appearance.

Abbreviations
DECT: Dual-energy computed tomography; kVp: peak kilovoltage; NCCT: Non-contrast enhanced computed tomography; PNL: Percutaneous nephrolithotomy; UA: Uric acid

Acknowledgments
None.

Authors' contributions
GM: Project development, Data collection and analysis, Manuscript writing. PB: Data collection and analysis. BK: Data collection and analysis. DN: Data collection and analysis. MDA: Data collection and analysis. AG: Data collection and analysis. PW: Data collection and analysis. FS: Data collection and analysis. CGS: Project development, Data collection and management. MS: Project development, Data collection and management. All authors read and approved the final manuscript.

Author details
[1]Department of Urology, Ludwig-Maximilians-University of Munich, Marchioninistrasse 15, 81377 Munich, Germany. [2]Department of Radiology, Ludwig-Maximilians-University of Munich, Munich, Germany. [3]Siemens Healthcare GmbH, Research and Development, Forchheim, Germany. [4]Gemeinschaftspraxis Radiologie München, Munich, Germany.

References
1. Curhan GC. Epidemiology of stone disease. Urol Clin North Am. 2007; 34(3):287–93.
2. Stamatelou KK, Francis ME, Jones CA, Nyberg LM, Curhan GC. Time trends in reported prevalence of kidney stones in the United States: 1976-1994. Kidney Int. 2003;63(5):1817–23.
3. Turk C, Petrik A, Sarica K, Seitz C, Skolarikos A, Straub M, et al. EAU guidelines on diagnosis and conservative Management of Urolithiasis. Eur Urol. 2016;69(3):468–74.
4. Niemann T, Kollmann T, Bongartz G. Diagnostic performance of low-dose CT for the detection of urolithiasis: a meta-analysis. AJR Am J Roentgenol. 2008;191(2):396–401.
5. Primak AN, Fletcher JG, Vrtiska TJ, Dzyubak OP, Lieske JC, Jackson ME, et al. Noninvasive differentiation of uric acid versus non-uric acid kidney stones using dual-energy CT. Acad Radiol. 2007;14(12):1441–7.
6. Spek A, Strittmatter F, Graser A, Kufer P, Stief C, Staehler M. Dual energy can accurately differentiate uric acid-containing urinary calculi from calcium stones. World J Urol. 2016;34(9):1297–302.
7. Boll DT, Patil NA, Paulson EK, Merkle EM, Simmons WN, Pierre SA, et al. Renal stone assessment with dual-energy multidetector CT and advanced postprocessing techniques: improved characterization of renal stone composition--pilot study. Radiology. 2009;250(3):813–20.
8. Eiber M, Holzapfel K, Frimberger M, Straub M, Schneider H, Rummeny EJ, et al. Targeted dual-energy single-source CT for characterisation of urinary calculi: experimental and clinical experience. Eur Radiol. 2012;22(1):251–8.
9. Eliahou R, Hidas G, Duvdevani M, Sosna J. Determination of renal stone composition with dual-energy computed tomography: an emerging application. Semin Ultrasound CT MR. 2010;31(4):315–20.
10. Graser A, Johnson TR, Bader M, Staehler M, Haseke N, Nikolaou K, et al. Dual energy CT characterization of urinary calculi: initial in vitro and clinical experience. Investig Radiol. 2008;43(2):112–9.
11. Hidas G, Eliahou R, Duvdevani M, Coulon P, Lemaitre L, Gofrit ON, et al. Determination of renal stone composition with dual-energy CT: in vivo analysis and comparison with x-ray diffraction. Radiology. 2010;257(2):394–401.
12. Lombardo F, Bonatti M, Zamboni GA, Avesani G, Oberhofer N, Bonelli M, et al. Uric acid versus non-uric acid renal stones: in vivo differentiation with spectral CT. Clin Radiol. 2017;72(6):490–6.
13. Knoll T, Schubert AB, Fahlenkamp D, Leusmann DB, Wendt-Nordahl G, Schubert G. Urolithiasis through the ages: data on more than 200,000 urinary stone analyses. J Urol. 2011;185(4):1304–11.
14. Turk C, Petrik A, Sarica K, Seitz C, Skolarikos A, Straub M, et al. EAU guidelines on interventional treatment for urolithiasis. Eur Urol. 2016; 69(3):475–82.
15. Zhang GM, Sun H, Xue HD, Xiao H, Zhang XB, Jin ZY. Prospective prediction of the major component of urinary stone composition with dual-source dual-energy CT in vivo. Clin Radiol. 2016;71(11):1178–83.
16. Jepperson MA, Thiel DD, Cernigliaro JG, Broderick GA, Parker AS, Haley WE. Determination of ureter stent appearance on dual-energy computed tomography scan. Urology. 2012;80(5):986–9.
17. Jepperson MA, Cernigliaro JG, Sella D, Ibrahim E, Thiel DD, Leng S, et al. Dual-energy CT for the evaluation of urinary calculi: image interpretation, pitfalls and stone mimics. Clin Radiol. 2013;68(12):e707–14.
18. Duan X, Li Z, Yu L, Leng S, Halaweish AF, Fletcher JG, et al. Characterization of urinary stone composition by use of third-generation dual-source dual-energy CT with increased spectral separation. AJR Am J Roentgenol. 2015; 205(6):1203–7.

14

Hypertension as a prognostic factor in metastatic renal cell carcinoma treated with tyrosine kinase inhibitors

Yu Liu†, Liang Zhou†, Yuntian Chen†, Banghua Liao, Donghui Ye, Kunjie Wang* and Hong Li

Abstract

Background: Conflicting evidence exists regarding the effect of hypertension on the prognosis of metastatic renal cell carcinoma (mRCC) patients treated with tyrosine kinase inhibitors (TKIs). This study aimed to assess the predictive value of TKIs-induced hypertension in patients with mRCC.

Methods: This study was registered in PROSPERO (CRD42019129593). PubMed, Embase, Web of Science and the Cochrane Library database were searched with terms: "renal cell carcinoma", "hypertension", "blood pressure", "tyrosine kinase inhibitor", "sunitinib", "axitinib", "sorafenib" and "pazopanib" until March 21, 2019. Hazard Ratios (HR) and 95% confidence intervals (CI) for progression-free survival (PFS) or overall survival (OS) were extracted and analyzed with Stata 15.0 software. Heterogeneity was assessed using the I^2 value. Meta-regression, subgroup analysis and sensitivity analysis were also performed to explore heterogeneity. Publication bias was assessed with funnel plots and precisely assessed by Egger's and Begg's tests. The quality of evidence of outcomes was generated according to the Grading of Recommendations Assessment, Development, and Evaluation (GRADE).

Results: A total of 4661 patients from 22 studies were included in the study. The results showed that the increase of blood pressure was an effective predictor for longer PFS (HR = 0.59, 95% CI: 0.48–0.71, $p < 0.001$; $I^2 = 77.3\%$) and OS (HR = 0.57, 95% CI: 0.45–0.70, $p < 0.001$; $I^2 = 77.4\%$) of patients with mRCC. Subgroup analysis revealed that patients receiving sunitinib and pazopanib could have longer PFS and OS.

Conclusions: This study indicated that TKIs-induced hypertension may be a good predictor for better prognosis of patients with mRCC receiving TKIs treatment, especially using sunitinib or pazopanib.

Keywords: Metastatic renal cell carcinoma, Tyrosine kinase inhibitors, Hypertension, Prognosis, Meta-analysis

Background

Renal cell carcinoma (RCC) is the 9th most common cancer in men and 14th most common cancer in women worldwide [1]. Its incidence (3–6/100,000) and mortality (1.2–2.5/100,000) are increasing rapidly, which has a great negative effect on our society [2, 3]. In addition, about 25–30% of patients have evidence of metastasis upon its diagnosis [4]. Now, vascular endothelial growth factor receptor tyrosine kinase inhibitors (TKIs), like sunitinib, pazopanib, sorafenib or axitinib, are the favored medicine for metastatic RCC (mRCC). Several clinical trials showed that response to TKIs was uncertain (objective response rate was 31–67.4%) [5–8], which indicated the existence of wide inter-individual variation and the lack of reliable factors for predicting the outcomes of mRCC patients. Therefore, a big challenge faced by urologists is how to predict the prognosis of mRCC patients receiving TKIs more precisely.

The occurrence of several adverse events (AEs) during TKIs therapy, such as hypertension, hand-foot syndrome or hypothyroidism, were shown to be correlated with the

* Correspondence: wangkj@scu.edu.cn
†Yu Liu, Liang Zhou and Yuntian Chen contributed equally to this work and should be considered as co-first authors
Department of Urology, Institute of Urology (Laboratory of Reconstructive Urology), West China Hospital, Sichuan University, No.37 Guo Xue Xiang, Chengdu, Sichuan 610041, People's Republic of China

longer median progression-free survival (PFS) and overall survival (OS) of mRCC patients [9]. Hypertension during TKIs therapy was very common, with incidence ranging from 22 to 81% [9, 10]. Recently, a study found that RCC patients with longer median PFS (>5.3 months) demonstrated a significantly higher incidence of high-grade hypertension (a treatment-associated adverse event) than those with shorter PFS [11]. It indicated that TKIs-induced hypertension may be associated with improved prognosis [12, 13]. However, others reported insignificant results [14, 15]. In 2014, a systematic review and meta-analysis reported that the occurrence of hypertension due to sorafenib therapy may be associated with improved prognosis of patients with cancer. However, this study did not specifically focus on the mRCC patients. Thus, the association between TKIs-induced hypertension and prognosis of mRCC is still controversial. In the present study, we attempt to conduct a systematic review and meta-analysis to assess the predictive value of the TKIs-induced hypertension for PFS and OS in patients with mRCC during TKIs therapy.

Methods

Data sources and literature search strategy

We conducted this meta-analysis in accordance with the Preferred Reporting Items for Systematic Reviews and Meta-Analysis statement. This study was registered in PROSPERO (CRD42019129593). A literature search was performed in the following databases: PubMed, Embase, Web of Science and the Cochrane Library database. The latest search was performed on March 21, 2019. The search keywords were (renal cell carcinoma) AND [(tyrosine kinase inhibitor) OR sunitinib OR axitinib OR sorafenib OR pazopanib] AND [hypertension OR (blood pressure). The resulted literatures were further scanned by Endnote X7 (Thomson Corporation, Canada) to exclude duplications followed by title and abstract screening. In addition, we manually searched the references of the literatures for additional eligible studies.

Inclusion and exclusion criteria

Studies were included in our meta-analysis if the following criteria were met: 1) mRCC patients were treated with TKIs; 2) studies compared Hazard Ratios (HR) between patients with or without TKIs-induced hypertension for PFS or OS.

Studies were excluded based on the following criteria: 1) reviews, meta-analysis, letters, comments, case reports or conference abstracts; 2) duplicated studies and repeated analysis; 3) studies lacking sufficient data for HR and their 95% confidence intervals (CI); 4) studies included mRCC patients received different therapeutic regimen, such as TKIs or radiotherapy.

Quality of original studies

We assessed the quality of the 22 included studies using the Newcastle-Ottawa Scale (NOS). The total score was 9 stars. Studies awarded 7–9 stars were rated as high-quality, 5–6 stars as moderate-quality, and < 5 stars as low-quality.

Data extraction

Eligible studies were read thoroughly and carefully to extract the following information, including first author, year, region, sample size, male/female ratio, mean age, histology, number of disease sites, prior nephrectomy, Memorial Sloan Kettering Cancer Center (MSKCC) score, Eastern Cooperative Oncology Group performance status (ECOG PS) score, definition of hypertension, type of analysis (univariate or multivariate), study design (prospective or retrospective), type of TKIs. The primary outcome was HR and 95% CI between patients with or without hypertension for PFS and secondary one for OS. The definition of PFS was time from initiation of TKIs therapy to disease progression or death. OS was defined as time from initiation of TKIs therapy to death. If a study provided both univariate and multivariate analysis results, the multivariate analysis would be selected to achieve higher accuracy. Any discrepancies were resolved by discussion with the third reviewer.

Data synthesis and statistical analysis

Data were extracted and analyzed with Stata 15.0 software (Stata Corporation, College Station, TX, USA). *P* value< 0.05 was considered statistically significant. A merged HR greater than 1 indicated a poorer prognosis for mRCC patients. Heterogeneity was assessed using the I^2. We considered $I^2 > 50\%$ as an indicator of substantial heterogeneity. A random effects model and a fixed effects model were applied for $I^2>50\%$ and $I^2<50\%$, respectively. Then, to determine which factors may contribute to heterogeneity, univariate and multivariate meta-regression analysis were performed. The possible factors were year, sample size, gender, mean age, country, ECOG PS, MSKCC score, histology, prior nephrectomy, Number of disease sites, type of analysis (univariate, multivariate), study design (retrospective, prospective), type of TKIs. Then, subgroup analysis was performed to investigate whether different sample size could explain the heterogeneity and whether relationship between hypertension and PFS or OS still exist in different TKIs subgroups. Factor with *P* value < 0.05 meant that it may be the source of heterogeneity. We did sensitivity analysis to find if some original studies may mainly contribute to the heterogeneity. Publication bias was assessed with funnel plots and precisely assessed by Egger's and Begg's tests.

Quality of evidence

The quality of evidence of the predictive effect of TKIs-induced hypertension for the outcomes in mRCC patients

Table 1 Baseline characteristics of eligible studies in the meta-analyses

Study	Year	Country	Study design	Sample size	Male/ Female ratio	Mean age	Histology (clear cell%)	Survival analysis	Definition of hypertension	Type of analysis	TKIs	Quality Assessment (NOS Score = 9)
Rini (a) [10]	2011	the USA	R	534	2.3	60.6	98%	PFS, OS	SBP ≥ 140 mmHg, DBP ≥ 90 mmHg	multivariate	SUN	7
Szmit [12]	2011	Poland	R	111	3.0	55.9	100%	PFS, OS	BP ≥ 140/90 mmHg	univariate	SUN	9
Bono [17]	2011	Finland	R	54	1.7	64	92%	PFS	BP > 150/100 mmHg OR blood pressure requiring intensifi cation of pre-existing anti-hypertensive medication.	multivariate	SUN	7
Fujita [18]	2012	Japan	R	41	2.7	64	100%	PFS	–	univariate	SUN	7
Eechoute [19]	2012	Netherlands	R	158	1.7	60	87%	PFS, OS	SBP > 140 mmHg, DBP > 90 mmHg, MAP > 110 mmHg	multivariate	SUN	7
Rini (b) [13]	2013	the USA	R	168	2.5	60	–	PFS, OS	DBP ≥90 mmHg	multivariate	AXI	7
Motzer (a) [20]	2013	the USA	P	350	2.8	61	100%	PFS, OS	SBP > 140 mmHg, DBP > 90 mmHg	multivariate	AXI	6
Motzer (b) [20]	2013	the USA	P	336	2.5	61	100%	PFS, OS	SBP > 140 mmHg, DBP > 90 mmHg	multivariate	SOR	6
Hong [21]	2013	China	R	136	2.0	56	93%	OS	Hypertension class III/IV	multivariate	SUN	7
Nakano [22]	2013	Japan	R	36	3.5	65.8	61%	PFS	grade 1–3 (NCI-CTCAE, version 3.0)	multivariate	SOR	7
Fujita [23]	2014	Japan	R	44	2.7	63.5	95%	PFS	–	multivariate	SUN	7
Eto [24]	2014	Japan	R	54	2.2	63	97%	OS	DBP ≥90 mmHg	–	AXI	7
Rini (c) [25]	2015	the USA	P	203	2.0	61.9	–	PFS	DBP change from baseline ≥10/15 mmHg	–	AXI	7
Zhang (a) [26]	2015	China	R	256	2.5	58	79%	OS	–	multivariate	SOR	7
Kucharz [27]	2015	Poland	R	28	2.1	65	–	PFS	office SBP ≥140 and/or DBP ≥90 mmHg; home SBP ≥135 and/or DPB ≥85 mmHg; pre-existing medication-controlled arterial hypertension and required additional antihypertensive medication during treatment	multivariate	SUN	7
Izzedine [28]	2015	France	R	212	3.4	57.7	86%	PFS, OS	–	multivariate	SUN	8
Donskov [29]	2015	the USA	R	770	2.6	60	98%	PFS	SBP ≥ 140 mmHg	multivariate	SUN	7
Zhang (b) [30]	2016	China	R	134	2.4	59.8	77%	OS	–	multivariate	SOR	7
Goldstein (a) [14]	2016	Australia	R	479	2.2	59.5	–	PFS, OS	MAP change from baseline>10 mmHg	univariate	PAZ	9
Goldstein (b) [14]	2016	Australia	R	506	2.6187	61	–	PFS, OS	SBP > 140 mm H, DBP > 90 mmHg, MAP change from baseline>10 mmHg, SBP change from baseline>10 mmHg	univariate	PAZ	9
Goldstein (c) [14]	2016	Australia	R	475	3.3394	60.9	–	PFS, OS	SBP > 140 mm H, DBP > 90 mmHg, MAP change from baseline>10 mmHg, SBP change from baseline>10 mmHg	univariate	SUN	9

Table 1 Baseline characteristics of eligible studies in the meta-analyses *(Continued)*

Study	Year	Country	Study design	Sample size	Male/ Female ratio	Mean age	Histology (clear cell%)	Survival analysis	Definition of hypertension	Type of analysis	TKIs	Quality Assessment (NOS Score = 9)
Cecere [31]	2016	Italy	R	38	1.375	61	84.2%	OS	grade ≥ 3 (NCI-CTCAE, version 4.0)	multivariate	PAZ	7
Miyake [32]	2016	Japan	R	50	4.0000	64	80%	PFS	SBP ≥ 140 or DBP ≥ 90 mmHg	multivariate	SUN	7
Fukuda [15]	2016	Japan	R	62	2.4444	66	92%	PFS, OS	–	univariate	SUN	7
Matias [33]	2017	France	P	106	2.3125	54	90%	PFS, OS	grade ≥ 3 (NCI-CTCAE, version 4.0)	univariate	AXI	7

R Retrospective, *P* Prospective, *PFS* Progression-free survival, *OS* Overall survival, *SBP* Systolic blood pressure, *DBP* Diastolic blood pressure, MAP ≈ 2/3 DBP + 1/3 SBP; *SUN* Sunitinib, *AXI* Axitinib, *SOR* Sorafenib, *PAZ* Pazopanib, *NCI-CTCAE* National Cancer Institute Common Terminology Criteria for Adverse Events

—: The data were not available in this study

was assessed according to the Grading of Recommendations Assessment, Development, and Evaluation (GRADE) [16].

Results

Study selection

The searching process is shown in Additional file 1: Figure S1. A total of 982 studies were searched in the database. We excluded 345 duplicated articles. After screening title and abstract, 26 relevant studies were identified. In addition, three relevant studies were obtained from the references and seven articles were excluded due to lack of HR and 95% CI for PFS or OS. Finally, 22 studies were selected for the meta-analysis.

Study characteristics and quality

The baseline characteristics of these studies were demonstrated in Table 1. All the studies were published between 2011 and 2017. Of them, 3 were prospective and 19were retrospective. The sample size ranged from 28 to 770 patients. The total number of included patients was 4661 and hypertension occurred in 2932 (62.9%). The male/female ratio included in each study ranged from 1.4 to 3.5%, and the median age of the study patients was between 54 years and 66 years. The histology of most RCC is clear cell (61–100%). Most patients had received nephrectomy, cytokine therapy, targeted therapy or radiation therapy. Among the 22 studies providing HR, four reported univariate HR, which did not adjust for the potential confounding factors. The standard of hypertension or BP increasement during TKIs therapy varied between studies, including systolic blood pressure (SBP) ≥140/135 mmHg, diastolic blood pressure (DBP) ≥90/85 mmHg, mean arterial blood pressure (MAP) > 110 mmHg, an increase in BP (SBP, DBP, MAP) > 10/15 mmHg from baseline, or grades of hypertension according to National Cancer Institute Common Terminology Criteria for Adverse Events Version 3.0 or 4.0 [34, 35]. The quality of the studies varied from a NOS score of 6 to 9, most of which were high-quality (Table 2).

Table 2 Newcastle-Ottawa scale score of the reviewed studies

Study	Selection (4 stars)				Comparability (2 stars)	Outcome (3 stars)			Total score
	Representativeness of the hypertensive cohort	Selection of the non-hypertensive cohort	Ascertainment of hypertension	Demonstration that outcome of interest was not present at start of study		Assessment of outcome	Was follow up long enough for outcomes to occur?	Adequacy of follow up of cohort	
Rini (a)	★	★	★	★	–	★	★	★	7
Szmit	★	★	★	★	★★	★	★	★	9
Bono	★	★	★	★	–	★	★	★	7
Fujita	★	★	★	★	–	★	★	★	7
Eechoute	★	★	★	★	–	★	★	★	7
Rini (b)	★	★	★	★	–	★	★	★	7
Motzer	–	★	★	★	–	★	★	★	6
Hong	★	★	★	★	–	★	★	★	7
Nakano	★	★	★	★	–	★	★	★	7
Fujita	★	★	★	★	–	★	★	★	7
Eto	★	★	★	★	–	★	★	★	7
Rini (c)	★	★	★	★	–	★	★	★	7
Zhang (a)	★	★	★	★	–	★	★	★	7
Kucharz	★	★	★	★	–	★	★	★	7
Izzedine	★	★	★	★	★	★	★	★	8
Donskov	★	★	★	★	–	★	★	★	7
Zhang (b)	★	★	★	★	–	★	★	★	7
Goldstein	★	★	★	★	★★	★	★	★	9
Miyake	★	★	★	★	–	★	★	★	7
Fukuda	★	★	★	★	–	★	★	★	7
Matias	★	★	★	★	–	★	★	★	7

—: The data were not available in this study

Relationship between TKIs-induced hypertension and PFS or OS of mRCC patients

HR of PFS and OS were quantitatively synthesized and data were shown in Figs. 1 and 2. Elevated blood pressure was positively correlated with better PFS (HR = 0.59, 95% CI: 0.48–0.71, $p < 0.001$; $I^2 = 77.3\%$) and OS (HR = 0.57, 95% CI: 0.45–0.70, $p < 0.001$; $I^2 = 77.4\%$). It meant that patients developing hypertension may have a lower mortality risk and live longer without progression of mRCC. The heterogeneity was obvious between studies.

Meta-regression analysis

Univariate meta-regression analysis was performed for PFS and results were showed in Table 3. Among the variables above mentioned, only sample size (Adjusted R^2 = 27.34%, P = 0.019) might contribute to the inter-study heterogeneity, while others did not (P = 0.052–0.942).

Multivariate meta-regression analysis revealed that P value of sample size changed to 0.025. The overall adjusted R^2 was 74.84% (P = 0.239), which meant that all these factors together could account for 74.84% of heterogeneity.

Subgroup analysis

Subgroup analysis for PFS revealed that sample size could not change the subgroup heterogeneity significantly (I^2 = 72.1 and 75%) (Table 3). In addition, for different TKIs, only patients with TKIs-induced hypertension in sunitinib subgroup (HR = 0.47, 95% CI: 0.34–0.64, p<0.001) and pazopanib subgroup (HR = 0.79, 95% CI: 0.66–0.94, p = 0.01) could have longer PFS. However, development of hypertension in four different TKIs subgroups could all predict longer OS, including sunitinib subgroup (HR = 0.48, 95% CI: 0.30–0.78, p = 0.003), pazopanib subgroup (HR = 0.73, 95% CI: 0.55–0.97, p = 0.032), axitinib subgroup (HR = 0.62, 95% CI: 0.43–0.88, p = 0.007) and sorafenib subgroup (HR = 0.66, 95% CI: 0.48–0.91, p = 0.010) (Figs. 1 and 2).

Sensitivity analysis

As shown in Fig. 3, study of "Szmit", "Motzer (a)" and "Donskov" could affect the heterogeneity for PFS. We excluded these studies and found that I^2 decreased to 44.6% (P = 0.03), with pooled HR = 0.665

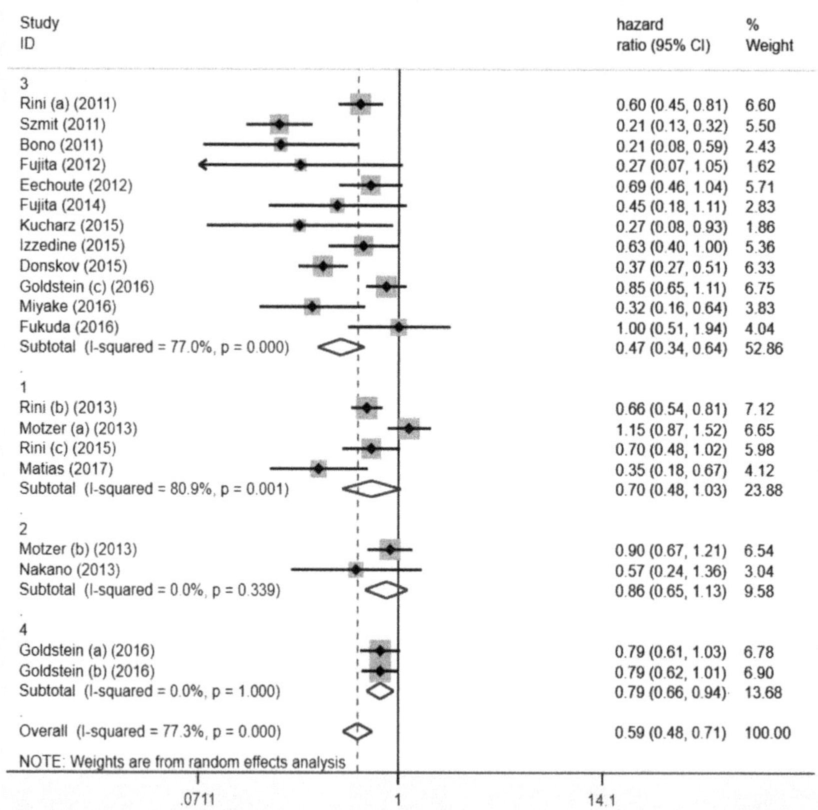

Fig. 1 Forest plot reflects the association between TKIs -induced hypertension and oncologic outcomes (progression free survival) in different TKIs subgroups (1: axitinib; 2: sorafenib; 3: sunitinib; 4: pazopanib)

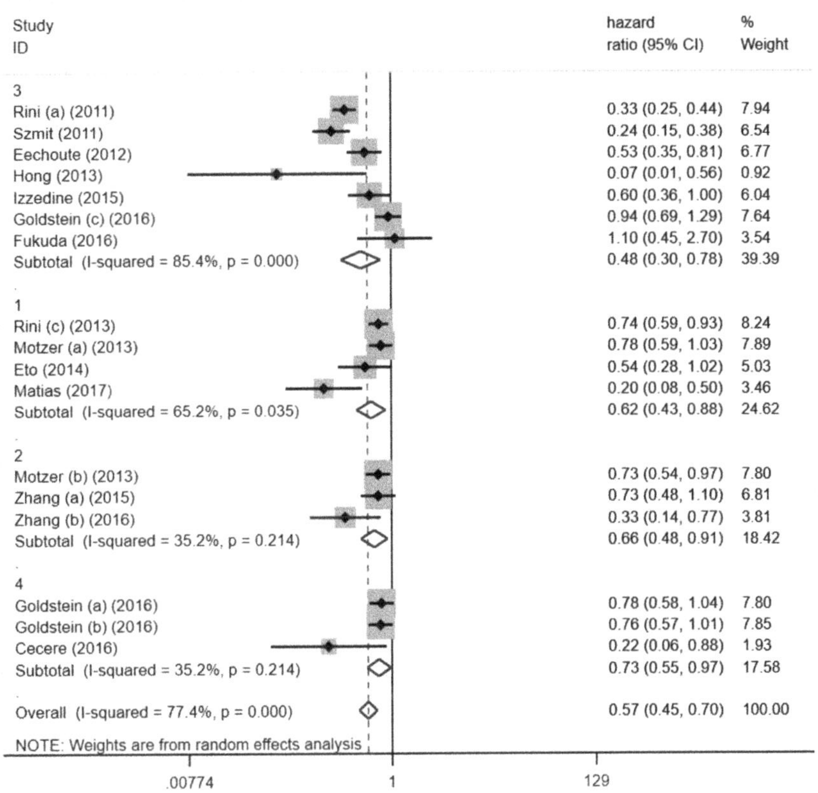

Fig. 2 Forest plot reflects the association between TKIs-induced hypertension and oncologic outcomes (overall survival) in different TKIs subgroups (1: axitinib; 2: sorafenib; 3: sunitinib; 4: pazopanib)

(0.579–0.764, P = 0.025). Then, we reviewed these studies carefully to find something they had in common. Interestingly, most of the mRCC patients in these three studies had failed one previous cytokine immunotherapy. Maybe it was the reason for high heterogeneity.

Publication bias

We assessed the publication bias with funnel plot and Egger's and Begg's tests (Fig. 4). The shape of funnel plots was not symmetric. The Egger's and Begg's tests were further performed. The results indicated significant publication bias for studies, with merged PFS (Begg's test, P = 0.015; Egger's test, P = 0.028) and merged OS (Begg's test, P = 0.026; Egger's test, P = 0.085).

Evaluation of the quality of evidence according to GRADE system

The assessment of the quality of evidence was performed for PFS and OS which were critical in evaluating the outcome of mRCC patients. The quality of evidence of PFS and OS was both "very low" due to retrospective studies, publication bias and high heterogeneity (Table 4).

Discussion

This meta-analysis and systematic review investigated whether TKIs-induced hypertension can predict the prognosis of patients suffering from mRCC. AEs, like hypothyroidism, though shown to be a good predictor of PFS or OS, was usually diagnosed later than hypertension [17, 36]. Thus, it would be better if we can predict the prognosis of mRCC patients based on the TKIs-induced hypertension. It will help urologists decide whether patients should continue this TKIs therapy or not, which may help patients get more suitable treatments as soon as possible. Based on 22 original studies, our results showed that the occurrence of hypertension during treatment may predict better survival for mRCC, with longer PFS and OS. Additionally, when it comes to different TKIs, sunitinib or pazopanib therapy were both associated with longer PFS and OS.

The mechanisms of hypertension induced by TKIs are complicated. First, activation of VEGF receptor-2 via

Table 3 Meta-regression and subgroup analyses of pooled hazard ratios for progression-free survival

Subgroup	Meta-regression							Pooled HR of PFS		Heterogeneity	
	No. of studies	Coefficient	Standard error	T value	*P* value	Tau^2	Adjusted R^2	HR (95% CI)	P value	I^2	*P* value
Year	20	0.060	0.228	0.26	0.795	0.182	−8.86%				
2011–2014								0.56 (0.40–0.77)	<0.001	83.00%	<0.001
2015–2017								0.61 (0.48–0.77)	<0.001	73.60%	<0.001
Sample size	20	0.507	0.197	2.57	0.019	0.122	27.34%				
<200								0.43 (0.30–0.61)	<0.001	72.10%	<0.001
≥200								0.73 (0.60–0.89)	0.002	75%	<0.001
Gender (male/female ratio)	20	−0.117	0.228	−0.51	0.614	0.177	−5.64%				
<2.5								0.66 (0.53–0.82)	<0.001	54.50%	0.025
≥2.5								0.55 (0.40–0.74)	<0.001	84.70%	<0.001
Mean age	20	0.320	0.264	2.21	0.241	0.156	6.69%				
<60								0.44 (0.23–0.86)	0.015	89.40%	<0.001
≥60								0.64 (0.53–0.78)	<0.001	69.70%	<0.001
Country	20	0.168	0.301	0.56	0.584	0.173	−3.31%				
the USA, Europe								0.60 (0.49–0.74)	<0.001	81.40%	<0.001
Asia								0.51 (0.31–0.83)	0.006	39.50%	0.158
ECOG PS (grade 0%)	20	0.036	0.133	0.27	0.79	0.182	−8.59%				
<0.5								0.35 (0.14–0.89)	0.028	87.20%	<0.001
≥0.5								0.64 (0.52–0.79)	<0.001	71.90%	<0.001
MSKCC score (favorable%)	20	0.231	0.111	2.08	0.052	0.123	26.74%				
<0.25								0.43 (0.21–0.87)	0.019	76%	0.002
≥0.25								0.86 (0.73–1.02)	0.076	40.30%	0.137
Histology (clear cell%)	20	−0.139	0.126	−1.11	0.283	0.166	1.11%				
<0.9								0.53 (0.39–0.71)	<0.001	29.30%	0.226
≥0.9								0.51 (0.33–0.79)	0.002	87.90%	<0.001
Prior nephrectomy (%)	20	−0.162	0.129	−1.25	0.226	0.166	1.16%				
<0.9								0.52 (0.40–0.67)	0.296	17.50%	<0.001
≥0.9								0.52 (0.33–0.81)	<0.001	89.30%	0.005
No. of disease sites (1%)	20	−0.253	0.139	−1.81	0.086	0.144	13.81%				
<0.2								0.41 (0.28–0.60)	<0.001	62.40%	0.047
≥0.2								0.52 (0.37–0.74)	<0.001	0	0.594
Type of analysis	20	−0.030	0.231	−0.13	0.898	0.182	−8.91%				
Univariate								0.59 (0.42–0.82)	0.002	82.70%	<0.001
Multivariate								0.58 (0.46–0.75)	<0.001	74.50%	<0.001
Study design	20	0.343	0.257	1.34	0.198	0.157	6.32%				
Retrospective								0.54 (0.44–0.67)	<0.001	74.90%	<0.001
Prospective								0.77 (0.53–1.12)	0.175	76.20%	0.006
Type of TKIs	20	−0.073	0.114	−0.64	0.942	0.178	−10.49%				
Axitinib								0.70 (0.48–1.03)	0.07	80.90%	0.001
Sorafenib								0.86 (0.65–1.13)	0.277	0	0.339
Sunitinib								0.47 (0.34–0.64)	<0.001	77.90%	<0.001
Pazopanib								0.79 (0.66–0.94)	0.010	0	1.000

No. number, *HR* hazard ratio, *PFS* progression-free survival, *ECOG PS* Eastern Cooperative Oncology Group performance status, *MSKCC score* Memorial Sloan Kettering Cancer Center score

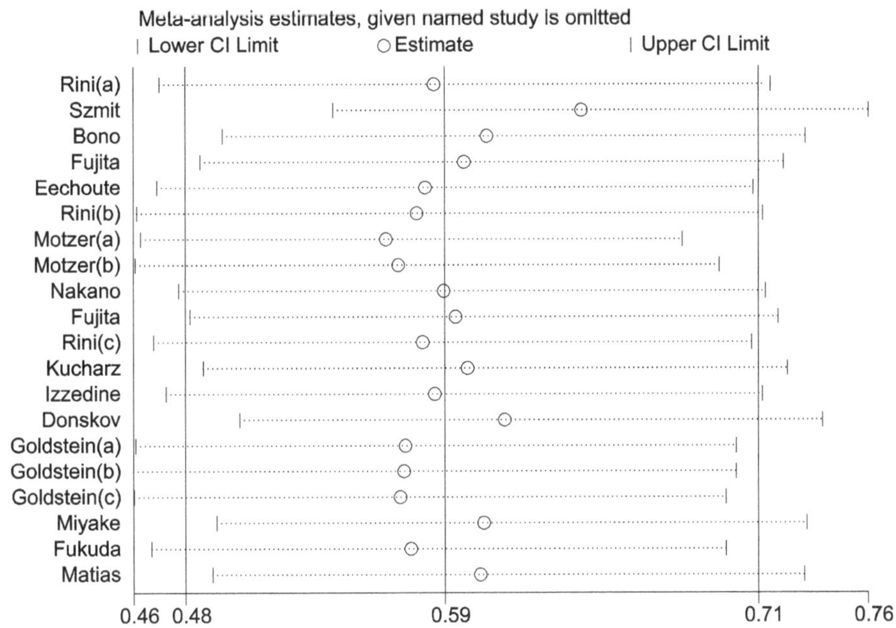

Fig. 3 Sensitivity analysis of progression free survival for the evaluation of potential heterogeneity

phosphoinositide 3-kinase and its downstream serine protein kinase Akt can stimulate endothelium-derived nitric oxide synthase, leading to the production of nitric oxide (NO). Therefore, the inhibition of VEGF receptor might lead to a decrease in NO bioavailability, followed by vasoconstriction and increased blood pressure (BP) [17, 37–39]. Second, plasma vasoconstrictor endothelin-1, a vasoconstrictor produced by the endothelium, also increased in patients or rats receiving sunitinib [40–42]. Third, NO is also involved in the control of renal and glomerular hemodynamics, tubuloglomerular feedback response, release of renin and sympathetic transmitters, tubular ion transport. As a result, reduction of NO can also result in renal water and sodium retention, leading to hypertension [43]. TKIs may also directly cause renal injury and proteinuria, which could play a role in long-lasting hypertension [44]. Finally, hypertension may also result from structural or functional vascular rarefaction [45–47]. VEGF is also crucial in the maintenance of endothelial viability [48, 49]. Therefore, the inhibition of VEGF and PDGF receptors can induce endothelial cell apoptosis, reduction in capillary density, vascular diameter and microvascular flow, and thus increase the blood pressure.

The reason why TKIs-induced hypertension might be a prognostic factor in patients with mRCC is still

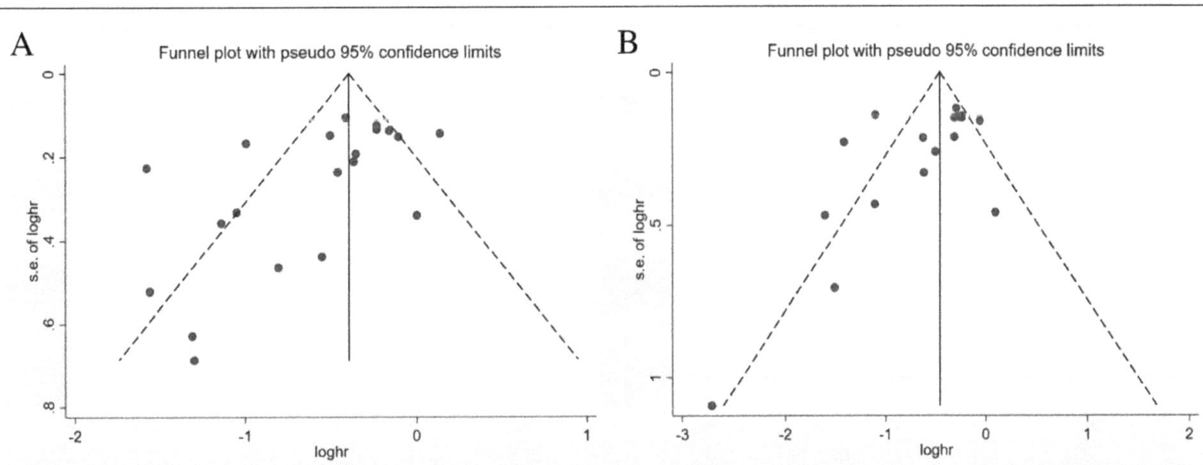

Fig. 4 Funnel plot for publication bias. **a** progression free survival, **b** overall survival

Table 4 Evaluation of the quality of evidence according to GRADE system

Quality assessment							No. of patients		Hazard Ratios (95% CI)	Quality	Importance
No of studies	Design	Risk of bias	Inconsistency	Indirectness	Imprecision	Other considerations	TKI-induced hypertension	Control			
Progression-free survival (follow-up median 5.6–43.2 years; measured with: follow-up)											
20	observational studies	no serious risk of bias	serious[1]	no serious indirectness	no serious imprecision	reporting bias[2]	3021	1327	0.59 (0.48–0.71)	Very low	Critical
Overall survival (follow-up median 5.2–61.8 months; measured with: follow-up)											
17	observational studies	no serious risk of bias	serious[1]	no serious indirectness	no serious imprecision	reporting bias[3]	2313	1804	0.57 (0.45–0.70)	Very low	Critical

[1]The heterogeneity of this outcome was obvious between studies

[2]The shape of funnel plots was not symmetric. The Egger's and Begg's tests were further performed. The results indicated significant publication bias for studies, with merged PFS (Begg's test, $P = 0.015$; Egger's test, $P = 0.028$).

[3]The shape of funnel plots was not symmetric. The Egger's and Begg's tests were further performed. The results indicated significant publication bias for studies, with merged OS (Begg's test, $P = 0.026$; Egger's test, $P = 0.085$)

not quite clear. The anticarcinogenic effect of TKIs relies on the block of VEGF receptor, which may also lead to hypertension as above mentioned. Thus, when TKIs inhibit the progress of mRCC and prolong the PFS or OS of patients, hypertension may occur at the same time. It may be the reason why the rise of blood pressure could indicate a better prognosis in mRCC patients.

Of note, the intention of therapy is not to drive all patients into a hypertensive state. On the contrary, when hypertension occurs, patients should receive antihypertensive therapy as soon as possible. Additionally, despite the PFS and OS of mRCC patients have prolonged because of TKIs therapy, few comparable benefits have been described in terms of the quality of life [50, 51]. An innovative study that compared sunitinib with pazopanib to evaluate patient preferences suggested that the toxicity profile may have an impact on quality of life and the choice of treatment when two comparable options are on offer [52]. In addition, sunitinib-induced hypertension may be associated with cardiotoxicity or reversible posterior leukoencephalopathy [53–55]. Thus, the panel of National Cancer Institute of the USA had several recommendations for mRCC patients received TKIs [56]. First, urologists should recognize the preexisting hypertension prior to therapy or actively monitor BP throughout treatment. Early use of antihypertensive medication is necessary when high blood pressure occurs, and it is critical for maintaining dose intensity and improving a patient's quality of life simultaneously [56]. If possible, the goal of management is to reduce BP below 140/90 mmHg. It was also suggested that there was no need to reduce the dose of antihypertensive medication because it did not compromise efficacy of TKIs [57]. Some evidence indicated that using Angiotensin receptor blockers (ARBs) or angiotensin-I-converting enzyme inhibitors may even protect against cancer [58–60]. ARBs were shown to induce apoptosis and inhibit the proliferation of RCC cells in vitro [28]. Thus, some randomized prospective studies could be carried out to see if it is better to use more than one drugs with different antihypertensive mechanisms, which may improve the prognosis [12]. Second, doctors should assess the risk of potential cardiovascular complications.

Several underlying limitations of the study should be presented. First, most eligible studies were retrospective, though with high NOS scores. Second, the reciprocal correlation between the hypertension and other AEs should be noted. Patients with more than one adverse event of any grade had longer PFS and OS [61]. Thus, further studies are needed to analyze the relationship between several adverse events and mRCC. Third, obvious inter-study heterogeneity was observed in this meta analysis, which may be due to different therapies mRCC patients had received before, such as cytokine immunotherapy. In addition, a publication bias was detected in this study. The potential reason may be that studies with non-significant results were not published. High heterogeneity and publication bias weakened the quality of evidence, which may be improved by more randomized prospective trials.

However, our analysis also has some advantages. First, we conducted this review with enough data available for extraction by a comprehensive and robust search strategy. Second, we applied a rigorous inclusion/exclusion criterion. Additionally, most of the studies operated multivariable analysis, which could eliminate the co-factors affecting the PFS and OS of mRCC patients.

Conclusions

In summary, our analysis of currently available clinical evidence suggests that TKIs-induced hypertension may predict longer PFS and OS in patients with mRCC during TKIs therapy, especially using sunitinib or pazopanib.

Additional file

Additional file 1: Figure S1. Flow chart showing literature searching process of meta-analysis. The search keywords are (renal cell carcinoma) AND [(tyrosine kinase inhibitor) OR sunitinib OR axitinib OR sorafenib OR pazopanib] AND [hypertension OR (blood pressure). (DOCX 140 kb)

Abbreviations

AEs: Adverse events; BP: Blood pressure; CI: Confidence intervals; DBP: Diastolic blood pressure; ECOG PS: Eastern Cooperative Oncology Group performance status; GRADE: Grading of Recommendations Assessment, Development and Evaluation; HR: Hazard Ratios; MAP: Mean arterial blood pressure; mRCC: Metastatic renal cell carcinoma; MSKCC: Memorial Sloan Kettering Cancer Center; NO: Nitric oxide; NOS: Newcastle-Ottawa Scale; OS: Overall survival; PFS: Progression-free survival; RCC: Renal cell carcinoma; SBP: Systolic blood pressure; TKIs: Tyrosine kinase inhibitors

Acknowledgements

Not applicable.

Authors' contributions

LY was mainly responsible for the design of the work, the acquisition and analysis of data and manuscript writing. ZL carried out the acquisition of data. CYT and YDH participated in the analysis of data. LBH, WKJ and LH revised the manuscript. All authors read and approved the final manuscript.

References

1. Znaor A, Lortet-Tieulent J, Laversanne M, Jemal A, Bray F. International variations and trends in renal cell carcinoma incidence and mortality. Eur Urol. 2015;67(3):519–30.
2. Wong MCS, Goggins WB, Yip BHK, Fung FDH, Leung C, Fang Y, Wong SYS, Ng CF. Incidence and mortality of kidney cancer: temporal patterns and global trends in 39 countries. Sci Rep. 2017;7(1):15698.
3. Rossi SH, Klatte T. Epidemiology and screening for renal. cancer. 2018;36(9): 1341–53.

4. Gupta K, Miller JD, Li JZ, Russell MW, Charbonneau C. Epidemiologic and socioeconomic burden of metastatic renal cell carcinoma (mRCC): a literature review. Cancer Treat Rev. 2008;34(3):193–205.
5. Naito S, Tsukamoto T, Murai M, Fukino K, Akaza H. Overall survival and good tolerability of long-term use of sorafenib after cytokine treatment: final results of a phase II trial of sorafenib in Japanese patients with metastatic renal cell carcinoma. BJU Int. 2011;108(11):1813–9.
6. Tomita Y, Shinohara N, Yuasa T, Fujimoto H, Niwakawa M, Mugiya S, Miki T, Uemura H, Nonomura N, Takahashi M, et al. Overall survival and updated results from a phase II study of sunitinib in Japanese patients with metastatic renal cell carcinoma. Jpn J Clin Oncol. 2010;40(12):1166–72.
7. Motzer RJ, Hutson TE, Tomczak P, Michaelson MD, Bukowski RM, Rixe O, Oudard S, Negrier S, Szczylik C, Kim ST, et al. Sunitinib versus interferon alfa in metastatic renal-cell carcinoma. N Engl J Med. 2007;356(2):115–24.
8. Rixe O, Bukowski RM, Michaelson MD, Wilding G, Hudes GR, Bolte O, Motzer RJ, Bycott P, Liau KF, Freddo J, et al. Axitinib treatment in patients with cytokine-refractory metastatic renal-cell cancer: a phase II study. Lancet Oncol. 2007;8(11):975–84.
9. Ravaud A, Schmidinger M. Clinical biomarkers of response in advanced renal cell carcinoma. Ann Oncol. 2013;24(12):2935–42.
10. Rini BI, Cohen DP, Lu DR, Chen I, Hariharan S, Gore ME, Figlin RA, Baum MS, Motzer RJ. Hypertension as a biomarker of efficacy in patients with metastatic renal cell carcinoma treated with sunitinib. J Natl Cancer Inst. 2011;103(9):763–73.
11. Li Y, Li S, Zhu Y, Liang X, Meng H, Chen J, Zhang D, Guo H, Shi B. Incidence and risk of sorafenib-induced hypertension: a systematic review and meta-analysis. J Clin Hypertens (Greenwich, Conn). 2014;16(3):177–85.
12. Szmit S, Langiewicz P, Zlnierek J, Nurzynski P, Zaborowska M, Filipiak KJ, Opolski G, Szczylik C. Hypertension as a predictive factor for survival outcomes in patients with metastatic renal cell carcinoma treated with sunitinib after progression on cytokines. Kidney Blood Press Res. 2012;35(1): 18–25.
13. Rini BI, Garrett M, Poland B, Dutcher JP, Rixe O, Wilding G, Stadler WM, Pithavala YK, Kim S, Tarazi J, et al. Axitinib in metastatic renal cell carcinoma: results of a pharmacokinetic and pharmacodynamic analysis. J Clin Pharmacol. 2013;53(5):491–504.
14. Goldstein D, Rosenberg JE, Figlin RA, Townsend RR, McCann L, Carpenter C, Pandite L. Is change in blood pressure a biomarker of pazopanib and sunitinib efficacy in advanced/metastatic renal cell carcinoma? Eur J Cancer (Oxford, England : 1990). 2016;53:96–104.
15. Fukuda H, Kondo T, Iida S, Takagi T, Tanabe K. Treatment-related deterioration of renal function is associated with the antitumor efficacy of sunitinib in patients with metastatic renal cell carcinoma. Urol Oncol. 2016; 34(8):338.e331–9.
16. Guyatt G, Oxman AD, Akl EA, Kunz R, Vist G, Brozek J, Norris S, Falck-Ytter Y, Glasziou P, DeBeer H, et al. GRADE guidelines: 1. Introduction-GRADE evidence profiles and summary of findings tables. J Clin Epidemiol. 2011;64:383–94.
17. Bono P, Rautiola J, Utriainen T, Joensuu H. Hypertension as predictor of sunitinib treatment outcome in metastatic renal cell carcinoma. Acta Oncol (Stockholm, Sweden). 2011;50(4):569–73.
18. Fujita T, Iwamura M, Ishii D, Tabata K, Matsumoto K, Yoshida K, Baba S. C-reactive protein as a prognostic marker for advanced renal cell carcinoma treated with sunitinib. Int J Urol. 2012;19(10):908–13.
19. Eechoute K, van der Veldt AA, Oosting S, Kappers MH, Wessels JA, Gelderblom H, Guchelaar HJ, Reyners AK, van Herpen CM, Haanen JB, et al. Polymorphisms in endothelial nitric oxide synthase (eNOS) and vascular endothelial growth factor (VEGF) predict sunitinib-induced hypertension. Clin Pharmacol Ther. 2012;92(4):503–10.
20. Motzer RJ, Escudier B, Tomczak P, Hutson TE, Michaelson MD, Negrier S, Oudard S, Gore ME, Tarazi J, Hariharan S, et al. Axitinib versus sorafenib as second-line treatment for advanced renal cell carcinoma: overall survival analysis and updated results from a randomised phase 3 trial. Lancet Oncol. 2013;14(6):552–62.
21. Hong YP, Yao XD, Zhu Y, Ye DW, Shi GH, Zhang SL, Dai B, Zhang HL, Shen YJ, Zhu YP, et al. Exploratory analysis of the effect of toxicity of sunitinib on the clinical outcome of patients with advanced renal cell carcinoma. Zhonghua Yi Xue Za Zhi. 2013;93(36):2880–3.
22. Nakano K, Komatsu K, Kubo T, Natsui S, Nukui A, Kurokawa S, Kobayashi M, Morita T. Hand-foot skin reaction is associated with the clinical outcome in patients with metastatic renal cell carcinoma treated with sorafenib. Jpn J Clin Oncol. 2013;43(10):1023–9.
23. Fujita T, Wakatabe Y, Matsumoto K, Tabata K, Yoshida K, Iwamura M. Leukopenia as a biomarker of sunitinib outcome in advanced renal cell carcinoma. Anticancer Res. 2014;34(7):3781–7.
24. Eto M, Uemura H, Tomita Y, Kanayama H, Shinohara N, Kamei Y, Fujii Y, Umeyama Y, Ozono S, Naito S, et al. Overall survival and final efficacy and safety results from a Japanese phase II study of axitinib in cytokine-refractory metastatic renal cell carcinoma. Cancer Sci. 2014;105(12):1576–83.
25. Rini BI, Melichar B, Fishman MN, Oya M, Pithavala YK, Chen Y, Bair AH, Grunwald V. Axitinib dose titration: analyses of exposure, blood pressure and clinical response from a randomized phase II study in metastatic renal cell carcinoma. Ann Oncol. 2015;26(7):1372–7.
26. Zhang HL, Qin XJ, Wang HK, Gu WJ, Ma CG, Shi GH, Zhou LP, Ye DW. Clinicopathological and prognostic factors for long-term survival in Chinese patients with metastatic renal cell carcinoma treated with sorafenib: a single-center retrospective study. Oncotarget. 2015;6(34):36870–83.
27. Kucharz J, Dumnicka P, Kuzniewski M, Kusnierz-Cabala B, Herman RM, Krzemieniecki K. Co-occurring adverse events enable early prediction of progression-free survival in metastatic renal cell carcinoma patients treated with sunitinib: a hypothesis-generating study. Tumori. 2015;101(5):555–9.
28. Izzedine H, Derosa L, Le Teuff G, Albiges L, Escudier B. Hypertension and angiotensin system inhibitors: impact on outcome in sunitinib-treated patients for metastatic renal cell carcinoma. Ann Oncol. 2015;26(6):1128–33.
29. Donskov F, Michaelson MD, Puzanov I, Davis MP, Bjarnason GA, Motzer RJ, Goldstein D, Lin X, Cohen DP, Wiltshire R, et al. Sunitinib-associated hypertension and neutropenia as efficacy biomarkers in metastatic renal cell carcinoma patients. Br J Cancer. 2015;113(11):1571–80.
30. Zhang Y, Li Y, Cai Y, Wang K, Li H. Efficacy of sorafenib correlates with Memorial Sloan-Kettering Cancer Center (MSKCC) risk classification and bone metastasis in Chinese patients with metastatic renal cell carcinoma. Cell Oncol (Dordr). 2016;39(1):15–21.
31. Cecere SC, Rossetti S, Cavaliere C, Della Pepa C, Di Napoli M, Crispo A, Iovane G, Piscitelli R, Sorrentino D, Ciliberto G, et al. Pazopanib in metastatic renal Cancer: a "real-world" experience at National Cancer Institute "Fondazione G. Pascale". Front Pharmacol. 2016;7:287.
32. Miyake M, Kuwada M, Hori S, Morizawa Y, Tatsumi Y, Anai S, Hosokawa Y, Hayashi Y, Tomioka A, Otani T, et al. The best objective response of target lesions and the incidence of treatment-related hypertension are associated with the survival of patients with metastatic renal cell carcinoma treated with sunitinib: a Japanese retrospective study. BMC Res Notes. 2016;9:79.
33. Matias M, Le Teuff G, Albiges L, Guida A, Brard C, Bacciarelo G, Loriot Y, Massard C, Lassau N, Fizazi K, et al. Real world prospective experience of axitinib in metastatic renal cell carcinoma in a large comprehensive cancer Centre. Eur J Cancer (Oxford, England: 1990). 2017;79:185–92.
34. Trotti A, Colevas AD, Setser A, Rusch V, Jaques D, Budach V, Langer C, Murphy B, Cumberlin R, Coleman CN, et al. CTCAE v3.0: development of a comprehensive grading system for the adverse effects of cancer treatment. Semin Radiat Oncol. 2003;13(3):176–81.
35. Chen AP, Setser A, Anadkat MJ, Cotliar J, Olsen EA, Garden BC, Lacouture ME. Grading dermatologic adverse events of cancer treatments: the common terminology criteria for adverse events version 4.0. J Am Acad Dermatol. 2012;67(5):1025–39.
36. Buda-Nowak A, Kucharz J, Dumnicka P, Kuzniewski M, Herman RM, Zygulska AL, Kusnierz-Cabala B. Sunitinib-induced hypothyroidism predicts progression-free survival in metastatic renal cell carcinoma patients. Med Oncol (Northwood, London, England). 2017;34(4):68.
37. Aparicio-Gallego G, Blanco M, Figueroa A, Garcia-Campelo R, Valladares-Ayerbes M, Grande-Pulido E, Anton-Aparicio L. New insights into molecular mechanisms of sunitinib-associated side effects. Mol Cancer Ther. 2011; 10(12):2215–23.
38. Hayman SR, Leung N, Grande JP, Garovic VD. VEGF inhibition, hypertension, and renal toxicity. Curr Oncol Rep. 2012;14(4):285–94.
39. Robinson ES, Khankin EV, Karumanchi SA, Humphreys BD. Hypertension induced by vascular endothelial growth factor signaling pathway inhibition: mechanisms and potential use as a biomarker. Semin Nephrol. 2010;30(6):591–601.
40. Merkus D, Sorop O, Houweling B, Boomsma F, van den Meiracker AH, Duncker DJ. NO and prostanoids blunt endothelin-mediated coronary vasoconstrictor influence in exercising swine. Am J Phys Heart Circ Phys. 2006;291(5):H2075–81.
41. Kappers MH, van Esch JH, Sluiter W, Sleijfer S, Danser AH, van den Meiracker AH. Hypertension induced by the tyrosine kinase inhibitor sunitinib is associated with increased circulating endothelin-1 levels. Hypertension (Dallas, Tex : 1979). 2010;56(4):675–81.
42. Kappers MH, Smedts FM, Horn T, van Esch JH, Sleijfer S, Leijten F, Wesseling S, Strevens H, Jan Danser AH, van den Meiracker AH. The vascular endothelial growth factor receptor inhibitor sunitinib causes a

preeclampsia-like syndrome with activation of the endothelin system Hypertension (Dallas, Tex : 1979). 2011;58(2):295–302.
43. Zou AP, Cowley AW Jr. Role of nitric oxide in the control of renal function and salt sensitivity. Curr Hypertens Rep. 1999;1(2):178–86.
44. Khan G, Golshayan A, Elson P, Wood L, Garcia J, Bukowski R, Rini B. Sunitinib and sorafenib in metastatic renal cell carcinoma patients with renal insufficiency. Ann Oncol. 2010;21:1618–22.
45. Lacouture ME, Reilly LM, Gerami P, Guitart J. Hand foot skin reaction in cancer patients treated with the multikinase inhibitors sorafenib and sunitinib. Ann Oncol. 2008;19(11):1955–61.
46. Steeghs N, Gelderblom H, Roodt JO, Christensen O, Rajagopalan P, Hovens M, Putter H, Rabelink TJ, de Koning E. Hypertension and rarefaction during treatment with telatinib, a small molecule angiogenesis inhibitor. Clin Cancer Res. 2008;14(11):3470–6.
47. Hubner N, Yagil C, Yagil Y. Novel integrative approaches to the identification of candidate genes in hypertension. Hypertension (Dallas, Tex: 1979). 2006;47(1):1–5.
48. Rees ML, Khakoo AY. Molecular mechanisms of hypertension and heart failure due to antiangiogenic cancer therapies. Heart Fail Clin. 2011;7(3):299–311.
49. Lee S, Chen TT, Barber CL, Jordan MC, Murdock J, Desai S, Ferrara N, Nagy A, Roos KP, Iruela-Arispe ML. Autocrine VEGF signaling is required for vascular homeostasis. Cell. 2007;130(4):691–703.
50. Cella D, Pickard AS, Duh MS, Guerin A, Mishagina N, Antras L, Neary MP, McCann L, Hodge R, Sternberg CN. Health-related quality of life in patients with advanced renal cell carcinoma receiving pazopanib or placebo in a randomised phase III trial. Eur J Cancer (Oxford, England: 1990). 2012;48(3):311–23.
51. Bukowski R, Cella D, Gondek K, Escudier B. Effects of sorafenib on symptoms and quality of life: results from a large randomized placebo-controlled study in renal cancer. Am J Clin Oncol. 2007;30(3):220–7.
52. Escudier B, Porta C, Bono P, Powles T, Eisen T, Sternberg CN, Gschwend JE, De Giorgi U, Parikh O, Hawkins R, et al. Randomized, controlled, double-blind, cross-over trial assessing treatment preference for pazopanib versus sunitinib in patients with metastatic renal cell carcinoma: PISCES study. J Clin Oncol. 2014;32(14):1412–8.
53. Chu TF, Rupnick MA, Kerkela R, Dallabrida SM, Zurakowski D, Nguyen L, Woulfe K, Pravda E, Cassiola F, Desai J, et al. Cardiotoxicity associated with tyrosine kinase inhibitor sunitinib. Lancet (London, England). 2007;370(9604): 2011–9.
54. Kapiteijn E, Brand A, Kroep J, Gelderblom H. Sunitinib induced hypertension, thrombotic microangiopathy and reversible posterior leukencephalopathy syndrome. Ann Oncol. 2007;18(10):1745–7.
55. Padhy BM, Shanmugam SP, Gupta YK, Goyal A. Reversible posterior leucoencephalopathy syndrome in an elderly male on sunitinib therapy. Br J Clin Pharmacol. 2011;71(5):777–9.
56. Maitland ML, Bakris GL, Black HR, Chen HX, Durand JB, Elliott WJ, Ivy SP, Leier CV, Lindenfeld J, Liu G, et al. Initial assessment, surveillance, and management of blood pressure in patients receiving vascular endothelial growth factor signaling pathway inhibitors. J Natl Cancer Inst. 2010;102(9):596–604.
57. Langenberg MH, van Herpen CM, De Bono J, Schellens JH, Unger C, Hoekman K, Blum HE, Fiedler W, Drevs J, Le Maulf F, et al. Effective strategies for management of hypertension after vascular endothelial growth factor signaling inhibition therapy: results from a phase II randomized, factorial, double-blind study of Cediranib in patients with advanced solid tumors. J Clin Oncol. 2009;27(36):6152–9.
58. Rao GA, Mann JR, Shoaibi A, Pai SG, Bottai M, Sutton SS, Haddock KS, Bennett CL, Hebert JR. Angiotensin receptor blockers: are they related to lung cancer? J Hypertens. 2013;31(8):1669–75.
59. Lever AF, Hole DJ, Gillis CR, McCallum IR, McInnes GT, MacKinnon PL, Meredith PA, Murray LS, Reid JL, Robertson JW. Do inhibitors of angiotensin-I-converting enzyme protect against risk of cancer? Lancet (London, England). 1998;352(9123):179–84.
60. Makar GA, Holmes JH, Yang YX. Angiotensin-converting enzyme inhibitor therapy and colorectal cancer risk. J Natl Cancer Inst. 2014;106(2):djt374.
61. Iacovelli R, Verri E, Cossu Rocca M, Aurilio G, Cullura D, de Cobelli O, Nole F. Prognostic role of the cumulative toxicity in patients affected by metastatic renal cells carcinoma and treated with first-line tyrosine kinase inhibitors. Anti-Cancer Drugs. 2017;28(2):206–12.

15

Does preoperative percutaneous nephrostomy insertion worsen upper-tract urothelial cancer oncological outcome?

Guan-Lin Huang[†], Hao-Lun Luo[†] and Po-Hui Chiang[*]

Abstract

Background: Physicians doubt percutaneous nephrostomy (PCN) insertion on cancer related hydronephrosis patients causes tumor seeding and worse cancer control. In this article, we attempted to determine if preoperative PCN alters cancer control in upper tract urothelial cancer (UTUC) patients.

Methods: Retrospective analysis of UTUC patients in a single center from 2005 to 2015. Exclusion criteria included lymph node metastasis, and patients underwent perioperative adjuvant chemotherapy or radiotherapy. There were 664 patients in this analysis, with clinico-pathological data being collected retrospectively for Cox-regression statistical analysis. Outcomes were measured by local recurrence, distant metastasis and cancer-specific death with Kaplan-Meier curves.

Results: There were respectively 25 and 639 UTUC cancers in the preoperative PCN and non-PCN insertion groups with mean follow-up duration of 37.9 and 48.6 months, respectively. The preoperative PCN group consisted of 17 patients (68%) with tumor located in the ureter, while the PCN-negative group included 236 patients (36%) with tumor located in the ureter being statistically significant. These two groups were comparable in gender, age, follow-up duration, tumor stage, and pathological features of the UTUC. As for the cancer control in the PCN group, 4(16%), 1(4%) and 1(4%) had local recurrence, distant metastasis and cancer-specific death respectively; in the non-PCN group, 101(15.8%), 96(15%) and 72(11.2%) exhibited local recurrence, distant metastasis and cancer-specific death respectively. Statistical analysis showed no difference in oncologic outcomes between these two groups.(p = 0.804, 0.201 and 0.254).

Conclusions: Preoperative percutaneous nephrostomy on upper-tract urothelial cancer poses little risk on tumor seeding and could be considered as part of treatment strategy if renal function preservation is needed.

Background

Hydronephrosis with compromised renal function is one manifestation of upper tract urothelial cancer [1]. Before definitive upper tract urothelial cancer diagnosis, percutaneous nephrostomy (PCN) may be undertaken for severe infective hydronephrosis or impending renal failure for temporary disease control. Although tumor seeding and invasion through the percutaneous nephrostomy tract has been reported on case reports [2, 3], there are no studies comparing locally or systemically driven cancer recurrence rates between preoperative PCN dwelling and non-PCN dwelling patients in preoperative upper-tract urothelial cancer patients. This study is the first study to analyze these two groups' of patients in the best of our knowledge.

Methods

We retrospectively collected upper-tract urothelial cancer patients receiving nephroureterectomy from 2005 to 2015 in single tertiary referring center. Procedures in the PCN group were initially intended for the preservation

* Correspondence: tuoa480713@yahoo.com.tw
Guan-Lin Huang and Hao-Lun Luo are Co-first authors.
Department of Urology, Kaohsiung Chang Gung Memorial Hospital and Chang Gung University College of Medicine, 123, Ta-Pei Road, Niaosung, Kaohsiung, Taiwan

of deteriorating renal function or medical failure infective hydronephrosis with information of possible malignant tumor seeding through the PCN tract to patients. Interventional radiologist performed whole PCN group patients with Fr 10. nephrostomy tube or pigtail. Radical nephroureterectomy procedure cases were enrolled in the study for definite UTUC treatment. Peri-operative positive lymph nodes and distant organ metastasis cases were excluded due to poor prognosis and possible need of further adjuvant treatment; besides, neo-adjuvant or adjuvant candidates were also excluded for comparability of the disease course. Patient basic characteristics and pathological features were collected, such as age, gender, follow up duration, pathological stage, tumor figuration, tumor site, lymphovascular invasion, carcinoma in situ, multifocal, tumor necrosis, smoking and end stage renal disease. The follow-up protocol after nephroureterecotmy was as follows: 1.Computed tomography (CT) abdomen scanning every 3–6 months in the first 2 years and annually thereafter. 2. Cystoscopy every 3 months until 2 years shifted to every 6 months if negative finding. 3. Physical examination over the surgical wound and PCN tract during outpatient clinics visits, and CT scanning if suspicion of disease recurrence. Outcome measurements were classified as bladder recurrence, local recurrence, and distant metastasis. Follow-up cystoscopy showed merely bladder recurrence residual bladder cuffing recurrence was deemed as bladder recurrence. In PCN group, local recurrence was defined as disease recurrence over ipsilateral retroperitoneal space or PCN sites. In PCN negative group, local recurrence was defined as disease over the ipsilateral retroperitoneal space. Distant metastasis was defined as regional/distant lymph nodes metastasis or organ metastasis. We used Cox-regression statistical analysis on comparability and significance of tumor recurrence between PCN (+) and PCN (−) groups. Kaplan-Meier survival curve was applied for time to recurrence between these two groups.

Results

In total, 25 patients in the PCN(+) group and 639 patients in the PCN(−) group had mean follow up duration of 37.9 and 48.6 months, respectively. The percentage of ureter tumor in the PCN(+) group(68%) was higher than the PCN(−) group(36%) with significant difference(p = 0.002). The median PCN dwelling time was 18 days [IOR: 5–26] Other basic characteristics such as gender, age, tumor stage, tumor grade, lymphovascular invasion, were collected with no significant difference between these two groups (Table 1.)

As for the cancer control in the PCN group, 4(16%), 1(4%) and 1(4%) had local recurrence, distant metastasis and cancer specific death respectively; in the non-PCN group, 101(15.8%), 96(15%) and 72(11.2%) had local recurrence, distant metastasis and cancer specific death respectively. Statistical analysis showed no cancer control difference between these two groups.(p = 0.804, 0.201 and 0.254)(Table 1.)

Table 1 Patient demography and oncological outcome

	Preop PCN(+) n = 25	Preop PCN(−) n = 639	
Gender(Male/Female)	11/14	366/273	0.189
Age(years)	70.8 ± 9.1	67.17 ± 10.8	0.098
Follow up duration	37.9 ± 27.8	48.6 ± 31.4	0.119
pT stage			0.353
pT0	6	181	
pT1	10	174	
pT2	5	122	
pT3	3	154	
pT4	1	8	
Papillary	18	506	0.378
Tumor location			
RP tumor	4	264	0.011
U tumor	17	236	0.002
RP + U tumor	4	138	0.790
High grade	23	578	0.796
LVI	6	97	0.232
CIS	7	226	0.449
Multifocal	9	189	0.491
TN	7	184	0.931
Smoking	5	65	0.116
ESRD	5	132	0.937
Prior bladder Ca	6	147	0.908
Oncological result			
Bladder recurrence	8	201	0.983
Local recurrence	4	101	0.804
Distant metastasis	1	96	0.201
Cancer specific death	1	72	0.254

RP tumor renal pelvis tumor, *U tumor* ureter tumor, *LVI* lymphovascular invasion
CIS carcinoma in situ, *TN* tumor necrosis, *ESRD* end stage renal disease

In the PCN group, no patients were found to have skin metastasis or PCN tract tumor invasion and the local recurrence pattern was over the ipsilateral retroperitoneal space, which is similar to PCN negative group. Besides, time to being local-recurrence free and time to being distant metastasis free in Kaplan-Meier survival curve showed no difference between these two groups.(p = 0.804 & 0.201)(Fig 1. & Fig 2.)

Discussion

Tumor seeding after the percutaneous nephrostomy insertion has been reported in case reports but no study

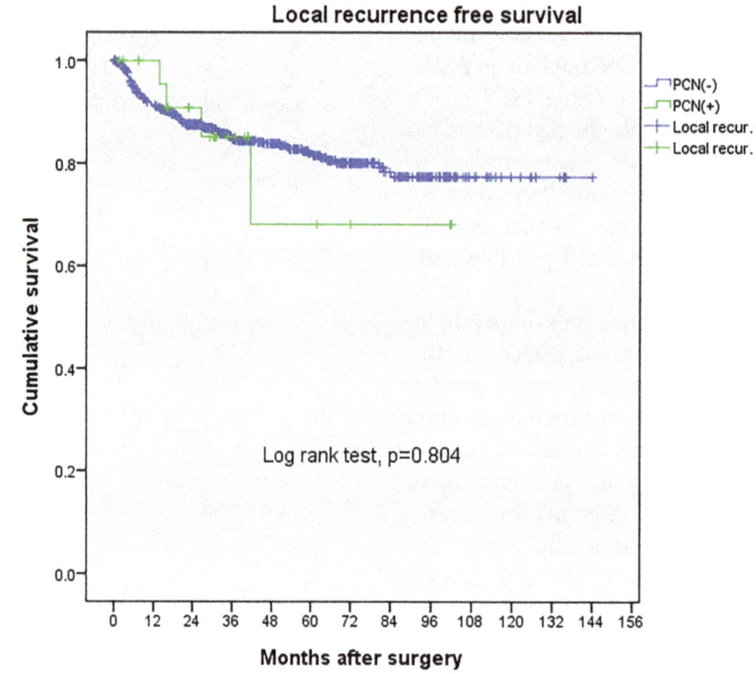

Fig. 1 Upper tract urothelial cancer local recurrence free survival after PCN

has evaluated if PCN procedure alter the risk of tumor seeding or cancer control [2–4]. In our study, the demographic and clinic-pathological data were similar between these two groups except for distribution of tumor location (17(68%) and 236(52%) ureter tumors in the PCN and non-PCN groups respectively, $p = 0.002$). It is reasonable that ureteral tumors are often associated with more event of hydronephrosis and sometimes external drainage was sometimes inevitable. Besides, relieving the post-renal obstruction may be considered earlier than urothelial cancer management when presenting as severe renal function impairment. After standard radical nephroureterectomy, comparable local

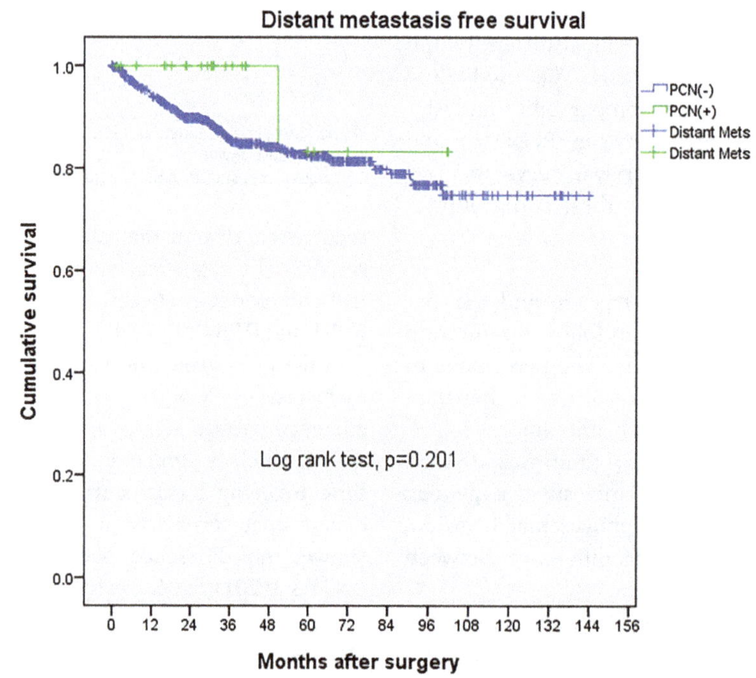

Fig. 2 Upper tract urothelial cancer distant metastasis free survival after PCN

recurrence (PCN group vs non-PCN group: 4/25 vs 101/639, 16% vs 15.8%, $p = 0.804$) and distant metastasis rate(PCN group vs non-PCN group: 1/25 vs 96/639, 4% vs 15%, $p = 0.201$) between these two groups were noted. Furthermore, there was no tumor dissemination along the PCN tract or skin metastasis observed in our study; hence, the risk of the worse oncological outcome related to the PCN procedure should not be over-emphasized especially for patients with need of salvaging residual renal function.

Table 2 Summarized the previous case reports of tumor seeding through the PCN tract [3–9]. Synchronous or metachronous urothelial cancer in upper urinary tract and bladder were the risk factors for tumor seeding [3–9]. Percutaneous endoscopic resection of the renal pelvis tumor seems another circumstance for tumor seeding [3–5, 8, 9]. However, Goel et al. reported long-term oncological outcomes of upper tract urothelial cancer status post percutaneous endoscopic resection, and concluded risk of tract seeding was low on low grade tumor [10]. Palou et al. also found percutaneous resection of superficial UTUC with good long term cancer outcome [11]. Roupret et al. retrospectively collected 24 patients receiving the percutaneous endoscopic resection of the tumor and reported 5-year disease-specific and tumor-free survival rates were 79.5 and 68%. There was none track seeding in the study as well [12]. Serrano et al. reviewed articles in Medline regarding the cancer disseminating in the PCN tracts and concluded that risk of tumor seeding is very low, and there were still other explanation rather than PCN tract manipulation, like blood stream or lymphatic metastasis [13]. Through the PCN tract, percutaneous resection of upper tract urothelial cancer was an alternative option for preservation renal function with comparable long-term cancer control in low-grade and limited tumor size patients. Meanwhile, risk for the tumor seeding through the PCN tract should be informed but downplayed [10–12, 14, 15]. In addition, Kiss et al. mentioned that internal drainage within urinary tract may increase the risk or urothelial recurrence [16]. According to the reviewed literature, the external drainage carried low risk of recurrence and should be considered for relieving urinary obstruction.

In our study, 25 preoperative PCN patients were initially performed for relieving urinary obstruction and clinical diagnosis instead of percutaneous endoscopic manipulation; hence, the risk of tumor seeding and altered oncological outcomes was minimal after standard nephroureterectomy. In addition, the evidences of neoadjuvant chemotherapy are getting more and more and the oncologic result is inspiring [17, 18]; however, impaired renal function is relatively contraindicated for cisplatin-based chemotherapy and such situation is not uncommon in clinical practice especially for UTUC patients [19, 20]. The PCN drainage may preserve residual renal function for UTUC patients with hydronephrosis and can be considered as a treatment strategy before neoadjuvant chemotherapy.

Limitation

The article is retrospective with relatively small-sized populations with short PCN dwelling time(Median: 18 days, IQR: 5–26). The prognostic effect of tumor site can not be fully assessed due to such small cohort by

Table 2 Case reports of tumor seeding through PCN track

Authors	Sex, M/F	Age, years	Concomitant with bladder cancer?	Tumor site	Histology	PCN function	Definite NUXBCE?	PCN dwelling time	Recurrence site	Time from PCN to recurrence
Sharma et al. 1994 [5]	M	56	Yes	RP, U	UC, high grade	PET	Yes	N.R.	Nephrectomy scar site	8 months
Huang et al. 1995 [6]	F	80	Yes	U	UC, high grade	Relief of obstruction, AP diagnosis	Yes	30 days	Nephrostomy track	1 month
Sengupta and Harewood,1998 [7]	M	78	Yes	RP	UC, high grade	Relief of obstruction	Yes	N.R.	Nephrostomy track	9 months
Yamada et al. 2002 [4]	M	63	Yes	RP	UC, low grade(G2)	PET	Yes	14 days	Nephrostomy track	3 months
Treuthardt et al. 2004 [8]	M	61	Yes	RP	UC, high grade(G2)	PET	No	6 weeks	Nephrostomy track	12 months
Wang et al. 2004 [9]	F	63	Yes	RP, U	UC, high grade(G3)	Relief of obstruction	Yes	7 days	Nephrostomy track	3 months
	M	52	No	RP	SCC, poor differentiated	PET	Yes	10 days	Nephrostomy track	4 months
Sorokin et al. 2013 [3]	M	76	Yes	RP	UC, high grade	PET	No	2 months	Nephrostomy track	5 months

UC urothelial cancer, *N.R.* not reported, *SCC* squamous cell carcinoma, *PCN* percutaneous nephrostomy, *NUXBCE* nephroureterectomy with bladder cuff excision, *PET* percutaneous endoscopic treatment, *AP* antegrade pyelography, *RP* renal pelvis, *U* ureter independent risk model. Further multi-center experience should be considered. Though the baseline asymmetry of ureteral tumor case between these two groups may cause of some bias, it reflect the real-world situation because that PCN was often used for preserving the residual function. The major size of PCN is eight to ten French in size and this study can further tell where if large size of PCN cause tumor seeding or not. However, this is the only study comparing PCN-related tumor seeding and oncological outcome, as we know.

Conclusion

Preoperative percutaneous nephrostomy on upper-tract urothelial cancer poses little risk on tumor seeding and could be considered as part of treatment strategy if renal function preservation is needed.

Abbreviations

AP: antegrade pyelography; CIS: carcinoma in situ; CT: computed tomography; ESRD: end stage renal disease; LVI: lymphovascular invasion; NUXBCE: nephroureterectomy with bladder cuff excision; PCN: percutaneous nephrostomy; PET: percutaneous endoscopic treatment; RP tumor: renal pelvis tumor; RP: renal pelvis; SCC: squamous cell carcinoma; TN: tumor necrosis; TURBT: transurethral resection of bladder tumor; U tumor: ureter tumor; U: ureter; UC: urothelial cancer; UTUC: upper tract urothelial cancer

Acknowledgements

Our team presented the preliminary abstract as poster on April 18 in 16th Urological Association of Asia Congress 2018 Kyoto, Japan. We are grateful to the poster participants giving directions for manuscript writing and precious clinical opinions.

Authors' contributions

GLH: data extract, manuscript and revision writing; HLL: statistical analysis, review data and revision writing direction; PHC: project development, revising and pictures production. All authors have read and approve of the final manuscript.

References

1. Yeh HC, Jan HC, Wu WJ, et al. Concurrent preoperative presence of Hydronephrosis and flank pain independently predicts worse outcome of upper tract urothelial carcinoma. PLoS One. 2015;10:e0139624.
2. Schwartzmann I, Pastore AL, Sacca A, et al. Upper urinary tract urothelial carcinoma tumor seeding along percutaneous nephrostomy track: case report and review of the literature. Urol Int. 2017;98:115–9.
3. Sorokin I, Welliver RC Jr, Elkadi O, et al. Tumor seeding of percutaneous nephrostomy tract from urothelial carcinoma of the kidney. Case reports in urology. 2013;2013:819470.
4. Yamada Y, Kobayashi Y, Yao A, et al. Nephrostomy tract tumor seeding following percutaneous manipulation of a renal pelvic carcinoma. Hinyokika kiyo Acta urologica Japonica. 2002;48:415–8.
5. Sharma NK, Nicol A, Powell CS. Track infiltration following percutaneous resection of renal pelvic transitional cell carcinoma. Br J Urol. 1994;73:597–8.
6. Huang A, Low RK, deVere White R. Nephrostomy tract tumor seeding following percutaneous manipulation of a ureteral carcinoma. J Urol. 1995;153:1041–2.
7. Sengupta S, Harewood L. Transitional cell carcinoma growing along an indwelling nephrostomy tube track. Br J Urol. 1998;82:591.
8. Treuthardt C, Danuser H, Studer UE. Tumor seeding following percutaneous antegrade treatment of transitional cell carcinoma in the renal pelvis. Eur Urol. 2004;46:442–3.
9. Wang SS, Ho HC, Su CK, et al. Seeding of malignant renal tumor through a nephrostomy tract. Journal of the Chinese Medical Association : JCMA. 2004;67:308–10.
10. Goel MC, Mahendra V, Roberts JG. Percutaneous management of renal pelvic urothelial tumors: long-term followup. J Urol. 2003;169:925–9 discussion 9-30.
11. Palou J, Piovesan LF, Huguet J, et al. Percutaneous nephroscopic management of upper urinary tract transitional cell carcinoma: recurrence and long-term followup. J Urol. 2004;172:66–9.
12. Rouprêt M, Traxer O, Tligui M, et al. Upper urinary tract transitional cell carcinoma: recurrence rate after percutaneous endoscopic resection. Eur Urol. 51:709–14.
13. Serrano Pascual A, Fernandez Gonzalez I, Gonzalez-Peramato P, et al. Is there a risk of carcinoma dissemination in the percutaneous access for endoscopical treatment of upper urinary tract urothelial tumors? Arch Esp Urol. 2004;57:283–90.
14. Fiuk JV, Schwartz BF. Upper tract urothelial carcinoma: paradigm shift towards nephron sparing management. World journal of nephrology. 2016;5:158–65.
15. Stewart GD, Tolley DA. What are the oncological risks of minimal access surgery for the treatment of urinary tract Cancer? Eur Urol. 46:415–20.
16. Kiss B, Furrer MA, Wuethrich PY, et al. Stenting prior to cystectomy is an independent risk factor for upper urinary tract recurrence. J Urol. 2017;198:1263–8.
17. Porten S, Siefker-Radtke AO, Xiao L, et al. Neoadjuvant chemotherapy improves survival of patients with upper tract urothelial carcinoma. Cancer. 2014;120:1794–9.
18. Kubota Y, Hatakeyama S, Tanaka T, et al. Oncological outcomes of neoadjuvant chemotherapy in patients with locally advanced upper tract urothelial carcinoma: a multicenter study. Oncotarget. 2017;8:101500–8.
19. Kaag MG, O'Malley RL, O'Malley P, et al. Changes in renal function following nephroureterectomy may affect the use of perioperative chemotherapy. Eur Urol. 2010;58:581–7.
20. Lane BR, Smith AK, Larson BT, et al. Chronic kidney disease after nephroureterectomy for upper tract urothelial carcinoma and implications for the administration of perioperative chemotherapy. Cancer. 2010;116:2967–73.

16

Evaluation of three stone-scoring systems for predicting SFR and complications after percutaneous nephrolithotomy

Kehua Jiang[1], Fa Sun[1*], Jianguo Zhu[1], Guangheng Luo[1], Peng Zhang[1], Yong Ban[1], Gang Shan[1] and Changxiang Liu[2]

Abstract

Background: Clinical studies assessing the feasibility and accuracy of three stone scoring systems's (SSSs: Guy's stone score, CROES nomogram and S.T.O.N.E nephrolithometry scoring system) have reported contradictory outcomes. This systematic evaluation was performed to obtain comprehensive evidence with regard to the feasibility and accuracy of three SSSs.

Methods: A systematic search of Embase, Pubmed, Medline, and the Cochrane Library was conducted to identify studies that compared three SSSs up to Mar 2018. Patients were categorized according to stone free (SF) and no-stone free (NSF), Outcomes of interest included perioperative variables, stone-free rate (SFR), and complications.

Results: Ten studies estimating three SSSs were included for meta-analysis. The results showed that SF patients had a significantly lower proportion of male (OR = 1.48, $P = 0.0007$), lower stone burden (WMD = -504.28, $P < 0.0001$), fewer No of involved calyces (OR = -1.23, $P = 0.0007$) and lower proportion of staghorn stone (OR = 0.33, $P < 0.0001$). Moreover, SF patients had significantly lower score of Guy score (WMD = -0.64, $P < 0.0001$), but, S.T.O.N.E. score (WMD = -1.23, $P < 0.0001$) and a higher score of CROES nomogram (WMD = 29.48, $P = 0.003$). However, the comparison of area under curves (AUC) of predicting SFR indicated that there was no remarkable difference between three SSSs. Nonetheless, Guy score was the only stone scoring system that predicted complications after PCNL (WMD = -0.29, 95% CI: − 0.57 to − 0.02, $P = 0.03$).

Conclusions: Our meta-analysis indicated that the three SSSs were equally, feasible and accurate for predicting SFR after PCNL. However, Guy score was the only stone scoring system that predicted complications after PCNL.

Keywords: Guy's score, S.T.O.N.E. score, CROES nomogram, Stone free rate, Meta-analysis

Background

The recommended treatment option for renal calculi and staghorn calculi is percutaneous nephrolithotomy (PCNL) according to the guidelines of the European Association of Urology (EAU) [1]. PCNL has increasingly been used over the past few decades and may continue in the future [2, 3]. However, PCNL outcomes among the authors are different, because of the vast heterogeneity in the methods for clinical and academic characterization of nephrolithiasis besides the evaluation of surgical outcomes. So assessing the preoperative factors that affect SFR and complications is critical.

The Guy's stone score, the Clinical Research Office of the Endourological Society(CROES) nomogram and the S.T.O.N.E.(stone size, tract length, obstruction, number of involved calices and essence) stone score are seen as predictors of stone-free status (SFS) and complications after PCNL [4–6]. The widespread use of a standardized stone scoring system is very precious for counseling patient, clinical decision, and

* Correspondence: sfgmc@sina.com
[1]Department of Urology, Guizhou Provincial People's Hospital, Guiyang, China
Full list of author information is available at the end of the article

assessment of outcomes, in addition to improving academic reporting [7]. However, no universally accepted stone scoring system for predicting SFR and complications after PCNL exists. Comparison of the SSSs in different clinical studies indicated some advantages as well as disadvantages of one nomogram to another for different variables. Hence, we performed a systematic review of the literature with a meta-analysis of the available published literature to compare the feasibility and accuracy of three SSSs in predicting PCNL outcomes concerning SFR and complications.

Methods

Study selection

According to the Cochrane Handbook recommendations, a systematic review of published literature was performed [8]. To identify all studies published up to Dec 31, 2018, which assessed the feasibility and accuracy of three SSSs. The following MESH search headings were used: "comparative studies", "Guy", "CROES", "S.T.O.N.E", "percutaneous nephrolithotomy", "stone free rate", and "complication".

Inclusion and exclusion criteria

All studies included in this meta-analysis satisfied the following requirements: (a) compare the two or three SSSs, (b) report the outcomes of two or three SSSs, (c) document the surgery as PCNL, (d) document indications for PCNL with renal stones. Studies were excluded if: (a) the article did not meet the inclusion criteria, (b) no outcomes were mentioned or the parameters were impossible to analyze the three SSSs from the published findings.

Data extraction and outcomes of interest

Two of the authors (JKH and SF) extracted data from the included studies including: author identification, country, publication years, study design, age, and the number of patients. All disagreements about eligibility were resolved by consensus through author discussions. The outcomes, including SFR and, overall complications, were extracted to compare between three SSSs. Overall complications were graded based on the Clavien-Dindo system [9].

Study quality assessment

In accordance with the criteria of Centre for Evidence-Based Medicine in Oxford, we evaluated the level of evidence (LOE) of the included ten studies. Furthermore, Jaded Score was applied to evaluate the methodological quality of RCTs [10]. while the Newcastle-Ottawa Scale (NOS) assessed the methodological quality of non-RCTs observational studies [11]. Besides, JKH and ZJG evaluated the quality of the articles and discrepancies were rechecked and resolved by discussion.

Statistical analysis

All analyses were conducted by Review Manager 5.3 (Cochrane Collaboration, Oxford, UK). Continuous and dichotomous variables were analyzed by weighted mean differences (WMDs) and odds ratios (ORs). All analysis results were reported with 95% CIs. I^2 and X^2 statistics were applied to evaluate the quantity of heterogeneity, and when $I^2>50\%$, the evidence was considered to have substantial heterogeneity, the random-effects (RE) model would be applied, otherwise, the fixed effects (FE) model was applied. Egger's test and funnel plot evaluated the publication bias. Sensitivity analyses estimated the influence of studies with a high risk of bias on the overall effect.

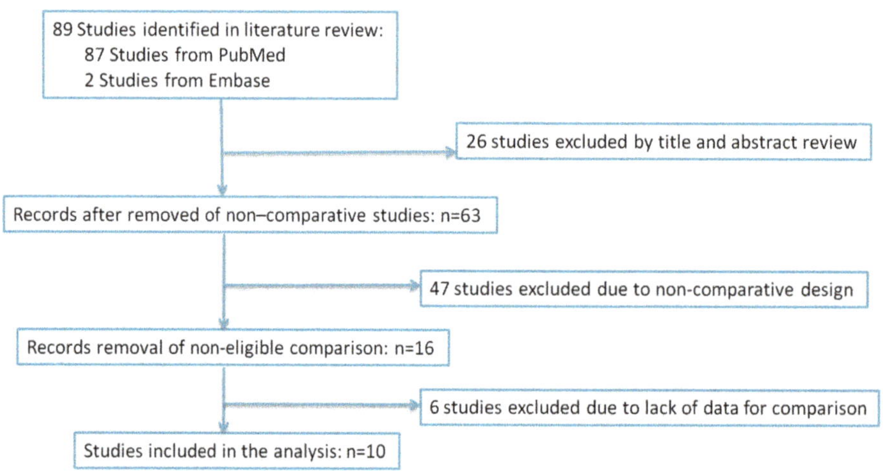

Fig. 1 PRISMA diagram. The search strategy and number of studies identified for inclusion in this meta-analysis

Table 1 Characteristics of included studies

First author year	Country	Study interval	Design	LOE	No.of patients	Matching/comparable[a]
Bozkurt, 2015 [12]	Turekey	2012–2015	Retrospective	3b	437	1,2,3,4,5
Choi, 2016 [13]	Korea	2003–2014	Retrospective	3b	217	1,2,3,4,5,6
Choi, 2016 [14]	Korea	2012–2015	Retrospective	3b	141	1,2,3,4, 5,6
Jaipuria, 2016 [15]	India	2014–2015	prospective	3b	606	1,3
Kocaaslan, 2016 [16]	Turekey	2010–2015	Retrospective	3b	137	1,2,3,4, 5,6
Labadie, 2015 [17]	USA	2009–2012	Retrospective	3b	246	1,2,3,4, 5,6
Noureldin, 2015 [18]	Canada	2009–2013	Retrospective	3b	185	1,2,3,5
Sfoungaristos, 2016 [19]	Israel	2010–2015	Retrospective	3b	73	1,3,4, 5,6
Tailly, 2016 [20]	Canada	2006–2013	Retrospective	3b	586	1,2,3,4, 5,6
Yarimoglu, 2016 [21]	Turekey	2012–2015	Retrospective	3b	262	1,2,3,4, 5

[a] Matching/comparable variable: 1 = age, 2 = BMI, 3 = gender, 4 = laterality(right/left), 5 = stone burden, 6 = stone density

Results

Characteristics of eligible studies

Ten studies [12–21] conformed to the inclusion criteria of this meta-analysis and were there included in the analysis of three SSSs (Fig. 1). The demographic and clinical characteristics of the included literature were shown in Table 1.

Quality of the studies and level of evidence(Table 1)

In this meta-analysis, the NOS quality assessment method of the observational studies [11], and the US Preventive Services Task Force grading system were applied to evaluate the quality of all studies [10]. Included studies were all level 3b. Also, the demographic variables of the three SSSs were extracted from included articles (Table 1).

Description of included studies and preoperative characteristics of the patients (Table 2)

Patients were categorized as stone free(SF) and no-stone free(NSF), and the pooled data of included studies [13, 14, 16, 17, 19, 20] showed that stone free patients had significantly lower proportion of male(OR = 1.48, 95% CI: 1.18 to 1.86, $P = 0.0007$) (Fig. 2), lower stone burden (WMD = -504.28, 95% CI: − 673.88 to − 334.67, $P < 0.0001$) (Fig. 2), fewer No of involved calyces (OR = -1.23, 95% CI: − 1.94 to − 0.52, $P = 0.0007$) (Fig. 2) and lower proportion of staghorn stone (OR = 0.33, 95% CI: 0.26 to 0.43, $P < 0.0001$) (Fig. 2). And stone free patients had significantly lower score of Guy score (WMD = -0.64, 95% CI: − 0.90 to − 0.37, $P < 0.0001$) (Fig. 2), lower score of S.T.O.N.E. score (WMD = -1.23, 95% CI: − 1.78 to − 0.67, $P < 0.0001$) (Fig. 2) and higher score of CROES nomogram (WMD = 29.48, 95% CI: 9.84 to 49.12, $P = 0.003$) (Fig. 2) (Table 2). However, there were no remarkable difference in terms of age, BMI, laterality and stone density between SF and NSF patients (Table 2, Additional file 1: Figure S1).

Outcomes of perioperative variables (Table 3)

With respect to perioperative variables, pooled data of 6 studies [13, 14, 16, 17, 20, 21] involving 1074 participants demonstrated that SF patients were associated

Table 2 Overall analysis of demographic and clinical characteristics compared stone-free with not stone-free after PCNL

Outcomes of interest	No. of studies	No. of patients SF/NSF	OR/WMD(95% CI) [a]	*p*-value	Study heterogeneity			
					Chi2	df	I^2	*p*-value
Age(year)	7	1101/559	0.02[−1.48,1.52] [a]	0.98	5.57	6	0%	0.47
BMI(kg/m^2)	6	1053/534	−0.59[− 1.80,0.63] [a]	0.34	21.87	5	77%	**0.0006**
Proportion/male	6	914/484	1.48[1.18,1.86]	**0.0007**	2.38	5	0%	0.80
Laterality(right/left)	6	914/484	1.10[0.88,1.38]	0.41	8.43	5	41%	0.13
Stone burden(mm2)	6	914/484	−504.28[−673.88,-334.67] [a]	**< 0.0001**	13.47	5	63%	**0.02**
No of involved calyces	3	560/316	−1.23[−1.94,-0.52]	**0.0007**	9.15	2	78%	**0.01**
Staghorn	6	914/484	0.33[0.26,0.43]	**< 0.0001**	6.58	5	24%	0.25
Stone density(HU)	4	777/377	−37.65[−81.95,6.65] [a]	0.10	4.90	4	18%	0.30
Guy score	5	777/377	−0.64[−0.90,-0.37] [a]	**< 0.0001**	26.42	4	85%	**< 0.0001**
CROES nomogram	6	964/452	29.48[9.84,49.12] [a]	**0.003**	57.50	5	91%	**< 0.0001**
S.T.O.N.E. score	6	964/452	−1.23[−1.78,-0.67] [a]	**< 0.0001**	35.04	5	86%	**< 0.0001**

SF stone free, *NSF* not stone free, *PCNL* percutaneous nephrolithotomy, *OR* odds ratio, *WMD* weighted mean difference, *CI* confidence interval, *BMI* body mass index, [a] WMD

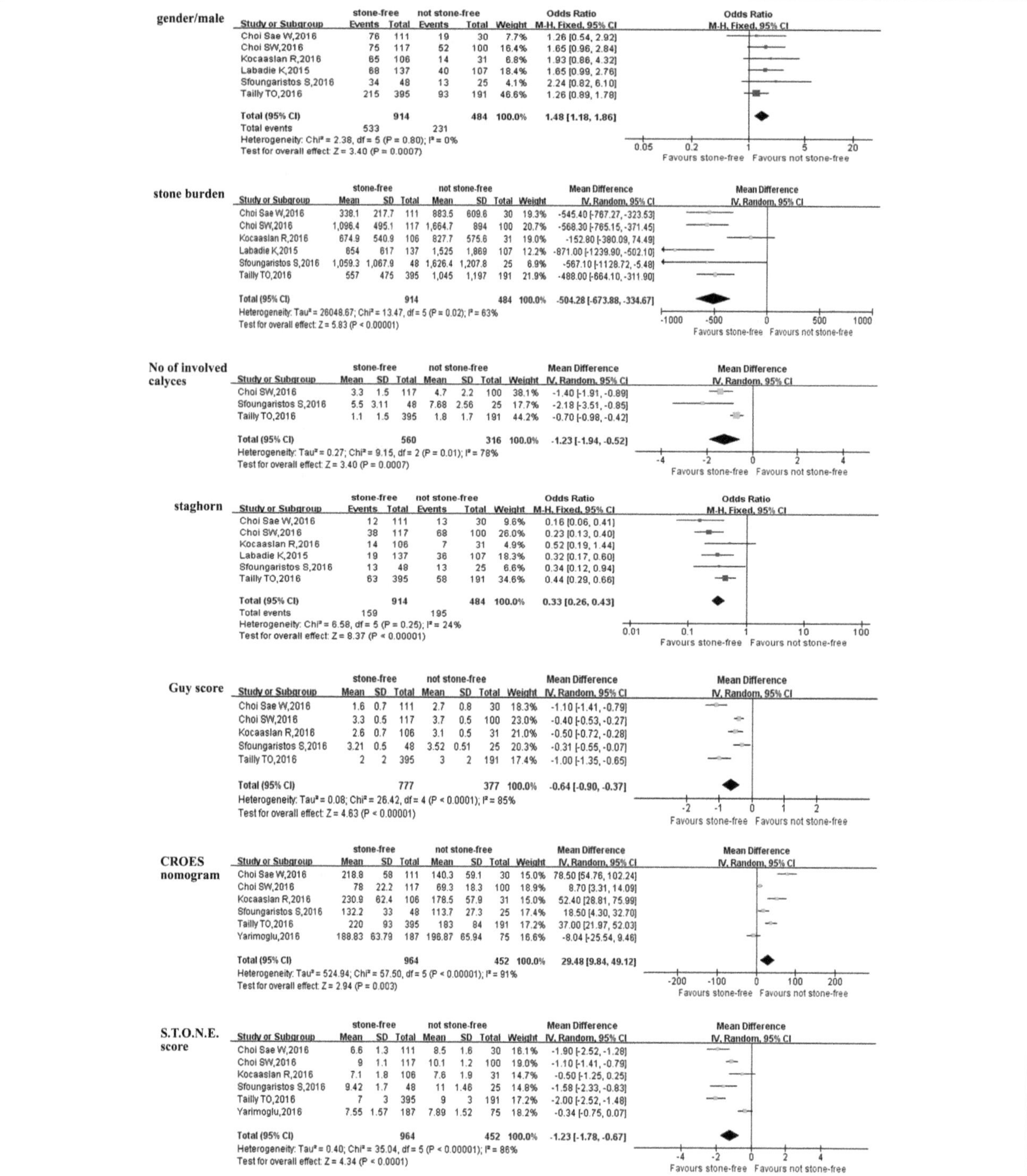

Fig. 2 Forest plot and meta-analysis of preoperative characteristics between the stone-free patients and not stone-free patients

with shorter operative time than NSF patients (WMD:- 19.85 min; 95% CI: − 25.52 to − 14.18; *P*<0.0001)(Fig. 3). SF patients were also associated with shorter length of hospital stay (LOS) (WMD: − 0.53 days; 95% CI: − 0.88 to − 0.17; *P* = 0.003) (Fig. 3) and lower transfusion rate (OR: 0.22; 95% CI: 0.08 to 0.55; *P* = 0.001) (Fig. 3) than NSF patients, respectively. However, there were no statistically difference between SF and NSF patients in term of No of tract (OR = -0.03; 95% CI: − 0.14 to 0.08; *P* = 0.62) (Fig. 3), mean tract length (WMD = 0.77; 95% CI: − 2.06 to 3.61; *P* = 0.59) (Fig. 3) and change in Hb level (WMD = − 0.21 g/mL; 95% CI: − 0.55 to 0.13; *P* = 0.22) (Fig. 3)(Table 3).

Table 3 Overall analysis of perioperative outcomes comparing stone free with not stone free after PCNL

Outcome of interest	No. of studies	No.of patients SF/NSF	OR/WMD(95%CI) [a]	*p*-value	Study heterogeneity			
					Chi^2	df	I^2	*p*-value
Operative time, min	6	706/368	−19.85[−25.52,-14.18]	**<0.0001**	8.62	5	42%	0.13
No of tract	3	618/322	−0.03[−0.14,0.08] [a]	0.62	4.76	2	58%	0.09
Mean tract length	3	623/321	0.77[−2.06,3.61]	0.59	1.92	2	0%	0.38
LOS, days	6	706/368	−0.53[−0.88,-0.17]	**0.003**	5.00	5	0%	0.42
Transfusion rate	2	228/130	0.22[0.08,0.55] [a]	**0.001**	0.34	1	0%	0.56
Change in Hb level(g/mL)	2	228/130	−0.21[−0.55,0.13]	0.22	0.01	1	0%	0.92

NS stone free, *NSF* not stone free, *LOS* length of stay, *PCNL* percutaneous nephrolithotomy, *OR* odds ratio, *WMD* weighted mean difference, *CI* confidence interval, [a] OR

Outcomes of three scoring systems for predicting SFR after PCNL (Table 4)

Pooled data of 7 studies [5, 12–14, 16, 17, 20] reported an accuracy of three SSSs in predicting post-PCNL SFR, the forest plot indicated that there was no statistical difference between Guy score and CROES nomogram with respect to area under curves(AUC) of prediction of SFR(WMD = 0.09; 95% CI:-0.12 to 0.29; $P = 0.41$) (Table 4, Fig. 4). There was also no significant difference between S.T.O.N.E. score and Guy score with respect to area under curves (AUC) of prediction of SFR (WMD = 0.00; 95% CI:-0.03 to 0.04; $P = 0.92$) (Table 4, Fig. 4) and no significant difference between CROES nomogram and S.T.O.N.E. score with respect to area under curves (AUC) of prediction of SFR (WMD = 0.00; 95% CI: − 0.05 to 0.04; $P = 0.94$) (Table 4, Fig. 4).

Outcomes of three scoring systems for predicting complications after PCNL (Table 5)

Pooled data of reported that the three SSSs in predicting post-PCNL complications, the forest plot indicated that Guy score was the only stone scoring system for predicting post-PCNL complications (WMD = -0.29, 95% CI: − 0.57 to − 0.02, $P = 0.03$) (Table 5, Fig. 5). No association between the two other scoring systems (CROES nomogram and S.T.O.N.E. score) and post-PCNL complications (Table 5, Fig. 5).

Discussion

Widely applicable and straightforward tools will highly improve patient counseling, clinical decision making, assessment of operation outcomes and academic study after PCNL for renal stones [22, 23]. These can allow reliable and accurate comparisons of treatment safety and efficacy, and facilitate the meaningful comparison of clinical studies [24]. We considered that the commonest and validated SSSs (Guy score, CROES nomogram, and S.T.O.N.E. score) could be predictive of SFR and complications after PCNL.

Both similar and divergent variables between the three SSSs has to be known. The Guy stone score consists of four grades based on stone burden and patient anatomy [7, 25]. The CROES nomogram is highly generalizable based on global data and uniquely grades risk across a continuous scale rather than dividing stones of varying complexity into discrete groups [7, 25]. The S.T.O.N.E. stone score stratifies patients into low-, moderate-, and high-risk groups, and it is more useful for decision making [7, 25]. The three SSSs included different parameters, however, the stone location, stone count and staghorn calculi were pivotal variables in the three SSSs [7].

On the other hand, Guy stone score included renal anatomy but not stone burden, and this was a difference from CROES nomogram and S.T.O.N.E. score. The CROES nomogram included prior treatment as well as operation volume, and these variables had remarkable relationships to the SFR. However, CROES nomogram lacked imageology information on hydronephrosis and calyceal abnormalities. The S.T.O.N.E. score comprised stone size, tract length, obstruction, number of involved calices and essence, and it had greater feasibility and accuracy than any of the individual variables alone. In our meta-analysis, the results showed preoperative variables gender, stone burden, number of involved calyces and staghorn calculi were remarkably correlating with SFR after PCNL for kidney calculi.

However, there is still no widely accepted stone scoring system for the prediction of outcomes after PCNL, and contradictions between different authors exist concerning the prediction of outcomes by the SSSs. Some experts reported that three SSSs were efficacy and equally predictive of SFR by estimating and comparing the three SSSs in 246 patients after PCNL [17]. Tailly et al. reported that three SSSs have similar predictive accuracy of SFS by comparing the three SSSs in 586 patients after PCNL, but no association between three SSSs and complications [20]. Moreover, Bozkurt et al. reported that both the Guy and CROES

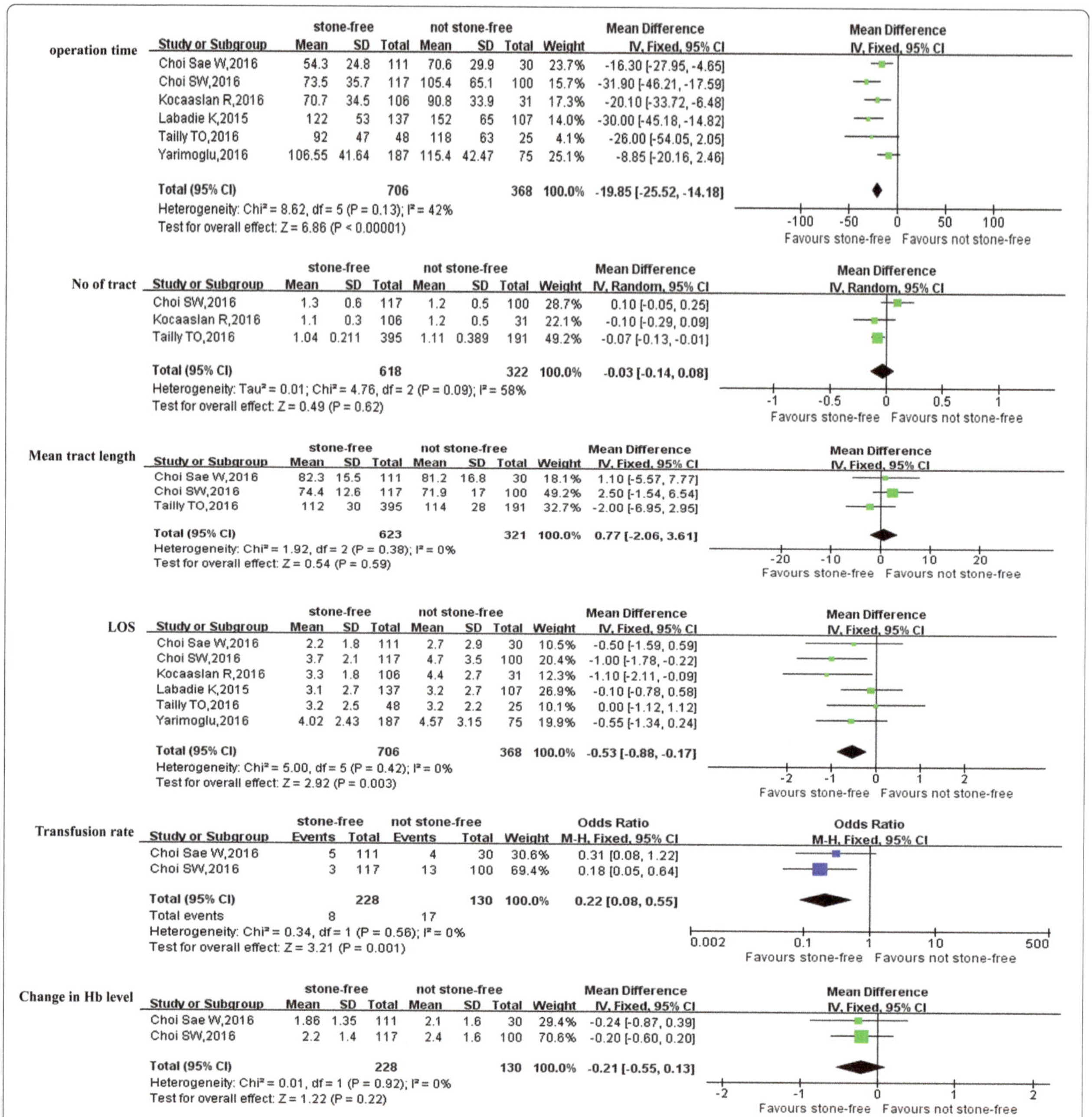

Fig. 3 Forest plot and meta-analysis of outcomes of perioperative variables between stone-free patients and not stone-free patients

nomogram had a remarkable relationship with SFS and complications [12]. Noureldin et al. also reported that the Guy score and S.T.O.N.E. score were equally associated with SFS, but there were no significant correlations with complications [18]. However, when other experts evaluated and compared three SSSs in predicting post-PCNL SFR and complications, the results showed that only S.T.O.N.E. score was a predictor of SFS after PCNL for renal stones [13]. Kocaaslan et al. reported that the CROES nomogram was well correlated with the success of PCNL in cases with anatomical abnormalities, and that the Guy score and S.T.O.N.E. score failed to predict the SFS and complications after PCNL [16]. Choi et al. compared the predictability and accuracy of the Guy score, CROES nomogram and S.T.O.N.E. score, the results showed that only Guy score could predict SFS and complications after PCNL [14]. Sfoungaristos et al. also compared three SSSs, and the results indicated that S.T.O.N.E. score was the only predictor of the

Table 4 Overall analysis of three stone-scoring systems for predicting SFR after PCNL

Outcome of interest	No.of studies	No. of patients	MD (95%CI)	*p*-value	Study heterogeneity			
					Chi^2	df	I^2	*p*-value
		CROES/Guy						
AUC	7	1837/1837	0.09[− 0.12,0.29]	0.41	14,350.0	6	100%	**<0.0001**
		STONE/Guy						
AUC	8	2191/2191	0.00[−0.03,0.04]	0.92	699.92	7	99%	**<0.0001**
		CROES/STONE						
AUC	7	1662/1662	−0.00[−0.05,0.04]	0.94	491.21	6	99%	**<0.0001**

SFR stone free rate, *PCNL* percutaneous nephrolithotomy, *AUC* area under curve, *CROES* clinical research office of the endourological society scoring system, *Guy* Guy scoring system, *S.T.O.N.E* S.T.O.N.E scoring system, *MD* mean difference, *CI* confidence interval

SFR for post-PCNL, and the three SSSs were not associated with complications [19]. In our meta-analysis, the results indicated that the three SSSs were remarkably associated with SFS and equally predictive of SFR, but only Guy score was a predictor of complications.

However, some critical limitations exist in the three SSSs. Firstly, stone burden and density as the important parameters dide not reflect in Guy's score. Moreover, it is also failed to describe procedure difficulties as well as clinical variability. Secondly, the CROES nomogram is also did not reflect stone density and lacked important variables affecting the outcomes, including imaging information on hydronephrosis and pelvicalyceal abnormalities [5, 26]. Moreover, the CROES

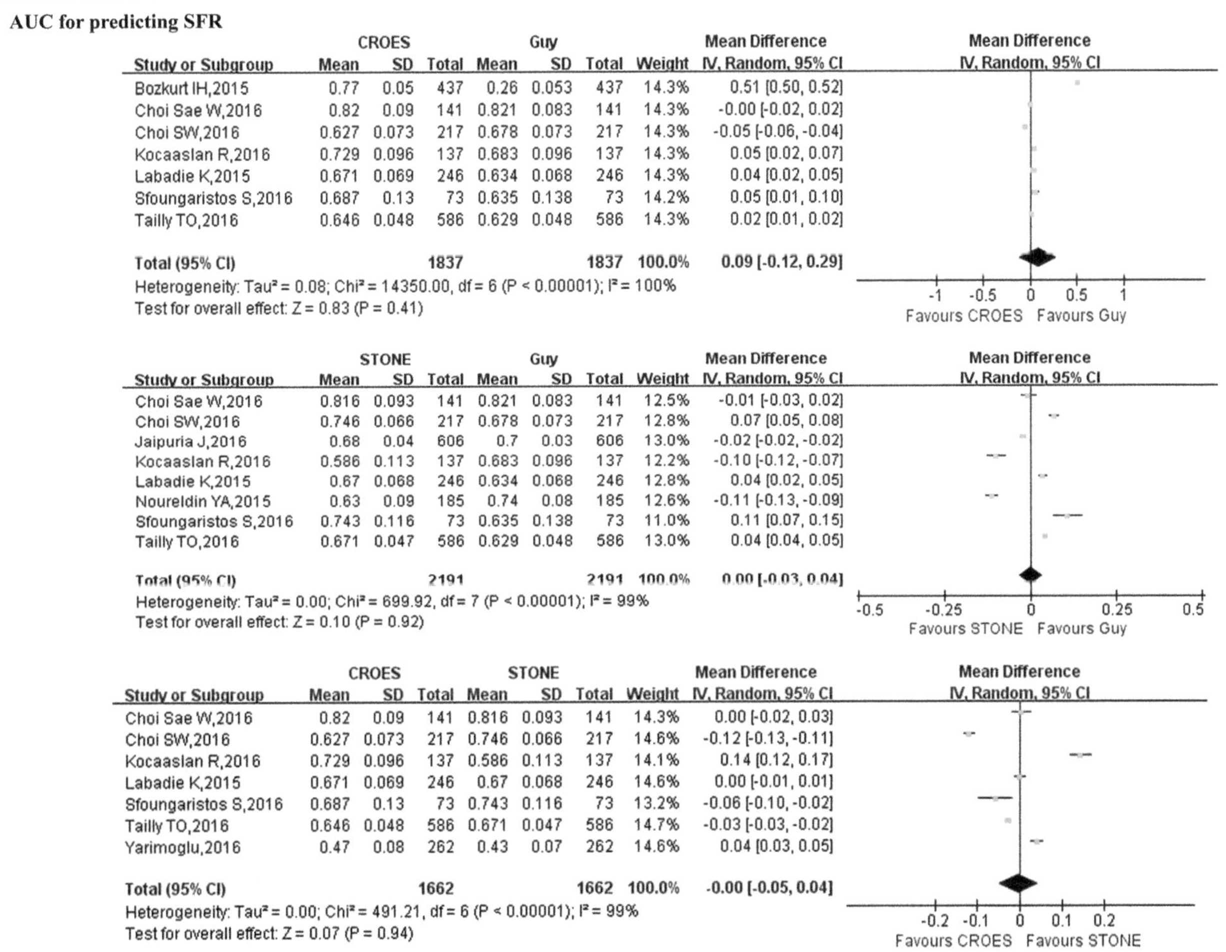

Fig. 4 Forest plot and meta-analysis of outcomes of three scoring systems for predicting SFR after PCNL. SFR = stone free rate

Table 5 Overall analysis of three scoring systems for predicting complications after PCNL

Outcome of interest	No. of studies	No.of patients Non-complicated/ complicated	OR/WMD(95%CI) [a]	*p*-value	Study heterogeneity			
					Chi^2	df	I^2	*p*-value
Guy score	2	263/95	−0.29[− 0.57,-0.02]	**0.03**	2.02	1	51%	0.15
CROES nomogram	2	263/95	1.97[−3.77,7.71]	0.50	0.00	1	0%	0.96
S.T.O.N.E. score	2	263/95	−0.27[−0.59,0.05]	0.10	0.20	1	0%	0.66

PCNL percutaneous nephrolithotomy, *CROES* clinical research office of the endourological society scoring system, *Guy* Guy scoring system, *S.T.O.N.E* S.T.O.N.E scoring system, *OR* odds ratio, *WMD* weighted mean difference, *CI* confidence interval, [a] OR

nomogram was complex in the clinical applications [17]. Thirdly, the limitations of S.T.O.N.E. score were validated with a small cohort which may limit its widespread usage [4, 7].

Similarly, several limitations existed while analyzing and interpreting results in our meta-analysis. Firstly, to identify prognostic factors, we acknowledge that other variables, such as surgeon experience and advanced surgical instruments, may need further investigation. These factors in the future may need to be incorporated in multicenter and larger samples clinical applications. Secondly, there existed heterogeneities of studies, some studies in this meta-analysis had the risk of selection bias. Lastly, all patients were evaluated for SFR after PCNL by KUB but not by CT, which may have overstated the SFR. Therefore, a need to develop more accurate and practical SSS to assess the relationship between the SSS and SFR, complications.In conjunction, our meta-analysis thus provides some up to date conclusions for the advantages and disadvantages of three SSSs in predicting of SFS and complications.

Conclusions

The Guy score, CROES nomogram and S.T.O.N.E. score were equally accurate predictive of SFR in patients undergoing PCNL, but the Guy score is the only SSS for predicting complications.

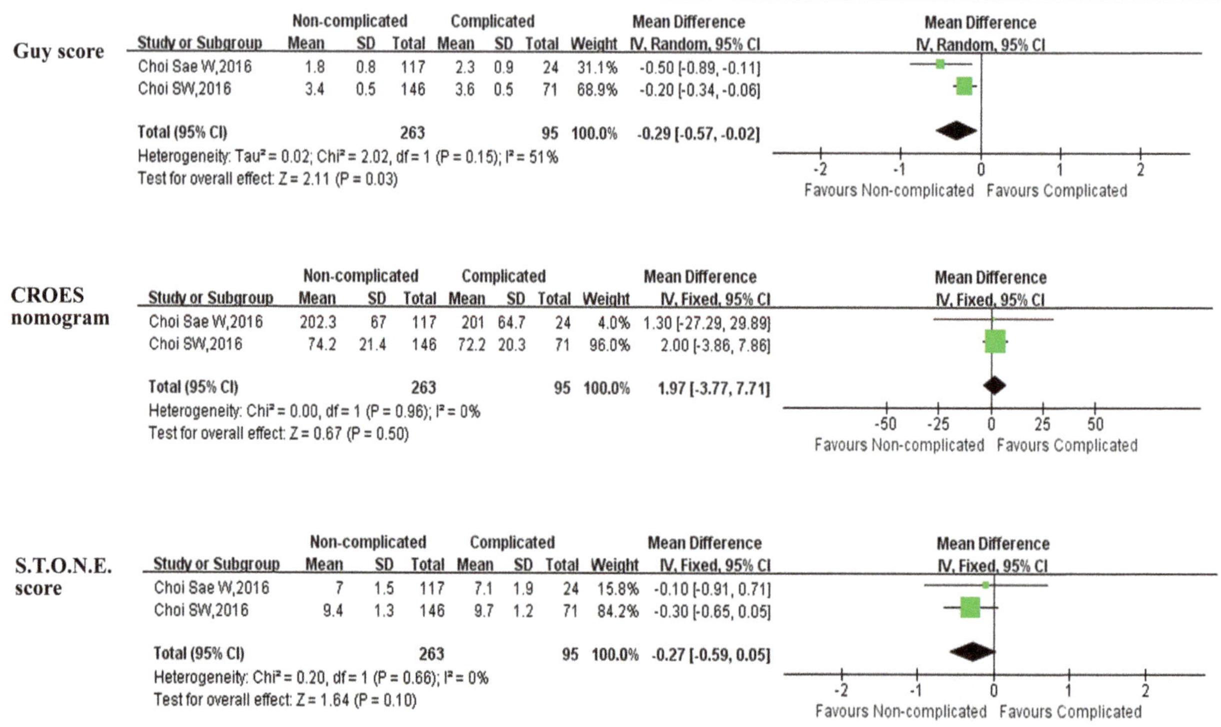

Fig. 5 Forest plot and meta-analysis of outcomes of three scoring systems for predicting complications after PCNL

Additional file

Additional file 1: Figure S1. Forest plot and meta-analysis of demographic and clinical characteristics compared stone-free with not stone-free after PCNL. (TIF 3058 kb)

Abbreviations

AUC: Area under curves; CROES: The Clinical Research Office of the Endourological Society nomogram; EAU: European Association of Urology; FE: Fixed effects; LOE: Level of evidence; NOS: The Newcastle-Ottawa Scale; ORs: Odds ratios; PCNL: Percutaneous nephrolithotomy; RE: Random-effects; SFR: Stone free rate; SSS: Three stone scoring systems; the S.T.O.N.E: stone size, tract length, obstruction, number of involved calices and essence; WMDs: Weighted mean differences

Acknowledgements

Not applicable.

Authors' contributions

Manuscript writing and editing: JKH, SF. Project development: SF. Data collection: ZP, BY, SG, data management/analysis: LGH, ZJG, LCX. All authors reviewed the manuscript. All authors read and approved the final manuscript.

Author details

[1]Department of Urology, Guizhou Provincial People's Hospital, Guiyang, China. [2]Department of Urology, The Affiliated Hospital of Guizhou medical University, Guiyang, China.

References

1. Turk C, Petrik A, Sarica K, Seitz C, Skolarikos A, Straub M, Knoll T. EAU guidelines on interventional treatment for urolithiasis. Eur Urol. 2016;69(3):475–82.
2. Ganpule AP, Vijayakumar M, Malpani A, Desai MR. Percutaneous nephrolithotomy (PCNL) a critical review. Int J Surg. 2016;36(Pt D):660–4.
3. Ghani KR, Andonian S, Bultitude M, Desai M, Giusti G, Okhunov Z, Preminger GM, de la Rosette J. Percutaneous Nephrolithotomy: update, trends, and future directions. Eur Urol. 2016;70(2):382–96.
4. Okhunov Z, Friedlander JI, George AK, Duty BD, Moreira DM, Srinivasan AK, Hillelsohn J, Smith AD, Okeke Z. S.T.O.N.E. nephrolithometry: novel surgical classification system for kidney calculi. Urology. 2013;81(6):1154–9.
5. Smith A, Averch TD, Shahrour K, Opondo D, Daels FP, Labate G, Turna B, de la Rosette JJ, Group CPS. A nephrolithometric nomogram to predict treatment success of percutaneous nephrolithotomy. J Urol. 2013;190(1):149–56.
6. Thomas K, Smith NC, Hegarty N, Glass JM. The Guy's stone score--grading the complexity of percutaneous nephrolithotomy procedures. Urology. 2011;78(2):277–81.
7. Vernez SLOZ, Motamedinia P, Bird V, Okeke Z, Smith A. Nephrolithometric scoring systems to predict outcomes of percutaneous Nephrolithotomy. Rev Urol. 2016;18(1):15–27.
8. Liberati A, Altman DG, Tetzlaff J, Mulrow C, Gotzsche PC, Ioannidis JP, Clarke M, Devereaux PJ, Kleijnen J, Moher D. The PRISMA statement for reporting systematic reviews and meta-analyses of studies that evaluate health care interventions: explanation and elaboration. J Clin Epidemiol. 2009;62(10):e1–34.
9. Dindo D, Demartines N, Clavien P-A. Classification of surgical complications. Ann Surg. 2004;240(2):205–13.
10. Clark HD, Wells GA, Huet C, McAlister FA, Salmi LR, Fergusson D, Laupacis A. Assessing the quality of randomized trials: reliability of the Jadad scale. Control Clin Trials. 1999;20(5):448–52.
11. Stang A. Critical evaluation of the Newcastle-Ottawa scale for the assessment of the quality of nonrandomized studies in meta-analyses. Eur J Epidemiol. 2010;25(9):603–5.
12. Bozkurt IH, Aydogdu O, Yonguc T, Yarimoglu S, Sen V, Gunlusoy B, Degirmenci T. Comparison of guy and clinical research Office of the Endourological Society Nephrolithometry Scoring Systems for predicting stone-free status and complication rates after percutaneous Nephrolithotomy: a single center study with 437 cases. J Endourol. 2015;29(9):1006–10.
13. Choi SW, Bae WJ, Ha US, Hong SH, Lee JY, Kim SW, Cho HJ. Prognostic impact of stone-scoring systems after percutaneous Nephrolithotomy for staghorn calculi: a single Center's experience over 10 years. J Endourol. 2016;30(9):975–81.
14. Choi SW, Bae WJ, Ha US, Hong SH, Lee JY, Kim SW, Cho HJ. Prediction of stone-free status and complication rates after tubeless percutaneous nephrolithotomy: a comparative and retrospective study using three stone-scoring systems and preoperative parameters. World J Urol. 2016;35(3):449-57.
15. Jaipuria J, Suryavanshi M, Sen TK. Comparative testing of reliability and audit utility of ordinal objective calculus complexity scores. Can we make an informed choice yet? BJU Int. 2016;118(6):958–68.
16. Kocaaslan R, Tepeler A, Buldu I, Tosun M, Utangac MM, Karakan T, Ozyuvali E, Hatipoglu NK, Unsal A, Sarica K. Do the urolithiasis scoring systems predict the success of percutaneous nephrolithotomy in cases with anatomical abnormalities? Urolithiasis. 2016;45(3):305-10.
17. Labadie K, Okhunov Z, Akhavein A, Moreira DM, Moreno-Palacios J, Del Junco M, Okeke Z, Bird V, Smith AD, Landman J. Evaluation and comparison of urolithiasis scoring systems used in percutaneous kidney stone surgery. J Urol. 2015;193(1):154–9.
18. Noureldin YA, Elkoushy MA, Andonian S. Which is better? Guy's versus S.T.O. N.E. nephrolithometry scoring systems in predicting stone-free status post-percutaneous nephrolithotomy. World J Urol. 2015;33(11):1821–5.
19. Sfoungaristos S, Gofrit ON, Pode D, Landau EH, Duvdevani M. Percutaneous nephrolithotomy for staghorn stones: which nomogram can better predict postoperative outcomes? World J Urol. 2016;34(8):1163–8.
20. Tailly TO, Okhunov Z, Nadeau BR, Huynh MJ, Labadie K, Akhavein A, Violette PD, Olvera-Posada D, Alenezi H, Amann J, et al. Multicenter external validation and comparison of stone scoring Systems in Predicting Outcomes after Percutaneous Nephrolithotomy. J Endourol. 2016;30(5):594–601.
21. Yarimoglu S, Polat S, Bozkurt IH, Yonguc T, Aydogdu O, Aydin E, Degirmenci T. Comparison of S.T.O.N.E and CROES nephrolithometry scoring systems for predicting stone-free status and complication rates after percutaneous nephrolithotomy: a single center study with 262 cases. Urolithiasis. 2016; 45(5):489-94.
22. Allen DOBT, Tiptaft R, Glass J. Defining the learning curve for percutaneous nephrolithotomy. J Endourol. 2005;19(3):279–82.
23. de la Rosette JJ, Laguna MP, Rassweiler JJ, Conort P. Training in percutaneous nephrolithotomy--a critical review. Eur Urol. 2008;54(5):994–1001.
24. Autorino RQG, Sio MD, Lima E, Quarto E, Damiano R, Oliviero R, Osorio L, Marcelo F, D'Armiento M. Fate of abstracts presented at the world congress of Endourology: are they followed by publication in peer-reviewed journals? J Endourol. 2006;20(12):996–1001.
25. Withington J, Armitage J, Finch W, Wiseman O, Glass J, Burgess N. Assessment of stone complexity for PCNL: a systematic review of the literature, how best can we record stone complexity in PCNL? J Endourol. 2016;30(1):13–23.
26. Akhavein A, Henriksen C, Syed J, Bird VG. Prediction of single procedure success rate using S.T.O.N.E. Nephrolithometry surgical classification system with strict criteria for surgical outcome. Urology. 2015;85(1):69–73.

17

Reducing kidney motion: Optimizing anesthesia and combining respiratory support for retrograde intrarenal surgery

Nariman Gadzhiev[1], Ullubiy Oibolatov[2], Leonid Kolotilov[2], Sergei Parvanyan[2], Gagik Akopyan[3], Sergei Petrov[1], Courtney M. Cottone[4], John Sung[4] and Zhamshid Okhunov[4*]

Abstract

Background: One of the greatest challenges presented with RIRS is the potential for movement of the stone within the operative field associated with diaphragm and chest respiratory excursions due to mechanical ventilation. To overcome this challenge, we propose in this pilot study a new general anesthesia technique combining high frequency jet ventilation (HFJV) with small volume mechanical ventilation (SVMV). Data regarding safety, feasibility and surgeons' impression was assessed.

Methods: Patients undergoing RIRS for kidney stones from November 2017 to May 2018 were prospectively recruited to participate in the study. In each case after the beginning of general anesthesia (GA) with mechanical ventilation (MV) surgeons were asked to assess the mobility of the operative field and conditions for laser lithotripsy according to the developed questionnaire scale. The questionnaire consisted of 5 degrees of assessment of kidney mobility and each question was scored from 1 to 5, 1 being very mobile (extremely poor conditions for dusting) and 5 completely immobile (Ideal conditions for dusting).

After the assessment GA was modified with combined respiratory support (CRS), reducing tidal volume and respiratory rate (small volume mechanical ventilation, SVMV) and applying in the same time transcatheter high frequency jet ventilation (HFJV) inside the closed circuit.

After beginning of CRS, surgeons were once again asked to assess the mobility of the operative field and the conditions for laser lithotripsy. Main ventilation parameters were recorded and compared in both regimens.

Results: A total of 38 patients were included in the study. The mean age was 49 (range 45–53) with a mean stone size of 10 mm (range 10–14) and Hounsfield unit of 1060 (range 930–1190). All patients underwent successful RIRS and no intraoperative complications occurred throughout the duration of the study. A statistically significant difference between ventilation parameters prior to and after CRS institution was detected in all cases, however their clinical impact was negligible. Despite this, assessment via the questionnaire scale point values varied significantly before and after the application of CRS and were 2.3 (2.1; 2.6) and 3.8 (3.7; 4.0) respectively ($p < 0.001$).

Conclusions: The novel combined respiratory approach consisting of HFJV and SVMV appears to provide better conditions for stone dusting through reduced respiratory kidney motion and is not associated with adverse health effects or complications.

(Continued on next page)

* Correspondence: zokhunov@uci.edu
[4]Department of Urology, University of California, Irvine, 333 City Boulevard West, Orange, CA 92868, USA
Full list of author information is available at the end of the article

(Continued from previous page)

Keywords: General anesthesia (GA), Retrograde intrarenal surgery (RIRS), Mechanical ventilation (MV), Periodic apnea (PA), High frequency jet ventilation (HFJV), Shockwave lithotripsy (SWL), Urolithiasis, Nephrolithiasis, Combined respiratory support (CRS)

Background

According to the currently established guidelines released by the European Association of Urology, retrograde intrarenal surgery (RIRS) via flexible ureterorenoscopy, is considered a well-established and effective procedure for the treatment of urolithiasis [1]. RIRS is most typically performed under general anesthesia (GA) with mechanical ventilation (MV) assistance, though can also be conducted under spinal or epidural anesthesia [2].

Regardless of anesthesia method one of the greatest challenges presented with RIRS is the potential for movement of the stone within the operative field associated with diaphragm and chest respiratory excursions due to MV. To overcome this impediment, Emiliani and Traxer suggested a technique known as periodic apnea (PA) to allow for momentary respites in respirations to facilitate stone removal and to minimize stone movements during laser lithotripsy [3]. However, surgeons may hesitate to induce PA due to relevant concerns of inducing hypercapnea. To circumvent these concerns, high frequency jet ventilation (HFJV) during GA has been suggested [4]. However, this method makes it impossible to use inhalational anesthetics and does not monitor end-tidal CO_2 levels nor the volume of exhaled air [5].

Thus, to provide stability of the operative field during RIRS, we propose a modified technique of GA, referred to as combined respiratory support (CRS). It implies HFJV with small volume mechanical ventilation (SVMV). The purpose of this study is to perform a pilot study to assess the safety and feasibility of this technique during RIRS.

Material and methods

After obtaining approval by the local ethics committee, we performed a prospective, single-center study in patients undergoing RIRS for renal stones from November of 2017 to May of 2018. Patients with kidneys stones with indications for RIRS, who were eligible to enroll in this study, were identified by the appropriate research personnel via diagnosis at an outpatient clinic visit. All patients provided written consent to participate in the study. Patients consented to publish the data obtained during the study. Thorough explanation of the study was provided to patients, after which all provided signed, informed consent. Patients with ASA class of greater than 3 and active urinary tract infection were excluded from the study. All procedures were performed by two experienced endourologists [6].

Questionnaire

The secondary outcome of the study was to implement a subjective questionnaire in order to assess surgeon's feedback on novel technique. The questionnaire consisted of 5 degrees of assessment of kidney mobility and each question was scored from 1 to 5, 1 being very mobile (extremely poor conditions for dusting), 2 being significantly mobile (unsatisfactory conditions for dusting), 3 being slightly mobile (satisfactory conditions for dusting), 4 almost immobile (good conditions for dusting) and 5 completely immobile (Ideal conditions for dusting) (Table 1). This was done in 2-step fashion in every patient and each patient served his own control: first, after the beginning of GA with MV in the mode of normal ventilation the questionnaire was implemented and surgeons were asked to assess the mobility of the operative field and the decency of conditions for laser lithotripsy. In addition to this assessment, anesthesia parameters including results of arterial blood gas analysis were recorded and evaluated in order to address safety concerns.

Second, novel CRS technique was then instituted and maintained throughout RIRS. Before lithotripsy itself surgeons were once again asked to assess the mobility of the operative field and conditions for laser lithotripsy according to the previously mentioned questionnaire. Monitoring of end-tidal carbon dioxide (EtCO2) level was carried out by intermittent capnography. Besides main anesthesia parameters with results of arterial blood gas analysis were recorded at the end of lithotripsy while on CRS for later comparison.

Table 1 Developed questionnaire scale assessing the mobility and conditions of the operative field

Classification	Description	Value
Very Mobile	Extremely poor conditions for dusting	1 point
Significantly Mobile	Unsatisfactory conditions for dusting	2 points
Slightly Mobile	Satisfactory conditions for dusting	3 points
Almost Immobile	Good conditions for dusting	4 points
Completely Immobile	Excellent conditions for dusting	5 points

CRS technique

The concentration of Sevoflurane was increased from 1.4–2.6 vol% to 8 vol%. The following changes were then made to alter ventilation patterns: the tidal volume (Vt) (6–8 ml/kg IBW) and the respiratory rate (8–15 per minute) (RR) were decreased by 2–3 times, the ratio of inhalation to exhalation (I:E) was increased from 1:2 to 1:3, the fraction of inspired oxygen (FiO_2) was decreased from 40 to 21% in the fresh gas flow (FGF) of 1.0 l/min. Transcatheter HFJV through tracheal tube was initiated with a ZisLINEJV-100 high frequency respirator (Triton-Electronics, Russia) with a respiratory cycle frequency (RCF) of 300 per minute, I:E = 1:3, FiO_2 = 1.0 and working pressure (WP) 0.3–0.6 bar. Depth of anesthesia was measured by BIS Monitor (Covidien AG, Zurich, Switzerland).

Surgical technique

RIRS was performed with the patient in the lithotomy position with 7.5 Flex X^2 ureteroscope (Karl Storz, Tuttlingen, Germany). Lithotripsy was performed with a holmium laser using 270 µm fibers at 0.3–0.5 J and 20–40 Hz (VersaPulse® PowerSuite™ 100 W) with patient under CRS. Dusting technique was utilized in all patients. A fragment was deliberately left to be extracted for stone analysis. Ureteral access sheath was used in 2 cases (stone size 14 mm).

Statistical analysis

Nonparametric resampling, permutation and randomization procedures (bootstrap and Monte Carlo) were applied for the statistical data analysis using software PAST [7]. Statistical significance of the observed effects was tested by *p*-values and confidence intervals (CIs). Threshold of 0.001 was considered as a critical significance level. For the expression of the clinical importance of findings, and their unification the so-called "standardized effect size" was used.

Results

A total of 38 patients were enrolled in the study with a mean age of 49 years (range 45–53). Mean body mass index was 27 kg/m^2 (range 25–28). Mean ASA score was 2 (range 1–3). Mean stone size was 10 mm (range 10–14). Mean stone density was 1060 (range 930–1190). All cases were successful. Mean duration of RIRS was 26 min (range 20–32). Stone free rate in the study confirmed by ultrasound and KUB at 8 weeks was 86% (Table 2).

A statistically significant difference between ventilation parameters prior and after CRS institution was detected in all cases (Table 3). End-tidal CO_2 with CRS implementation was ${}_{40}\,42\,{}_{43}$ mmHg during RIRS which is in the range of normocapnia. No intraoperative complications occurred for any patients throughout the duration of the study. There was statistical significance in surgeons' subjective questionnaire assessment points before and after the application of CRS 2.3 (2.1; 2.6) and 3.8 (3.7; 4.0) $p < 0.0001$, respectively (Table 2).

Table 2 Patient and stone characteristics

Feature	Mean (range)
Sample size, *n*	38
Age, years	49 (45; 53)
Body mass index, kg/m2	27 (25; 28)
ASA, scores	2 (1; 3)
Maximum diameter of the stone, mm	10 (10; 14)
Density of the stone, HU	1060 (930; 1190)
Stone location	
Upper calyx	16
Middle calyx	11
Lower calyx	7
Pyelus	4
Duration of RIRS, min	26 (14; 32)
Stone free rate	86%

Surgeon's impression assessed with the proposed questionnaire scale demonstrated that CRS leads to extremely high improvement in the stability of operative field (Fig. 1).

Discussion

Retrograde Intrarenal surgery is being increasingly used in renal stones. This is partly due to advancements in surgical and endoscopic technology. Although RIRS is less technically challenging then PCNL, laser lithotripsy can be challenging. Respiratory renal movement and proper laser settings are the two main contributing components of successful lithotripsy [8]. In order to minimize kidney displacement due to respiratory motion, several methods have been previously suggested including high frequency ventilation [9], PA [3], abdominal compression [10], and general anesthesia with low ventilation [11]. There have been many modifications suggested, but each technique has its own advantages and limitations.

Öberg and Sjöstrand were first to describe the HFJV in 1967 [9]. Initially it was utilized in otolaryngology, bronchial and lung surgery [12]. In the past decade, an increasing interest in HFJV's advantages in keeping target organs relatively motionless during surgery to optimize surgical precision has grown. In regards to stone treatment, in 1988 Warner and colleagues were the first to demonstrate the potential benefits of HFJV for shock wave lithotripsy (SWL) and since then several studies have confirmed the benefits of HFJV in SWL [4, 13, 14].

Table 3 Ventilation parameters and points without and with CRS technique

Features	Mean (95% *CI*)		Mean difference ($d = Ma - Mb$) (95% *CI*)	*p*-value
	Without CRS (*Mb*)	*With CRS* (*Ma*)		
V_E (l/min)	6.1 (5.8; 6.5)	9.3 (8.9; 9.7)	3.2 (2.6; 3.7)	< 0.001
P_{peak} (cm H_2O)	18.2 (17.5; 18.8)	19 (18; 20)	0.7 (0.4; 1.0)	< 0.001
P_{mean} (cm H_2O)	7.9 (7.7; 8.1)	6.7 (6.5; 6.9)	−1.2 (−1.4; −1.0)	< 0.001
SpO_2 (%)	98 (97; 99)	99 (98; 100)	1.0 (0.2; 1.5)	< 0.001
$EtCO_2$ (mm Hg)	36 (35; 37)	42 (40; 43)	6 (4; 7)	< 0.001
PaO_2 (mm Hg)	180 (170; 190)	320 (300; 340)	170 (160; 190)	< 0.001
$PaCO_2$ (mm Hg)	39 (38; 40)	43 (41; 45)	4.0 (0.4; 7.6)	< 0.001
Fi_{sev} (vol%)	2.2 (2.1; 2.3)	7.3 (7.0; 7.6)	5.1 (4.9; 5.3)	< 0.001
Et_{sev} (vol%)	1.8 (1.7; 2.0)	1.0 (0.9; 1.1)	−0.8 (−0.9; −0.7)	< 0.001
MAC	0.91 (0.87; 0.95)	0.52 (0.48; 0.56)	−0.39 (−0.44; −0.34)	< 0.001
BIS	44 (42; 47)	53 (49; 56)	9 (5; 13)	< 0.001
Points	2.3 (2.1; 2.6)	3.8 (3.7; 4.0)	1.6 (1.3; 1.8)	< 0.001

Notations: *CI* – confidence intervals; Mb and *Ma* – mean values *before and after the application of the CRS technique*, respectively; *d* – mean difference

Popiolek et al. was the first to present high frequency positive pressure ventilation in RIRS during the 2017 World Congress of Endourology, demonstrating the true necessity of stabilization of the operative field [15]. However, while high frequency ventilation may facilitate quicker stone removal via the occurrence of less adverse stone movements, this method also makes it impossible to use inhalational anesthetics and does not monitor end-tidal CO_2 levels nor the volume of exhaled air [5]. Therefore in our opinion, high frequency ventilation remains a suboptimal approach toward anesthesiological support during RIRS.

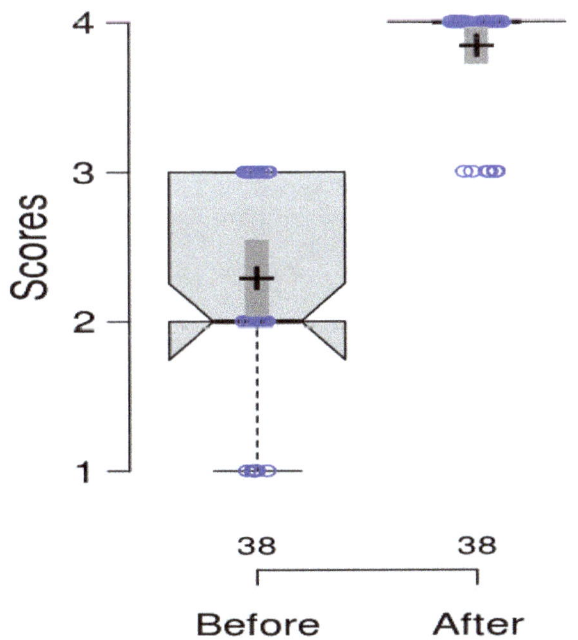

Fig. 1 Boxplots with notches corresponding to the scores developed through the surgeon questionnaire scale before and after the application of the CRS technique

The periodic apnea technique has been presented as useful during RIRS to minimize adverse motion of target organs [3]. This method uses preoxygenation with FiO_2 of 1.0, followed by a MV pause. The criterion for starting over the ventilation was the SpO_2 drop below 93%. However, there is a possible delay between the true SpO_2 drop and the pulse oximeter readings [16, 17]. Prolonged apnea leads to an inevitable hypercapnea which, in turn, results in adverse effects in patients with compromised cardiovascular status, increased intracranial pressure, metabolic acidosis or hyperkalemia [18]. The hypoxemia tolerance varies highly depending on the patient's individual condition. SpO_2 decrease is usually accompanied by a compensatory circulatory system response, which requires shorter ventilation pauses in aged patients, while younger patients can tolerate up to 6 min apnea [19].

Abdominal compression in the form of belts or plates was previously described in SWL. Belt compression in a group of 50 patients provided reduction of the kidney motion amplitude by an average of 32% detected by fluoroscopy control [20]. Plate compression in a group of 10 volunteers and 10 patients reduced kidney motion by 4 mm on average and increased SWL efficacy by 23% detected by ultrasound control [10]. Currently, no information regarding the applicability of abdominal compression in RIRS exists. The technique of general anesthesia with low ventilation (LV) was previously described by Kourmpetis et al. who suggested the following settings of GA during RIRS: respiratory rate ≤ 8/min and tidal volume < 500 ml [11]. According to the results of their study, LV was associated with better fragmentation, removal, and processing rates but not operating rate.

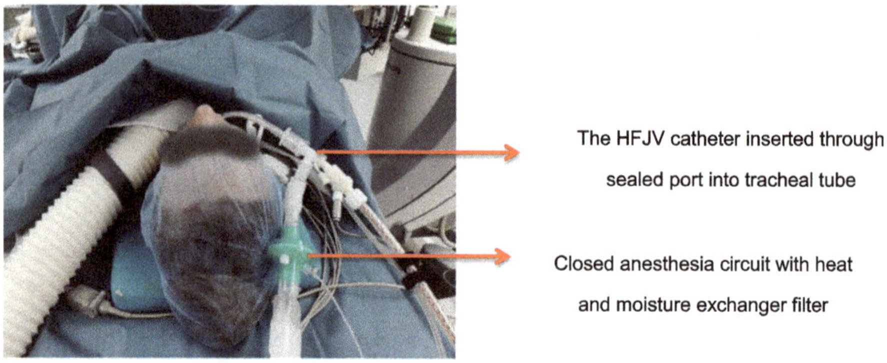

Fig. 2 Tubing and connections in CRS

Although end-tidal CO2 in the LV group was 50 mmHg this finding was not associated with clinical side effects. However, this level of end-tidal CO2 is defined as mild hypercapnia and may cause possible negative health consequences [21].

Our technique of combined two respiratory approaches, consisting of HFJV and SVMV, which thereby provided significantly better conditions for stone dusting assessed by expert urologists, all while precluding the development of hypercapnea. No CRS associated complications developed during or after the operation. In order to avoid any the following preventive measures were undertaken: the insufflation catheter was inserted through a sealed adapter into the tracheal tube thus, direct contact of the catheter with the trachea was excluded; development of tracheitis described in the literature is more attributed to the use of machines without gas conditioning option and the use of high pressure. We used "ZisLINEJV-100" machine with the air conditioning option and low working pressure of 0.3–0.6 bar; the heat and moisture exchanger filter was used in a closed respiratory circuit (Fig. 2).

Worth to mention disadvantages of CRS: expenditures associated with the cost of one insufflation catheter per patient; the necessity of purchasing HFJV machine; the inability to control the concentration of oxygen (FiO2) in some HFJV machines.

Our study has several limitations. First, our sample size was restricted to 38 patients. Despite this, we were able to demonstrate a statistically significant difference using the developed surgeon questionnaire scale; indicating that the use of CRS was beneficial. Secondly, our study lacks objective criteria for evaluation such as operating or fragmentation and dusting rates. However, we have deliberately simplified our study protocol due to the fact that variables such as fragmentation and dusting rates are inherently dependent on factors such as stone size, stone density, renal anatomy, the surgeon's expertise, where the main factor being assessed in this study was operative field stability. Lastly, we didn't corroborate our findings with the stone free rates of patients since we sought only to assess the feasibility and safety of reducing respiratory kidney motion and thus providing better conditions for intracorporeal lithotripsy. Due to the limitations of this pilot study, additional investigation will be needed to address the aforementioned concerns.

Conclusions

Our impression is that according to the urologist assessment the novel combined respiratory approach consisting of HFJV and SVMV provides better conditions for stone dusting through reduced respiratory kidney motion and is not associated with adverse health effects or complications. Further larger sample studies are needed to confirm these findings and elucidate its effect on stone free rates.

Abbreviations

CRS: Combined respiratory support; GA: General anesthesia; HFJV: High frequency jet ventilation; MV: Mechanical ventilation; PA: Periodic apnea; RIRS: Retrograde intrarenal surgery; SVMV: Small volume mechanical ventilation; SWL: Shockwave lithotripsy

Acknowledgements

Not applicable.

Authors' contributions

NG - Study conception & design and manuscript writing. UO - Study conception & design and manuscript writing. LK - Data collection and analysis. SPa - Study conception & design and manuscript writing. GA - Data collection and analysis. SPe - Study conception & design and manuscript writing. CMC - Manuscript writing and editing. ZO - Study conception & design, and manuscript writing. All authors read and approved the final manuscript.

Author details

[1]Department of Urology, Pavlov First Saint Petersburg State Medical University, Lva Tolstogo 17, Saint-Petersburg, Russian Federation197342. [2]Department of Anesthesiology, The Nikiforov Center of Emergency Medicine, Optikov 54, Saint-Petersburg, Russian Federation197448. [3]Department of Urology, Sechenov First Moscow State Medical University, Optikov 54, Saint-Petersburg, Russian Federation197448. [4]Department of Urology, University of California, Irvine, 333 City Boulevard West, Orange, CA 92868, USA.

References

1. Turk C, Petrik A, Sarica K, Seitz C, Skolarikos A, Straub M, Knoll T, Türk C, Knoll T, Petrik A. EAU Guidelines on Urolithiasis. Eur Assoc Urol. 2018;69(3):475–82.
2. Zeng G, Zhao Z, Yang F, Zhong W, Wu W, Chen W. Retrograde intrarenal surgery with combined spinal-epidural vs general anesthesia: a prospective randomized controlled trial. J Endourol. 2015;29(4):401–5.
3. Emiliani E, Talso M, Baghdadi M, Ghanem S, Golmard J, Pinheiro H, Gkentzis A, Butticè S, Traxer O. The use of apnea during Ureteroscopy. Urology. 2016;97:266–8.
4. Mucksavage P, Mayer WA, Mandel JE, Van Arsdalen KN. High-frequency jet ventilation is beneficial during shock wave lithotripsy utilizing a newer unit with a narrower focal zone. Can Urol Assoc J. 2010;4(5):333–5.
5. Galm En K, Harbut P, Freedman J, Jakobsson JG. High frequency jet ventilation for motion management during ablation procedures, a narrative review. Acta Anaesthesiol Scand. 2017;61(9):1066–74.
6. Skolarikos A, Gravas S, Laguna MP, Traxer O, Preminger GM, De La Rosette J. Training in ureteroscopy: a critical appraisal of the literature. BJU Int. 2011;108(6):798–805.
7. Hammer Ø, Harper DAT, Ryan PD. Paleontological statistics software package for education and data analysis. Palaeontol Electron. 2001;4:9–18.
8. Matlaga B, Chew B, Eisner B, Humphreys M, Knudsen B, Krambeck A, ... Shah O. Ureteroscopic Laser Lithotripsy: A Review of Dusting vs Fragmentation with Extraction. Journal of Endourology. 2018;32(1):1-6. https://doi.org/10.1089/end.2017.0641.
9. Sjöstrand U. Review of the physiological rationale for and development of high-frequency positive-pressure ventilation--HFPPV. Acta Anaesthesiol Scand Suppl. 1977;64:7–27.
10. Bohris C, Stief CG, Strittmatter F. Improvement of SWL efficacy: reduction of the respiration-induced kidney motion by using an abdominal compression plate. J Endourol. 2016;30(4):411–6.
11. Kourmpetis V, Dekalo S, Levy N, Nir T, Bar-Yosef Y, Beri A, Yossepowitch O, Sofer M. Toward respiratory-gated retrograde intrarenal surgery: a prospective controlled randomized study. J Endourol. 2018;32(9):1–19.
12. Galmén K, Harbut P, Freedman J, Jakobsson JG. The use of high-frequency ventilation during general anaesthesia: an update. F1000Research. 2017;6:756.
13. Warner MA, Warner ME, Buck CF, Segura JW. Clinical efficacy of high frequency jet ventilation during extracorporeal shock wave lithotripsy of renal and ureteral calculi: a comparison with conventional mechanical ventilation. J Urol. 1988;139(3):486–7.
14. Cormack JR, Hui R, Olive D, Said S. Comparison of two ventilation techniques during general anesthesia for extracorporeal shock wave lithotripsy: high-frequency jet ventilation versus spontaneous ventilation with a laryngeal mask airway. Urology. 2007;70(1):7–10.
15. Popiolek M, Al-Rammahi D, Swartz R. The impact of high frequency positive-pressure ventilation on operation time in retrograde intrarenal surgery for stones <1 cm. J Endourol 2017;31:MP3-17.
16. Smith RA, Fu ES, Downs JB, Schweiger JW, Miguel RV. Hypoventilation by Pulse Oximetry; 2008.
17. Cacho G, Pérez-Calle JL, Barbado A, Lledó JL, Ojea R, Fernández-Rodríguez CM. Capnography is superior to pulse oximetry for the detection of respiratory depression during colonoscopy. Rev Esp Enferm Dig. 2010;102(2):86–9.
18. Wong DT, Yee AJ, Leong SM, Chung F. The effectiveness of apneic oxygenation during tracheal intubation in various clinical settings: a narrative review. Can J Anesth Can d'anesthésie. 2017;64(4):416–27.
19. Ramkumar V, Umesh G, Philip FA. Preoxygenation with 20° head-up tilt provides longer duration of non-hypoxic apnea than conventional preoxygenation in non-obese healthy adults. J Anesth. 2011;25(2):189–94.
20. Honey RJD, Healy M, Yeung M, Psihramis KE, Jewett MAS. The use of an abdominal Compression Belt to reduce stone movement during extracorporeal shock wave lithotripsy. J Urol. 1992;148(3):1034–5.
21. Pantazopoulos C, Xanthos T, Pantazopoulos I, Papalois A, Kouskouni E, Iacovidou N. A review of carbon dioxide monitoring during adult cardiopulmonary resuscitation. Hear Lung Circ. 2015;24(11):1053–61.

18

Ureteric stent versus percutaneous nephrostomy for acute ureteral obstruction: Clinical outcome and quality of life

O. Shoshany[1,2*†], T. Erlich[2,3†], S. Golan[1,2], N. Kleinmann[2,3], J. Baniel[1,2], B. Rosenzweig[2,3], A. Eisner[2,3], Y. Mor[2,3], J. Ramon[2,3], H. Winkler[2,3] and D. Lifshitz[1,2]

Abstract

Background: To compare quality of life (QoL) indices between ureteral stent (DJS) and nephrostomy tube (PCN) inserted in the setting of acute ureteral obstruction.

Methods: Prospective bi-centered study. Over the span of 2 years, 45 DJS and 30 PCN patients were recruited. Quality of life was assessed by 2 questionnaires, EuroQol EQ-5D and 'Tube symptoms' questionnaire, at 2 time points (at discharge after drainage and before definitive treatment).

Results: Patients' demographics and pre-drainage data were similar. There were no clinically significant differences in patient's recovery between the groups, including post procedural pain, defeverence, returning to baseline renal function, and septic shock complications.

More DJS patients presented to the emergency room with complaints related to their procedure compared to PCN patients. At first, DJS patients complained more of urinary discomfort while PCN patients had worse symptoms relating to mobility and personal hygiene, with both groups achieving similar overall QoL score. At second time point, PCN patients' symptoms ameliorated while symptoms in the DJS group remained similar, translating to higher overall QoL score in the PCN group.

Conclusions: The two techniques had a distinct and significantly different impact on quality of life. Over time, PCN patients' symptoms relieve and their QoL improve, while DJS patients' symptoms persist. Specific tube related symptoms, and their dynamics over time, should be a major determinant in choosing the appropriate drainage method, especially when definitive treatment is not imminent.

Keywords: Double J stent, Nephrostomy tube, Acute ureteral obstruction, Quality of life

Background

The decision which drainage method, when indicated, should be used in a patient presenting with an obstructing ureteral stone is significantly influenced by the clinician's and patient's perception of the risks, complexity and quality of life (QoL) issues related to the different drainage methods. In certain health systems, such as the public health system in Israel, the waiting time for stone removal surgery is long. We often observed that an expected long period time for definitive treatment biased the treating urologist to prefer a ureteral stent over a nephrostomy tube, assuming the patient would be less bothered by the stent during the waiting period. There are few studies comparing the efficacy of ureteral double J stent (DJS) vs a percutaneous nephrostomy tube (PCN) in the setting of obstructive ureteral stones. Two prospective studies [1, 2], both published in 2001, incorporated QoL questionnaires

* Correspondence: ohadsh10@gmail.com

Shoshany O and Erlich T are authors consider that the first two authors should be regarded as joint First Authors

†O. Shoshany and T. Erlich contributed equally to this work.

[1]Urology Department, Rabin Medical Center, Hasharon Hospital, 7 Keren Kayemet St, 49372 Petah Tikva, Israel

[2]Sackler School of medicine, Tel Aviv University, Tel Aviv, Israel

Full list of author information is available at the end of the article

and compared patients' perception of the two drainage methods while awaiting definitive stone treatment. The results of these studies are not conclusive regarding the gross impact of each drainage method on the patient's QoL. The study by Joshi et al. [1] was conducted at a single time point, upon patients' admission for lithotripsy. No significant difference was found in the overall health state, suggesting similar patient's preference for either modality treatment. Conversely, in the study by Mokhmalji et al. [2] QoL was assessed at two time points, immediately following drainage and 2–4 weeks thereafter. Although not statistically significant, a tendency in favor of PCN was evident, particularly in males and patients younger than 40. The QoL progressively improved in the PCN group but deteriorated in the DJS group. Another recent prospective non-randomized study [3] evaluated QoL before and after the drainage procedure. DJS patients demonstrated worse QoL after drainage while PCN patients had similar ratings. DJS patients had worse urinary symptoms and a higher need of painkillers as well. Likewise, in a prospective study, albeit in a different setting, comparing nephrostomy vs ureteral stent following percutaneous nephrolithotomy (PCNL), Zhao et al. [4] found that despite the literature advocating "tubeless" PCNL, the QoL is significantly worse with stent placement in comparison to nephrostomy drainage. Similarly, Jiang et al. [5] compared PCN, an open-ended ureteral catheter and a DJS following PCNL, and found that patients in the first two groups reported a better QoL. Contrarily, in the setting of malignant obstruction, similar QoL was achieved in both PCN and DJS groups [6].

The aim of the present study was to evaluate whether these two renal drainage techniques truly have similar impact on the patient's QoL, in the setting of acute ureteral obstruction, and whether their effect changes over time during the waiting period for definitive treatment. Such data is important for the shared decision between the physician and the patient as to the preferred drainage technique.

Methods

Over a 2 year period, 75 consecutive patients presenting to the emergency room of two hospitals with an obstructing ureteral stone necessitating drainage were asked to participate in this study by an on-call urologist involved in the study. Estimated recruitment rate was 42%. The study is an Institutional Review Board approved, bi-center, prospective study comparing the impact on QoL of PCN and retrograde ureteral catheterization. Patients were offered renal drainage when definitive therapy was not available immediately or was contraindicated and when a two-stage procedure was considered a safer approach. Entry criteria included an obstructing ureteral stone with either fever (> 38°c), acute renal failure (estimated glomerular filtration rate [eGFR] ≤ 60 ml/min) or intractable pain. Diagnosis of the obstructing ureteral stone was made by either a non-contrast CT or a combination of renal ultrasound and abdominal X-ray. Exclusion criteria were age < 18 years, pregnant women and patients with a contraindications to either form of drainage (e.g. uncorrected coagulopathy excluding percutaneous drainage, hemodynamic instability precluding anesthesia required for DJS placement, or abnormalities of the urinary tract). Patients received either a DJS or a PCN according to the surgeon's preference. Practical issues such as the availability of an operating room or the interventional radiologist often dictated the choice of drainage, particularly in patients with fever as it is our policy to reduce time to drainage to the minimum in this high risk group.

PCN was performed in the angiographic suite by certified interventional radiologists. Local anesthesia (1% Lidocaine, 5–10 cc) was used routinely and when required additional parenteral analgesia with Meperidine (50-75 mg) and Midazolam (3 mg) was administrated. A percutaneous pigtail polyurethane 8.5-french, 25 cm catheter (Cook medical) was used. Ureteral stents were placed by the urologist in the operating room under general anesthesia. Initially, a guide wire was inserted into the kidney followed by a ureteral 5FR catheter. A urine culture was taken and contrast was injected at the same volume that was withdrawn for urine culture. Finally, a 6 FR, Percuflex (Boston Scientific) stent of the appropriate length was used. Most commonly, stent length of 24 to 28 cm was utilized. The ureteral length between the ureteropelvic and ureterovesical junctions was determined either by preoperative CT or by intraoperative retrograde and ureteral catheter placement.

Demographic and preoperative data were obtained included age, gender, body mass index (BMI), baseline and post drainage eGFR, urine culture and stone parameters. Post-procedural pain was measured on the day of the procedure, using a verbal visual analogue scale (VAS). QoL was assessed twice: at post-operative day 1–2 ("time 0") and at the day of (prior to) definitive treatment ("time 1"). Patients were requested to fill out two dedicated questionnaires: EuroQol EQ-5D and a 'Tube symptoms' questionnaire. EuroQol EQ-5D is a validated tool of general health assessment, consisting of 5 QoL questions and a thermometer indicating general well-being [1, 7]. A higher questionnaire score is associated with lower QoL, while a higher thermometer score is associated with better QoL. The 'Tube symptoms' questionnaire was based on several of the questions in the "Intervention-specific" questionnaire described by Joshi [8] with some modifications to allow uniformity of the questions between the groups. For example, patients were not asked about 'urine incontinence' or 'Bag leak/ slippage'. Alternatively, they were asked about 'personal hygiene problems' due to indwelling tube. The modified questionnaire includes six questions regarding pain, analgesics use, hematuria, urinary discomfort, discomfort associated with movement, and discomfort associated with personal hygiene. Answers to these questions were based on a four-point rating scale, and a higher score is associated with worse symptoms (see Additional file 1).

Statistical analysis

The association between different groups was assessed using the chi-square, 2-tailed Student t test and Mann-Whitney U tests, as appropriate. All statistical tests were 2-sided and for all comparisons $P < 0.05$ was considered significant. Statistical analysis was done using SPSS®, version 20.0.

Results

Pretreatment parameters

Overall, 45 patients underwent a DJS insertion and 30 patients had PCN drainage. Patients' demographics and pre-drainage data are presented in Table 1. Pretreatment differences in age, male to female ratio, and BMI were not significant. Stone parameters were also comparable, and the proportion of stone location (either proximal or distal ureter) was similar between the groups ($p > 0.05$). There were no cases of bilateral treatment. The indications for drainage were similar between the groups. Patients presenting with acute renal failure amounted to 57.8% in the DJS group and 60% in the PCN group. The only significant difference between the groups was pre-drainage eGFR: patients in the PCN group were found to have lower baseline eGFR and lower eGFR at presentation. Patients with fever had median temperatures of 38.1°c (range 38–39.5 °c) and 38.6 °c (range 38–39.6 °c) in the DJS and PCN groups, respectively.

Table 1 Patients' characteristics and outcomes

	DJS ($n = 45$)	PCN ($n = 30$)	p value
Pre-drainage patients' characteristics			
Age (years)	55 (39.5–70.5)	54 (46.5–61)	0.787
Gender- Female	15 (33%)	13 (43%)	0.467
BMI (kg/m^2)	27.6 (24.8–30.1)	27.7 (23.3–31)	0.944
Hypertension	24 (53.3%)	13 (43.3%)	0.683
Diabetes mellitus	14 (31.1%)	7 (23.3%)	0.622
Ischemic heart disease	8 (17.7%)	7 (23.3%)	0.775
Previous endourological procedures	14 (31.1%)	9 (30%)	1
Baseline eGFR (MDRD, mL/min/1.73 m^2)	85.5 (69.3–90.6)	69 (58.1–80.4)	**0.001**
eGFR at presentation (MDRD, mL/min/1.73 m^2)	60.3 (41.3–75.6)	41.2 (33–59)	**0.011**
Positive urine cultures	25.6%	40.7%	0.199
Indication for drainage – Fever≥30°c	15 (33.3%)	16 (53.3%)	0.099
Indication for drainage - Renal Failure (eGFR≤60 mL/min/1.73 m^2)	10 (22.2%)	10 (33.3%)	0.301
Stone diameter (mm)	8 (7–11)	8 (6–12.3)	0.872
Stone location-Proximal	55%	64%	0.469
Stone location-Distal	45%	36%	0.469
Post drainage outcomes			
Post procedure hospitalization Days	1 (1–3)	4 (2–6)	**< 0.001**
Post Procedural Pain (VAS)	1.02 ± 2.04	1.19 ± 1.52	0.283
Days to baseline eGFR [@]	1 (1–2)	2 (1–3)	**0.005**
Days to Temp ≤37.5 [@@]	1 (1–1.5)	1 (1–1.75)	1
Time to WBC ≤10,000 white blood cells per microliter (Days) [@@@]	1.5 (1–2)	2 (1–4)	0.167
Complications 1st procedure	6 (11%)	1 (3.3%)	0.226
Time from 1st to 2nd operation (Days)	47 (29–71)	20 (12–27)	**< 0.001**

Data presented as Median (IQR 25–75) or Mean ± STD as appropriate
MDRD The Modification of Diet in Renal Disease Study equation
[@] For patients with renal failure at presentation
[@@] For patients with fever at presentation
[@@@] For patients with leukocytosis at presentation
In bold - statistically significant result

Post-treatment parameters

Post renal drainage outcomes are presented in Table 1. Post procedural pain was similar in both groups as measured with VAS. The median length to defeverence was 1 day in both groups, while the median length of white blood count (WBC) normalization was 1.5 and 2 days, respectively. Three patients in the DJS group and one patient in the PCN group developed post drainage septic shock ($p = 0.646$). The median time to baseline eGFR level was found to be significantly higher in the PCN group (1 and 2 days respectively, $p < 0.01$). After discharge, none of the patients required readmission to the hospital. Although not statistically significant, more DJS patients presented to the emergency room with complaints related to their procedure compared to PCN patients (20% vs. 3.7% respectively, $p = 0.056$), mostly complaining of flank pain and dysuria. During the study period there were no cases of failed procedures or conversion from one technique to the other, and post-procedural complication rate was similar between the groups. The majority of patients in both groups underwent ureteroscopy as the definitive procedure. The length of time between the urgent drainage procedure and the definitive procedure was significantly higher in the DJS group compared to the PCN group (median 47 vs. 20 days respectively, $p < 0.001$).

Quality of life results

'Tube symptoms' questionnaire

Table 2 details the patients' scores in the 'Tube symptoms' questionnaire at time0 (shortly after the drainage procedure) and time1 (presenting for their definitive procedure). For each symptom, data is presented as percentage of patients reporting the presence of the symptom and an estimation of the frequency of the symptom using a 4 points scale. At both time points, the two groups reported similar pain, analgesics use, and presence of hematuria. However, other domains were remarkably different between the two groups. At time0, DJS patients had significantly higher urinary discomfort. Symptoms in this domain were much more prevalent and frequent compared to PCN patients. Pronounced urinary discomfort persisted in the DJS group, remaining significantly higher than the PCN group at time1. On the other hand, PCN patients had worse symptoms relating to mobility and personal hygiene. However, the severity of these symptoms decreased over time, and at time1 there were no significant differences between the groups in these domains. Interestingly, women reported using pain killers more frequently at time0 in both groups ($p = 0.022$ and $p = 0.04$ for DJS & PCN respectively), but not at time1.

EQ-5D questionnaire

EQ-5D questionnaire outcomes are presented in Table 3. At time0, PCN patients demonstrated more difficulties to self-care and resume usual activities ($p < 0.05$). Twice as many PCN patients reported difficulties in mobility compared to DJS patients, which was in accordance with the 'Tube symptoms' questionnaire results, but this did not reach statistical significance (16.6% vs. 34.5% for the DJS and PCN groups respectively, $p > 0.05$). In league with the trend observed in the 'Tube symptoms' questionnaire, symptoms which were higher in PCN patients decreased over time, and at time1 we observed no significant difference in patients' estimation of their ability to self-care or perform usual activities. Additionally, more DJS patients reported anxiety or depressed mood compared to PCN patients (19.4% vs. 0%, $p < 0.05$). It is important to note that both procedures caused pain or discomfort to a large portion of patients in both groups at both time points: 47.6% vs. 53.6% at time0 and 67.7% vs. 42.9% at time1, respectively. These proportions were not significantly different, although there were opposing trends in the different groups: over time the number of patients complaining about pain increased in the DJS-treated group, and decreased in the PCN-treated group. While in the PCN group there were no differences between the genders, in the DJS group women scored worse in the self-care domain at time0 ($p = 0.025$), and in pain / discomfort domain at both time points ($p = 0.049$ & $p = 0.048$ at time0 & time1, respectively).

On comparison of the thermometer rating (Table 3), representing overall health state as assessed subjectively

Table 2 QoL outcomes - 'Tube symptoms' questionnaire

	At discharge after urgent drainage						Upon arrival for definitive stone treatment					
	DJS		PCN		p value		DJS		PCN		p value	
Q1 Pain	45.5%	1.73 ± 0.94	48.3%	1.83 ± 1	1	0.755	76.7%	2.13 ± 0.9	50%	1.73 ± 0.88	0.076	0.082
Q2 Need of analgesia	40.1%	1.55 ± 0.74	62.1%	1.86 ± 0.79	0.164	0.138	50%	1.8 ± 1	40.1%	1.59 ± 0.85	0.581	0.461
Q3 Urinary discomfort	80.1%	2.71 ± 1.1	31%	1.59 ± 0.98	**0.0006**	**< 0.001**	80.6%	2.55 ± 1.06	45.5%	1.91 ± 1.15	**0.017**	**0.034**
Q4 Hematuria	54.5%	2 ± 1.15	37.9%	1.62 ± 0.9	0.268	0.216	48.4%	1.87 ± 1.02	27.3%	1.45 ± 0.91	0.159	0.104
Q5 Mobility	42.9%	1.71 ± 0.96	86.2%	2.66 ± 1.04	**0.0019**	**0.002**	32.3%	1.55 ± 0.89	45.5%	1.82 ± 1.05	0.395	0.317
Q6 Personal hygiene	33.3%	1.43 ± 0.68	60.7%	2.18 ± 1.09	0.084	**0.014**	25.8%	1.35 ± 0.66	40.1%	1.77 ± 1.07	0.371	0.155

Data presented as percentage of symptomatic patients (reporting any symptoms) and frequency score as reported using a 4 points scale
In bold - statistically significant result

Table 3 QoL outcomes - EQ-5D questionnaire

	At discharge after urgent drainage			At definitive stone treatment		
	DJS	PCN	p value	DJS	PCN	*p* value
Q1 Mobility	16.60%	34.50%	0.102	25.80%	18.20%	0.51
Q2 Self-care	7.10%	37.90%	**0.004**	9.70%	9.10%	0.944
Q3 Usual activities	19%	57.70%	**0.005**	38.70%	28.60%	0.39
Q4 Pain/discomfort	47.60%	53.60%	0.632	67.70%	42.90%	0.082
Q5 Anxiety/depression	35.70%	20.70%	0.199	19.40%	0%	**0.012**
"Health state" score	72.6 ± 22	68.6 ± 20	0.44	68.6 ± 25	83.2 ± 12.1	**0.016**

In bold - statistically significant result

by the patients, scores were similar in both groups at time0 (72.6 ± 22 vs. 68.6 ± 20, $p > 0.05$). In line with other reported QoL assessments, DJS patients score deteriorated over time, and they had a significant lower score compared to PCN patients at time1 (68.6 ± 25 vs. 83.2 ± 12.1 respectively, $p < 0.05$). On univariate analysis, drainage by PCN method, higher age, and decreased length of time to definitive procedure, were associated (all $p < 0.05$) with higher thermometer rating score at time1 (measured at presentation for definitive procedure). BMI, gender, mean thermometer score at time0, post-procedural pain, previous endourological procedure, stone load, and length of hospitalization were not associated with overall health score at time1. On multivariate analysis, no variable remained significantly associated with time1 overall health score.

Discussion

Urgent decompression of obstructed collecting systems due to a ureteral calculus is a daily practice in every urology department in cases of infection, renal failure or intractable pain. Despite the commonness of this situation, there are only a few studies comparing renal drainage methods, including clinical and QoL aspects [1–3, 9, 10]. This study prospectively compared 45 DJS procedures to 30 PCN procedures. Selection criteria ensured that all patients were potential candidates for both procedures, and analysis revealed similar patients' characteristics in both groups. QoL was evaluated with EuroQol EQ-5D and a 'Tube symptoms' questionnaire at two time points, in order to evaluate symptoms dynamics over time.

Clinical course

In face of opposing results in former studies [1, 2], we found no distinct difference in post-procedural in-hospital pain, with patients in both groups reporting low VAS scores. The finding of higher post-operative pain for DJS in Mokhmalji et al. study [2] might be explained by the fact that retrograde placement was achieved by using a rigid cystoscope with prior transurethral administration of local anesthetic sedation, and had a 80% success rate. Procedure complication rate was also comparable between the methods, and consistent with other reports [11]. Ramsey at el. [11] reported in their review that there appears little evidence to suggest that retrograde stent insertion leads to increased bacteremia or is significantly more hazardous in the setting of acute obstruction. In league with this report, few patients at each group developed post drainage sepsis, with no clear advantage for any method. Moreover, post procedural recuperation was equivalent in both groups, as supported by similar time to defeverence and time of leukocytosis returning to normal range. However, it should be mentioned that we excluded patients presenting with septic complications or shock, which may benefit from PCN drainage in comparison to DJS. Although time of eGFR return to baseline was found to be longer in the PCN group vs. the DJS group (2 days vs. 1 day respectively), this finding could be explained by the lower baseline eGFR of the PCN group, and is probably not clinically significant. The longer hospitalization is probably associated with a slower recovery to baseline GFR in the PCN group, as patients were kept under observation to assess the kidney recovery. The apparent difference in time to second procedure was also noted in other studies [2]. DJS patients were summoned for their definitive treatment approximately twice as long as the nephrostomy patients. This substantial difference can be explained to some extent by a misguided perception that a patient with a DJS is less debilitated compared to a patient with a nephrostomy tube (an apparent external tube). Overall, our study supports similar clinical outcomes in both drainage methods.

Quality of life

QoL outcomes in our study corresponded well with the only other prospective study comparing QoL at two time points after urgent renal drainage [2]. Both procedures caused pain or discomfort to a significant amount of patients. While the number of PCN patients complaining of pain remained similar over time, and analgesic use even lowered, more patients in the DJS group reported of pain, and analgesics use grew in prevalence and frequency as well. Clearly, the most troublesome symptoms in the DJS group are the urinary bother symptoms [3, 12]. These symptoms inflicted 80% of the patients in our DJS study group, much more frequent compared to other symptoms. Furthermore, there was no alleviation over time, the prevalence and severity of these symptoms did not change, translating to a higher number of emergency room visits. In distinct opposition, PCN patients suffered at first mostly from discomfort involving "movement", "self-care" and "personal hygiene". However, over time, these patients adjusted to the nephrostomy tube. The number of patients experiencing symptoms in these domains dropped by half, or more, reaching similar discomfort level with the DJS group at time1. These trends are manifested in the overall health state results. At first, both groups suffered from bothering symptoms, albeit different, amounting to similar overall disturbance. This result is corroborated by the recent study of de Sousa Morais N. et al [3]. Over time, PCN patients improved their symptoms, while DJS patients suffered similarly or worsened. This was reflected by significantly higher overall health state scores in the PCN group at time1. Of note, studies comparing PCN drainage vs DJS in other clinical scenarios [4, 5], such as following PCNL, also found that patients with DJS suffered significantly from pain and irritative symptoms that decreased the overall QoL. Interestingly, in the DJS group women reported higher level of pain / discomfort at both time points, and higher use of pain medications post operatively. In the PCN group, higher use of pain medications post operatively in women was also noted.

Is there a preferred approach for urgent decompression of obstructed collecting systems?

The decision on the appropriate method of drainage is multifactorial, including factors such as stone parameters, patient's characteristics, patient's and urologist preferences, the expected definitive approach for stone treatment and procedure availability. In their summary of 15 years outcomes, Goldsmith et al. [10] reported a tendency to prefer nephrostomy drainage in patients with larger stones and patients who are more acutely ill. Often, clinical judgment is exercised, and opinions may vary considerably [13]. When both procedures are available, and the patient is a potential candidate for either procedure, the expected clinical benefit and the expected QoL are major determinants in the decision. It appears that both methods result in similar good clinical result, with no significant benefit for the one over the other. Thus, the implications of the drainage on patient's QoL should not be overlooked or disregarded, but rather become a factor in the decision on the preferred rout. A thorough discussion with the patient is extremely important, explaining the pros and cons of each procedure, not only clinically, but of what is expected regarding tube symptoms and QoL. In general, for proximal ureteral stones the advantages of pre-stenting probably outweigh the discomfort associated with the stent. However, for patients with a distal ureteral stone requiring drainage, a nephrostomy tube may be the best choice as it would allow possible spontaneous passage and would avoid the stent discomfort.

There are several limitations to our study. The "tube symptoms" questionnaire was based on a validated DJS symptoms questionnaire, adjusted to be relevant for both DJS and PCN groups, but was not validated in itself or to local language, and might induce recall bias. As both hospitals are public, at no cost to the patient, procedural or hospitalization cost did not introduce bias. However, selection bias may have been introduced through choice of drainage procedure according to surgeon's preference, recruitment rate, possibly influenced by severity of eGFR, hydronephrosis, or other unmeasured parameters. Therefore patients suspected of long standing impaction probably had a higher chance of receiving a PCN, thus explaining the lower GFR in this group. Furthermore, as different imaging modalities were used, we could not assess hydronephrosis severity as a possible confounder. Finally, we did not assess a third time point, after tube removal, to confirm symptoms resolution. Nevertheless, we believe our study, supported by other past reports, demonstrate an overlooked truth. To quote Dr. Louis R Kavoussi [14], "Traditionally, urologists have placed stents because ... that's what we do", but his experience is that "patients are more comfortable with a nephrostomy than a stent". Interestingly, superior QoL of PCN over DJS placed after PCNL was also recently reported [4, 5]. The results of this study support superior QoL of nephrostomy tube over time, and may cause some urologists to reconsider their choice of renal drainage, especially in health systems in which definitive treatment might be delayed. Undoubtedly, the specific tube symptoms, and their influence of the patient over time, should be given a serious consideration in the deliberation for the right drainage method for a specific patient.

Conclusions

No significant clinical difference was found in the outcomes and morbidity indices, in a prospective comparison between retrograde and antegrade renal drainage approaches in cases of acute ureteral obstruction by stone. The two techniques had a distinct and significantly different impact on quality of life. However, post-drainage symptoms improved with time only in patients treated with PCN. At the time of definite treatment, nephrostomy patients had significantly higher overall health state scores. Specific tube related symptoms, and their dynamics over time, should be a major determinant in choosing the appropriate drainage method, especially when definitive treatment is not imminent.

Additional file

Additional file 1: Tube symptoms questionnaire. (DOCX 12 kb)

Abbreviations

BMI: Body mass index; DJS: Ureteral double J stent; eGFR: Estimated glomerular filtration rate; PCN: Percutaneous nephrostomy tube; PCNL: Percutaneous nephrolithotomy; QoL: Quality of life; VAS: Visual analogue scale

Acknowledgements

We thank Tzippy Shochat for her assistance with the statistical analysis.

Authors' contributions

OS made substantial contributions to the conception and design of the study, participated in the acquisition, analysis, and interpretation of data, and drafted the paper. TE participated in the acquisition, analysis, and interpretation of data, and substantively revised the paper. SG made substantial contributions to the conception and design of the study and substantively revised the paper. NK made substantial contributions to the conception and design of the study, participated in the acquisition of data, and substantively revised the paper. JB participated in the acquisition of data, and substantively revised the paper. BR participated in the acquisition, analysis, and interpretation of data, and substantively revised the paper. AE participated in the acquisition, analysis, and interpretation of data, and substantively revised the paper. YM participated in the acquisition, analysis, and interpretation of data, and substantively revised the paper. JR participated in the acquisition, analysis, and interpretation of data, and substantively revised the paper. HW made substantial contributions to the conception and design of the study, participated in the acquisition, analysis, and interpretation of data, and substantively revised the paper. DL made substantial contributions to the conception and design of the study, participated in the acquisition, analysis, and interpretation of data, and substantively revised the paper.

All authors read and approved the final manuscript.

Author details

[1]Urology Department, Rabin Medical Center, Hasharon Hospital, 7 Keren Kayemet St, 49372 Petah Tikva, Israel. [2]Sackler School of medicine, Tel Aviv University, Tel Aviv, Israel. [3]Urology Department, Chaim Sheba Medical Center, Ramat Gan, Israel.

References

1. Joshi HB, Adams S, Obadeyi OO, Rao PN. Nephrostomy tube or 'JJ' ureteric stent in ureteric obstruction. Assessment of patient perspectives using quality-of-life survey and utility analysis. Eur Urol. 2001;39:695.
2. Mokhmalji H, Braun PM, Martinez Portillo FJ, Siegsmund M, Alken P, Köhrmann KU. Percutaneous nephrostomy versus ureteral stents for diversion of hydronephrosis caused by stones: a prospective, randomized clinical trial. J Urol. 2001;165:1088.
3. de Sousa Morais N, Pereira JP, Mota P, Carvalho-Dias E, Torres JN, Lima E. Percutaneous nephrostomy vs ureteral stent for hydronephrosis secondary to ureteric calculi: impact on spontaneous stone passage and health-related quality of life-a prospective study. Urolithiasis. 2018. https://doi.org/10.1007/s00240-018-1078-2 Epub ahead of print.
4. Zhao PT, Hoenig DM, Smith AD, Okeke Z. A randomized controlled comparison of nephrostomy drainage vs ureteral stent following percutaneous Nephrolithotomy using the Wisconsin StoneQOL. J Endourol. 2016;30(12):1275–84.
5. Jiang H, Huang D, Yao S, Liu S. Improving drainage after percutaneous Nephrolithotomy based on health-related quality of life: a prospective randomized study. J Endourol. 2017;31(11):1131–8.
6. Monsky WL, Molloy C, Jin B, Nolan T, Fernando D, Loh S, et al. Quality-of life assessment after palliative interventions to manage malignant ureteral obstruction. Cardiovasc Intervent Radiol. 2013;36(5):1355–63.
7. Rabin R, de Charro F. EQ-5D: a measure of health status from the EuroQol group. Ann Med. 2001;33:337.
8. Joshi HB, Newns N, Stainthorpe A, MacDonagh RP, Keeley FX Jr, Timoney AG. Ureteral stent symptom questionnaire: development and validation of a multidimensional quality of life measure. J Urol. 2003;169:1060.
9. Pearle MS, Pierce HL, Miller GL, Summa JA, Mutz JM, Petty BA, et al. Optimal method of urgent decompression of the collecting system for obstruction and infection due to ureteral calculi. J Urol. 1998;160:1260.
10. Goldsmith ZG, Oredein-McCoy O, Gerber L, Bañez LL, Sopko DR, Miller MJ, et al. Emergent ureteric stent vs percutaneous nephrostomy for obstructive urolithiasis with sepsis: patterns of use and outcomes from a 15-year experience. BJU Int. 2013;112:E122.
11. Ramsey S, Robertson A, Ablett MJ, Meddings RN, Hollins GW, Little B, et al. Evidence-based drainage of infected hydronephrosis secondary to ureteric calculi. J Endourol. 2010;24:185.
12. Dellis A, Joshi HB, Timoney AG, Keeley FX Jr. Relief of stent related symptoms: review of engineering and pharmacological solutions. J Urol. 2010;184:1267.
13. Lynch MF, Anson KM, Patel U. Current opinion amongst radiologists and urologists in the UK on percutaneous nephrostomy and ureteric stent insertion for acute renal unobstruction: results of a postal survey. BJU Int. 2006;98:1143.
14. Practice update, comment by Kavoussi, L. R. 2016: http://www.practiceupdate.com/content/inferior-wisconsin-stoneqol-results-observed-with-ureteral-stent-vs-nephrostomy-drainage-following-percutaneous-nephrolithotomy/47216, Accessed 21 July 2018.

Practice patterns of ureteral access sheath during ureteroscopy for nephrolithiasis: A survey among endourologists worldwide

Dorit Esther Zilberman*, Alon Lazarovich, Harry Winkler and Nir Kleinmann

Abstract

Background: The use of ureteral access sheath (UAS) during ureteroscopy is controversial. We aimed to explore practice patterns of UAS during ureteroscopy for nephrolithiasis among endourologists worldwide.

Methods: A 15-question survey was designed using the SurveyMonkey® platform. The questions covered the background and professional experience of the potential respondents, indications for UAS insertion, UAS caliber and possible complications associated with its use.
The questions were anonymously tabulated in order to determine practice patterns of UAS during ureteroscopy for nephrolithiasis among endourologists.
The survey was then distributed via e-mail to all the Endourological Society members.

Results: 216 members responded. 99.53% of the respondents practice as endourologists, 63.4% are fellowship trained and 74.4% are at least 6 years post-fellow. 73.2% practice in an academic facility. 77.3% perform at least 100 ureteroscopies annually. 46 and 76% routinely use UAS for the treatment of ureteral and kidney stones, respectively. In both cases, the 12/14 access sheath is the most common. 42% use UAS in primary ureteroscopy. 90.3% believe that a double J stent insertion is not mandatory prior to UAS insertion. 79.1% think the use of UAS does not increase postoperative complications rate, and if the latter does encounter, then most likely it is either a ureteral stricture (93.2%) or pain (48%).

Conclusions: UAS is commonly used by highly skilled endourologists during ureteroscopy. 12/14 UAS is mostly used. Ureteral stricture and post-operative pain are proposed as possible complications following UAS introduction, however pre-stenting is not mandatory as overall low complication rate is expected.

Keywords: Endourology, Nephrolithiasis, Practice patterns, Ureteral access sheath, Ureteroscopy

Background

The ureteral access sheath (UAS) was first introduced in 1974 [1]. The stiff and hollow tube that literally paved the road to the upper urinary tract had carried the promise to smoother and easier surgical manipulations in a territory considered by then as difficult to inspect.

Despite its tremendous potential, an ongoing controversy still exists in the literature as regards to UAS safety and necessity during ureteroscopy.

* Correspondence: dorit1e@yahoo.com
Department of Urology , Chaim Sheba Medical Center, Affiliated to Sackler School of Medicine, Tel-Aviv University, Tel-Hashomer, Ramat-Gan, 52621 Tel-Aviv, Israel

The supporters, on one hand, point out its advantages, such as: better visibility [2], increased stone free rates (SFR) [3], decreased likelihood of infection [4] and bleeding [5], decreased intra-pelvic irrigation pressure [6–8], decreased wear of the flexible ureteroscope [2, 9] and shortening of total operative time [10].

The critics, on the other hand, emphasize traumatic insertion and the pressure the UAS poses over the ureteric tissue that in turn may result in ischemic injury and ureteric strictures [11–14].

Moreover, per their doctrine, UAS has no influence neither on SFR [4, 15] nor on total operative time [4]. However, it might contribute to higher rates of postoperative complications [16] and longer hospital stay [4].

In light of this controversy we sought to explore practice patterns of ureteral access sheath during ureteroscopy for nephrolithiasis among endourologists worldwide.

Methods

The current urological literature regarding UAS utilization was reviewed.

A 15-question survey was then designed using the SurveyMonkey® platform to cover practice patterns and known controversies which currently exist as regards to the application of UAS during ureteroscopy.

The questionnaire entitled " Practice Patterns Of Ureteral Access Sheath During Ureteroscopy For Nephrolithiasis", consisted of multi-choice answers varied between 2 (i.e: yes/no) to 5 answers options. In one question the respondents were allowed to check more than one box.

The questions covered the background and professional experience of the potential respondents, indications for UAS insertion, UAS caliber and possible complications associated with its insertion.

The questions were anonymously tabulated in order to determine practice patterns of UAS during ureteroscopy among endo-urologists.

The survey was subsequently distributed with the assistance of the Endourological Society office via e-mail to all the Endourological Society members.

Descriptive statistics and survey analysis were executed using the SurveyMonkey® platform.

If a respondent skipped a question, the response for that question was not included in the analysis.

Results

Out of estimated 2000 registered Endourological Society members who received the questionnaire, 216 responded.

Questions and responses are detailed in Table 1.

99.53% of the respondents practice as endourologists, almost two thirds of whom are fellowship trained endourologists and 74.4% are at least 6 years post-fellow. 73.2% practice in an academic facility, either in a university hospital or both university hospital and private practice.

77.3% perform at least 100 ureteroscopies annually.

Almost 46% routinely use UAS for the treatment of ureteral stone, and the rate further increases into 75.7% when it comes to treating kidney stones.

In both cases, the 12/14 access sheath is the most common (44.5 and 46%, respectively).

42% use UAS in primary ureteroscopy. 90.3% believe that a double J stent insertion is not mandatory prior to UAS insertion.

79.1% believe the application of UAS does not increase postoperative complications rate, and if the latter does occur, then most likely it is either a ureteral stricture (93.2%) or pain (48%).

Discussion

In 2007, Auge et al. distributed a 26-question survey to 570 urologists worldwide [17]. The aim of the survey was to assess practice patterns of ureteral stenting after routine ureteroscopic stone surgery.

Of the 173 respondents, only 21% dilated the ureteral orifice 90% of the time, and only 34.5% of those who did so used an access sheath either alone or in combination with ureteral balloon.

Clearly, ever since that time the endourology has become an established sub specialty, and the penetrance of designated devices has increased accordingly.

The present survey reflects highly skilled and trained endourologists:

99% of the respondents define themselves as endourologists; 63% graduated an established endourology fellowship program; most respondents have at least 6 years post-fellow seniority; 73% are affiliated to academic centers and 77% maintain high annual volume of at least 100 procedures.

This highly skilled study population uses access sheath in higher percentages than described earlier: 46 and 76% use access sheath for ureteral stones and kidney stones treatment, respectively, rates that are even higher than the 67% reported elsewhere [4].

In a study evaluating different UASs available in the international market and their compatibility with different available flexible ureteroscopes, the 12/14 access sheath was found to be the device that accepts all scopes [18].

Another study assumed that this sheath decreases the likelihood of infection compared to smaller caliber UAS [5].

This may explain the popularity of the 12/14 UAS in the present survey, as 44.5 and 46% of the endourologists use it for the treatment of ureteral and kidney stones, respectively.

Apparently, the rate of UAS introduction in ureteral stones treatment is relatively low (42%). The present survey did not split stone location in accordance with different portions of the ureter. By doing so, we would have probably been seeing higher percentages of UAS introduction mainly for proximal ureteral stones treatment.

Yet, the relatively low popularity of the UAS for ureteral stone treatment can be explained by the small caliber semi-rigid ureteroscopes which currently exist in the market, that in turn enable atraumatic exploration of the ureter even in its upper portions.

The latter may also explain why 90.3% of the survey respondents believe pre-stenting prior to UAS introduction is not mandatory, a finding that stands in line with another study observation [4], whereby of the 1494 patients who underwent UAS introduction, only 36% were pre-stented.

Both the present study and Traxer et al. study [4] contradict other studies which support pre-stenting

Table 1 Survey's questions and responses

Q1: Do you practice as an Endourologist?		
Answer Choices	Responses	
Yes	99.53%	213
No	0.47%	1
Total		214
Q2: Are you a fellowship-trained Endourologist?		
Answer Choices	Responses	
Yes	63.43%	137
No	36.57%	79
Total		216
Q3: How many years have passed since you graduated from your fellowship?		
Answer Choices	Responses	
0–5	25.59%	54
6–10	17.54%	37
> 10	56.87%	120
Total		211
Q4: Where do you practice?		
Answer Choices	Responses	
University hospital	54.46%	116
Private practice	26.76%	57
Combination university hospital and private practice	18.78%	40
Total		213
Q5: What is your yearly volume of ureteroscopy?		
Answer Choices	Responses	
< 100	22.69%	49
100–199	33.33%	72
200–299	23.61%	51
300–400	12.96%	28
> 400	7.41%	16
Total		216
Q6: Do you routinely use ureteral access sheath (UAS) for the treatment of ureteral stones?		
Answer Choices	Responses	
Yes	45.83%	99
No	54.17%	117
Total		216
Q7: In what percentage of cases do you use UAS?		
Answer Choices	Responses	
0–20%	4.55%	5
20–40%	6.36%	7
40–60%	26.36%	29
60–80%	30.91%	34
80–100%	31.82%	35
Total		110
Q8: What is the UAS size that you commonly use?		
Answer Choices	Responses	
9.5/11.5 F	11.82%	13
10/12 F	26.36%	29
12/14 F	44.55%	49
14/16 F	2.73%	3
Other	14.55%	16
Total		110
Q9: Do you routinely use UAS for the treatment of kidney stones?		
Answer Choices	Responses	
Yes	75.71%	159
No	24.29%	51
Total		210
Q10: In what percentage of cases do you use UAS?		
Answer Choices	Responses	
0–20%	5.03%	8
20–40%	6.92%	11
40–60%	15.72%	25
60–80%	25.79%	41
80–100%	46.54%	74
Total		159
Q11: What is the UAS size that you commonly use?		
Answer Choices	Responses	
9.5/11.5 F	14.01%	22
10/12 F	24.2%	38
12/14 F	45.86%	72
14/16 F	4.46%	7
Other	11.46%	18
Total		157
Q12: Do you use UAS in primary ureteroscopy?		
Answer Choices	Responses	
Yes	42.03%	87
No	57.97%	120
Total		207
Q13: Is a double J stent insertion mandatory prior to UAS insertion?		
Answer Choices	Responses	
Yes	9.66%	20
No	90.34%	187
Total		207
Q14: Do you think the use of UAS increases complications rate?		
Answer Choices	Responses	
Yes	20.87%	43
No	79.13%	163
Total		206
Q15: Which of the following? (you can choose more than one)		
Answer Choices	Responses	
Ureteral strictures	93.18%	41
Hydronephrosis	13.64%	6
Infection	6.82%	3
Pain	47.73%	21
Total respondents: 44		

prior to ureteroscopy and UAS insertion in order to decrease the likelihood of ureteral injury [12] and UAS insertion failure rates [19–21].

Overall, 79% of the survey respondents believe UAS insertion does not increase post operative complications rate. When a complication arises, the highest likelihood it is of a stricture kind (93%).

Delvecchio et al. [14] reviewed ureteral stricture rates following UAS insertion in 62 patients with at least 3 months post-operative follow up. In this study, a 12/14 UAS was applied in 79% of the cases. Only one case demonstrated a UPJ stricture that was not attributed to the UAS. Their conclusion was, therefore, that large caliber UAS should be used with caution especially when long operative time and ureteric ischemic injury are expected.

Risk factors for ureteral wall injuries resulting from insertion of UAS during retrograde intrarenal surgery, as declared by one study [12] are as follows: older age, male gender, absent ureteral double J stenting before procedure.

Another potentially commom complication the respondents mentioned in the present survey was pain (48%).

Lildal et al. [11], in a benchtop trial, inserted UASs in 44 porcine ureters for 2 min on one side and for 2 h on the contra-lateral side.

The ureters were excised and tissue samples from the proximal and the distal ureters were detected for mRNA of the inflammatory mediators COX-2 and TNF-α.

After UAS insertion for 2 min, mRNA expression levels of COX-2 and TNF-α in the distal ureters increased 6.5 and 8 fold, respectively, and after 2 h the levels further increased to as high as 9 and 9.5 fold, respectively.

Expression levels were significantly higher in the distal than in the proximal portion of the UAS treated ureters, and significantly higher in UAS treated ureters compared to controls.

These findings may explain the relatively high percentage of supposedly pain in the survey, which presumably reflects individual observation and personal experience of each respondent with his or her own cases.

Over the past 15 years, the endourological field has been evidencing technological advancements that have led to the introduction of numerous devices with various physical properties, that have made the lives of many urologists worldwide easier.

The UAS, from this standpoint, is of no exception.

The present survey does not come up with substantial recommendations as regards to when and where to use UAS.

It does not define practice patterns of UAS in different parts of the world either.

Another limitations that should be mentioned are the relatively low response rate (10.8%) as well as unknown number of manufacturers and substances involved in UASs' production.

Notwithstanding, the additional scientific value of this survey is the contemporary perspective it provides as regards to UAS introduction among high number (the highest so far) of highly skilled endourologists.

Moreover, it emphasizes the significant role UAS plays in the urologists' current armamentarium.

Conclusions

UAS is commonly used by highly skilled endourologists during ureteroscopy. 12/14 UAS is mostly used. Ureteral stricture and post-operative pain are proposed as possible complications following UAS introduction, however pre stenting is not mandatory as an overall low complication rate is expected .

Abbreviations

SFR: Stone Free Rates; UAS: Ureteral Access Sheath; URS: Ureteroscopy

Acknowledgements

The authors would like to thank Mrs. Yvonne Telner for her valuable assistance in manuscript proofreading.

Authors' contributions

DEZ: Manuscript writing; AL: Data collection and analysis; HW: Manuscript review; NK: Study design and manuscript review. All authors read and approved the final manuscript.

References

1. Takayasu H, Aso Y. Recent development for pyeloureteroscopy: guide tube method for its introduction into the ureter. J Urol. 1974;112:176–8.
2. Breda A, Territo A, Lopez-Martinez JM. Benefits and risks of ureteral access sheaths for retrograde renal access. Curr Opin Urol. 2016;26:70–5.
3. L'esperance JO, Ekeruo WO, Scales CD, et al. Effect of ureteral access sheath on stone-free rates in patients undergoing ureteroscopic management of renal calculi. Urology. 2005;66(2):252–5.
4. Traxer O, Wendt-Nordahl G, Sodha H, et al. Differences in renal stone treatment and outcomes for patients treated either with or without the support of a ureteral access sheath: the clinical research office of the endourological society ureteroscopy global study. World J Urol. 2015;33: 2137–44.
5. Zhong W, Leto G, Wang L, et al. Systemic inflammatory response syndrome after flexible ureteroscopic lithotripsy: a study of risk factors. J Endourol. 2015;29:25–8.
6. Rehman J, Monga M, Landman J, et al. Characterization of intrapelvic pressure during ureteropyloscopy with ureteral access sheath. Urology. 2003;61(4):713–8.
7. Auge BK, Pietrow PK, Lallas CD, et al. Ureteral access sheath provides protection against elevated renal pressures during routine flexible ureteroscopic stone manipulation. J Endourol. 2004;18(1):33–6.
8. Monga M, Bodie J, Ercole B. Is there a role for small-diameter ureteral access sheaths? Impact on irrigant flow and intrapelvic pressures. Urology. 2004; 64(3):439–41.
9. De Coninck V, Keller EX, Rodríguez-Monsalve M, et al. Systemic review of ureteral access sheaths: facts and myths. BJUI. 2018. https://doi.org/10.1111/bju.14389.
10. Kourambas J, Byrne RR, Preminger GM. Does a ureteral access sheath facilitate ureteroscopy ? J Urol. 2001;165:789–93.
11. Lildal SK, Nørregaard R, Andreassen KH, et al. Ureteral access sheath influence on ureteral wall evaluated by cyclooxygenase-2 and tumor necrosis factor-α in a porcine model. J Endourol. 2017;31(3):307–13.
12. Traxer O, Thomas A. Prospective evaluation and classification of ureteral wall injuries resulting from insertion of a ureteral access sheath during retrograde intrarenal surgery. J Urol. 2013;189(2):580–4.

13. Stern JM, Yiee J, Park S. Safety and efficacy of ureteral access sheaths. J Endourol. 2007;21(2):119–23.
14. Delvecchio FC, Auge BK, Brizuela RM, et al. Assessment of stricture formation with the ureteral access sheath. Urology. 2003;61(3):518–22.
15. Berquet G, Prunel P, Verhoest G, et al. The use of a ureteral access sheath does not improve stone-free rate after uteteroscopy for upper urinary tract stones. World J Urol. 2014;32(1):229–32.
16. Huang J, Zhao Z, AlSmadi JK, et al. Use of the ureteral access sheath during ureteroscopy: a systemic review and meta-analysis. PLoS One. 2018;13(2): e0193600. https://doi.org/10.1371/journal.pone.0193600.
17. Auge BK, Sarvis JA, L'esperance JO, et al. Practice patterns of ureteral stenting after routine ureteroscopic stone surgery: a survey of practicing urologists. J Endourol. 2007;22(11):1287–91.
18. Al-Qahtani SM, Letendre J, Thomas A, et al. Which ureteral access sheath is compatible with your flexible ureteroscope ? J Endourol. 2014;28(3):286–90.
19. Mogilevkin Y, Sofer M, Margel D, et al. Predicting an effective ureteral access sheath insertion: a bicenter prospective study. J Endourol. 2014;28(12):1414–7.
20. Kawahara T, Ito H, Terao H, et al. Preoperative stenting for ureteroscopic lithotripsy for a large renal stone. Int J Urol. 2012;19(9):881–5.
21. Viers BR, Viers LD, Hull NC, et al. The difficult ureter: clinical and radiographic characteristics associated with upper urinary tract access at the time of ureteroscopic stone treatment. Urology. 2015;86(5):878–84.

20

Robotic stereotactic ablative radiotherapy for renal cell carcinoma in patients with impaired renal function

C. Senger[1,2*], A. Conti[2,3], A. Kluge[1,2], D. Pasemann[1,2], M. Kufeld[2], G. Acker[2,4,5], M. Lukas[6], A. Grün[1,2], G. Kalinauskaite[1,2], V. Budach[1,2], J. Waiser[7] and C. Stromberger[1,2]

Abstract

Background: Robotic stereotactic ablative radiotherapy (SABR) is currently under investigation as a noninvasive treatment option for patients with renal cell carcinoma (RCC). For radiation therapy of RCC, tumor motion and the need for high ablative doses while preserving the remaining renal parenchyma is a challenge. We aimed to analyze the safety and efficacy of robotic radiosurgery in RCC in a specific difficult subgroup of patients with impaired renal function.

Methods: We retrospectively identified all patients with RCC, treated with robotic SABR and motion compensation in our institution between 2012 and 2017. Either single fraction SABR of 24 or 25 Gy or 3 fractions of 12 Gy prescribed to the 70% isodose line was applied. Local control, overall survival, radiation side effects were evaluated together with renal function and tumor motion.

Results: We analyzed data of 13 lesions treated in 10 patients with clear cell RCC and a mean age of 70.5 ± 13.6 years (range: 48–87). Prior to SABR, 8 patients underwent previous complete and/or partial nephrectomy, 7 patients presented with chronic kidney disease ≥ stage 3. The median of minimum, mean and maximum planning target volume doses were 23.2, 29.5 and 35.0 Gy for single fraction and 24.4, 42.5 and 51.4 Gy for the three fractions regime. Persistent local control by robotic SABR was achieved in 9 out of 10 patients (92.3% of all lesions) within a median follow-up period of 27 month (range: 15–54). One patient underwent nephrectomy due to progressive disease and sufficient renal function of the contralateral kidney. Renal function remained stable with a mean estimated glomerular filtration rate (eGFR) of 51.3 ± 19.7 ml/min at baseline and 51.6 ± 25.8 ml/min at follow-up. The largest respiratory-induced tumor motion was seen in superior-inferior direction, compensated by the CyberKnife with mean targeting errors of maximal 2.2 mm.

Conclusions: Robotic SABR is technically feasible for the treatment of RCC in preexisting kidney disease with good local tumor control at about 2 years follow-up. Robotic SABR with motion tracking offers a valid treatment option for patients, who are at increased risk for progression to end-stage renal disease due to partial nephrectomy or ablative techniques.

Keywords: CyberKnife, Radiosurgery, SABR, Renal cell carcinoma, Kidney, Motion tracking

* Correspondence: carolin.senger@charite.de
[1]Department of Radiation Oncology, Charité - Universitätsmedizin Berlin, Augustenburger Platz 1, 13353 Berlin, Germany
[2]Charité CyberKnife Center, Charité - Universitätsmedizin Berlin, Augustenburger Platz 1, 13353 Berlin, Germany
Full list of author information is available at the end of the article

Background

Renal cell carcinoma (RCC) is the most common form of kidney cancer and its incidence has risen in recent years [1]. Due to increased incidental detection rates of kidney tumors, more RCC are still confined to the kidney at the time of diagnosis. The standard treatment for Stage I RCC is a partial renal resection. Radical nephrectomy is only performed for centrally located tumors or when partial resection is not feasible. Patients with bilateral tumors, contralateral recurrent tumor after unilateral nephrectomy, metastases from RCC in the contralateral kidney or preexisting chronic kidney disease are special candidates for partial nephrectomy. In these patients preserving renal parenchyma is essential to avoid chronic kidney disease.

As a possible therapeutic approach robotic stereotactic ablative radiotherapy (SABR) is currently under investigation as a non-invasive treatment option for patients with RCC. Renal cell carcinoma is frequently reported as a radio-resistant tumor. However, pathologic complete responses have been described after ablative radiotherapy previously [2]. Tumor motion and the need for high ablative radiation doses while preserving the remaining renal parenchyma, poses a major challenge. Robotic radiosurgery allows continuous tumor tracking under free breathing and therefore minimal gross tumor volume (GTV) to planning target volume (PTV) margins are needed. Robotic SABR for moving tumors is already established as a standard treatment option for patients with early stage non-small cell lung cancer [3, 4].

Although current data seem to demonstrate that SABR provides good tumor control while preserving the renal function [5, 6], most studies are limited to patients with normal renal function. In this study, we analyzed the safety and efficacy of image-guided CyberKnife (Accuray Inc., Sunnivale, USA) radiosurgery in RCC in a specific subgroup of patients with preexisting impaired renal function. Feasibility and technical aspects of robotic SABR will be provided as well.

Methods

Study design

Retrospective analysis of patient data was approved by the Ethics Committee Campus Charité Mitte (EA1/233/18). We identified all histology proven RCC patients, who were treated with robotic SABR in our center between June 2012 and April 2017. We collected data on patient characteristics regarding disease stage, preexisting kidney disease, estimated glomerular filtration rate (eGFR), clinical outcome, complications, local tumor control and overall survival. Dose-volume parameters were analyzed including prescription dose, fractionation, treatment dose (D_{min}, D_{mean}, D_{max}), GTV, PTV, new conformity index (nCI), PTV coverage, tumor motion and tracking accuracy.

Robotic SABR planning and delivery

The patients were referred to CyberKnife irradiation from the nephrology department, all at increased risk for progression to end-stage renal disease caused by further invasive treatment. The decision to perform a robotic SABR was recommended by a multidisciplinary urology board review for patients who are at increased risk for progression to end-stage renal disease due to partial nephrectomy or other ablative techniques.

One gold fiducial marker (1.0 mm × 5.0 mm) was implanted within or close to each tumor using an 18-G needle under computed tomography (CT)-guidance in local anesthesia. A tissue sample was taken in the same procedure if there was no prior pathology report available. High-resolution native thin-slice (1.0 mm) planning CT was performed within a median of 8 days (range: 1–21) after fiducial insertion to allow for fiducial settlement [7]. For accurate tumor delineation, magnetic resonance images (MRI) were co-registered with the planning CT and contouring was performed on all axial slices. The GTV was defined as the tumor volume based on CT and MR images. The clinical target volume (CTV) was equivalent to the GTV. The PTV was obtained by adding in median a 3 mm (range: 0–5 mm) isotropic margin to the GTV. Depending on tumor size or organs at risk (OAR) two different dose concepts were used, either single fraction SABR of 24 or 25 Gy, or 36 Gy in 3 fractions (12 Gy/fraction) prescribed each to the 70% isodose covering the PTV. Treatment planning and dose calculations were obtained by MultiPlan 4.6 (Accuray Inc., Sunnyvale, USA) using the Ray-tracing algorithm.

The linear-quadratic model, assuming an a/ß ratio of 2.6–6.9 Gy for RCC [8], was used to calculate the biologically equivalent dose (BED) and the equivalent dose in 2 Gy fractions (EQD2). The calculated $BED_{6.9}$ and $EQD2_{6.9}$ encompassing the PTV for single fraction were 107.5 Gy and 83.3 Gy, and 98.6 Gy and 76.4 Gy for the 3-fraction treatment.

Dose constraints for OAR for single fraction treatments were as follows: < 5 cm^3 of small bowel loops could receive up to 10.0 Gy with a maximum point dose of 19.0 Gy; for the extratumoral kidney parenchyma < 200 cm^3 could receive up to 8.0 Gy. The normal tissue constraints for three fractions were: < 5 cm^3 could receive up to 16.0 Gy with a maximum point dose of 27.0 Gy for small bowel, and less than 33% of the remaining kidney parenchyma could receive a total of 15.0 Gy. The dose constraints for spinal cord, liver, stomach and large intestine were set according to published standard limits [9]. The nCI $[(V70\% \cdot V_{PTV})/V70\%_{PTV}{}^2]$, which describes the conformity between the prescription isodose and the volume and shape of the PTV, was also used for treatment plan evaluation.

Technical aspects

The CyberKnife System installed in July 2011 in Berlin combines two systems, a lightweight linear accelerator mounted on a robotic arm with 6-MV photon energy and an image guidance system consisting of two orthogonally positioned x-ray cameras. For patient positioning, an automatic tracking algorithm compares live x-rays with digital reconstructed images from planning CT. For respiratory motion compensation, the CyberKnife Synchrony® Respiratory Motion Tracking System (MTS) was used. Thereby, the external motion of LED markers located on the chest of the patient was correlated with the internal tumor motion represented by the fiducial position and determined by the x-ray images. The individually measured correlation model is continuously updated and synchronizes the radiation beam in real time such that the beam always remains aligned with the target. An accuracy of less than 1.0 mm is technically achieved and allows clinicians to reduce safety margins significantly, while eliminating the need for gating or breath-hold techniques. During treatment, the motion patterns for each patient were recorded in logfiles.

Follow-up and statistics

Clinical and radiological follow-up with CT or MRI was frequently performed after robotic SABR and the latest available follow-up was used in this analysis. For local control the MRI scans were evaluated by the senior physician in charge to verify treatment response. Tumor response was analyzed using response evaluation criteria in solid tumors (RECIST version 1.1). The treatment response of each RCC was categorized using OsiriX MD 10.0 (Pixmeo SARL, Bernex, Switzerland) to compare baseline MRI and planning CT with the latest available follow up images in 1) complete remission (CR): no measurable lesion; 2) partial remission (PR) defined as a volume reduction ≥ 30%; 3) stable disease (SD); 4) progressive disease (PD) defined as a ≥ 20% increase in volume or ≥ 5 mm increase in size. Local control (LC) was calculated from the end of SABR until last available follow-up or PD.

Overall survival (OS) was calculated from the end of SABR until last follow-up or death. LC and OS were estimated using Kaplan-Meier curves. Common Terminology Criteria for Adverse Event V4.03 (CTCAE) for acute and late radiosurgery related side effects were recorded separately. Renal function at baseline and latest available follow up was calculated according to the chronic kidney disease epidemiology collaboration (CKD-EPI) formula at baseline and last available follow up.

Due to respiratory induced kidney motion, the motion patterns and total targeting errors between the predicted and the actual position of the tumor were evaluated. Overall, the motion pattern and targeting accuracy of 19 out of 21 treatment sessions could be extracted. Motion pattern evaluation and statistical analysis were done with MATLAB 9.3 (The MathWorks, Inc., Natick, USA).

Results

Patient characteristics

Data of 13 lesions treated in 10 patients histologically confirmed as clear cell RCC grade 1 or 2 were collected. The mean age of patients who underwent robotic SABR was 70.5 ± 13.6 years (range: 48–87). The female/male ratio was 1:1. All patients treated with robotic SABR had an ECOG performance status 1 or 2 and suffered from chronic kidney disease (CKD). The median and mean time interval between the first histological diagnosis of RCC and SABR was 7.5 and 8.4 ± 6.0 years, respectively, with a large range of 2 months to 19.7 years. Tumor characteristics are summarized in Table 1. Seven patients had T1a (≤ 40 mm) and 3 patients had larger tumors (T3a). In 3 patients it remained unclear whether the treated tumor was a metachronous RCC or a metastasis from a previously occurred contralateral RCC. The subsites of the 13 lesions were the upper, mid or lower pole in 53.8%, close to the renal pelvis or extending to the perinephric tissue in 15.4% each and infiltrating the renal vein or close to the hilum in 7.7% each.

Prior to SABR, 8 out of 10 patients underwent surgery or radiofrequency ablation (RFA) for their renal tumors, 6 of them had procedures done on both sides. Nephrectomy was carried out in 5 patients, partial ipsilateral resection in 4 patients and contralateral resection in 3 patients. Previous RFA of the SABR treated kidney was performed in 2 patients. Von Hippel-Lindau disease was diagnosed in 2 patients. One patient had a RCC in his kidney transplant. Three patients had a diabetes mellitus type 2. CKD stage 2, 3 and 4 with an eGFR level below 90, 60, 45 ml/min was diagnosed in 3, 6 and one patient, respectively (see Table 1 for preexisting kidney disease).

Treatment and Dosimetric analysis

The tumors had a median diameter of 28.8 mm (range: 9–70). Two patients had tumors larger than 40 mm with RCC extension into the renal vein or perinephric tissue. The median GTV volume was 13.3 cm^3 (range: 1.3–108.4), the resulting median PTV was 22.1 cm^3 (range: 3.8–190.3). Five patients received single fraction SABR of 24 or 25 Gy, 4 patients received 3 fractions of 12 Gy every other day and one patient with three lesions received both regiments. The patient's median of minimum, mean and

Table 1 Tumor characteristics and preexisting kidney disease in patients with renal cell carcinoma

Case	Size (mm)	Primary tumor	Tumor location	Baseline CKD stage	First line treatment / Preexisting kidney disease
#1	32	cT1a/DD metastasis	close to renal pelvis	3b	Nephrectomy, RFA and embolisation ipsilateral
#2	30	cT1a/DD metastasis	mid pole	2	Nephrectomy, partial resection ipsilateral /DM type 2
#3	14 10	cT1a	upper pole mid pole	3b	Nephrectomy, partial resection ipsilateral / short term dialysis, DM type 2
#4	26	cT1a	upper pole	2	RPGN, kidney transplant
#5	70	cT3a	infiltrating renal vein	2	Partial resection contralateral
#6	36	cT1a	mid pole	4	Nephrectomy
#7	36	cT1a	lower pole	3a	partial resection contralateral, multiple RFA ipsilateral / VHL
#8	39	cT1a	close to renal pelvis	3a	partial resection ipsi- and contralateral / VHL
#9	47	cT3a	extends to perinephric tissue	3b	-
#10	9 10 15	cT3a/DD metastasis	lower pole extends to perinephric tissue close to hilum	3b	Nephrectomy, partial resection ipsilateral

RFA Radiofrequency ablation, *CKD* chronic kidney disease, *DM* diabetes mellitus, *RPGN* rapidly progressive glomerulonephritis, *VHL* von Hippel-Lindau disease

maximum PTV dose was 23.2, 29.5 and 35.0 Gy for single fraction and 24.4, 42.5 and 51.4 Gy for the three fractions regimen, respectively. Dose-volume parameters and further treatment characteristics including nCI and percentage of the PTV coverage are summarized in Table 2.

Each robotic SABR treatment was done as an outpatient procedure with delivery times between 46 min and 86 min per session. For single session treatments, the mean total treatment time was 62 ± 15 min, fractionated treatments took in total 184 ± 33 min (61 ± 11 min per fraction). All patients completed their treatment.

Tumor response

Local control (CR, PR and SD) by robotic SABR therapy was achieved in 9 out of 10 patients and 92.3% of all lesions within the median follow-up period of 27 month (range: 15–54). A representative example of the tumor response and treatment plan is shown in Fig. 1. Whereas SD was observed in 38.5% of the treated lesions, PR was observed in 30.8% and CR in 23.1% (Table 2). However, there was no difference in SD or PR between the one fraction or three fractions regiment. The only local treatment failure occurred in one lesion (7.7%) 5 month after SABR.

Four patients with metastases to other organs at time of radiosurgery or during follow-up had additional adjuvant systemic treatment. Out of 10 patients 8 were alive at the last available follow-up. Two patients with progressive metastatic disease died 15 and 16 months after SABR. Kaplan-Meier Curves for local control and overall survival are shown in Fig. 2.

Renal function and toxicity

Typical normal tissue dose constraints were within the range mentioned. Over a median follow-up period of 22

Table 2 Dose-volume and follow-up parameters for robotic stereotactic ablative body radiotherapy

Case	GTV (cm^3)	PTV (cm^3)	Margin (mm)	Dose (Gy)	PTV coverage (%)	nCI	Follow-up (month)	Local control
#1	8.2	17.9	4	1 × 24	97.8	1.07	54	SD
#2	20.4	31.0	3	1 × 25	97.8	1.06	23	PR
#3	13.5 17.0	13.5 17.0	0 0	1 × 24 1 × 24	96.8 98.5	1.13 1.13	47	CR PR
#4	14.3	24.6	3	1 × 25	99.9	1.06	33	SD
#5	108.4	190.3	5	3 × 12	92.0	1.23	25	SD
#6	13.2	22.7	3	1 × 25	99.5	1.13	15	SD
#7	9.2	17.4	3	3 × 12	98.3	1.14	32	SD
#8	45.5	88.4	5	3 × 12	86.0	1.40	30	PD
#9	44.2	66.2	3	3 × 12	98.7	1.21	23	PR
#10	1.3 9.0 2.3	3.8 21.4 5.6	3 4 3	1 × 25 3 × 12 1 × 25	99.7 82.0 98.4	1.09 1.50 1.20	16	CR PR CR

GTV Gross tumor volume, *PTV* planning target volume, *nCI* new conformity index, *SD* stable disease, *PR* partial remission, *CR* complete remission, *PD* progressive disease

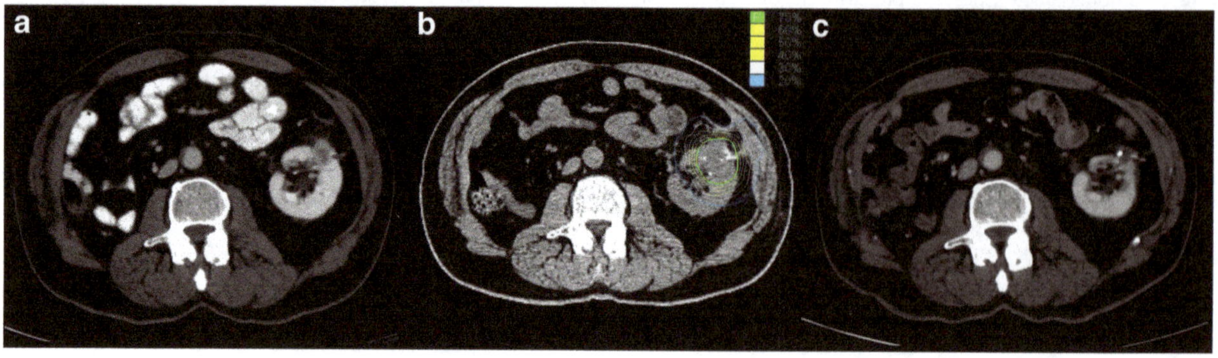

Fig. 1 A representative case of a renal cell carcinoma. **a** Demonstrates a representative image before radiotherapy and **b** the treatment plan with exemplary planning computed tomography image in axial view with the treatment plan. Single fraction 25 Gy was prescribed to 70% isodose line (in green) to treat planning target volume shown in red line. The yellow and white circle lines represent the remaining isodose lines until 20% in blue. **c** shows an image 2 years after robotic stereotactic ablative radiotherapy

month (range: 4–51) renal function remained stable with a mean serum creatinine of 1.4 ± 0.5 mg/dl (eGFR 51.3 ± 19.7 ml/min) at baseline and 1.5 ± 0.8 mg/dl (eGFR 51.6 ± 25.8 ml/min) at follow-up (Fig. 3). One patient underwent nephrectomy due to progressive disease after SABR with three fractions of 12 Gy and sufficient renal function of the contralateral kidney. One patient developed mild abdominal pain (grade 1) and another one diarrhea and abdominal distension (grade 1). All symptoms occurred in the two patients with tumors larger than 40 mm. No patient developed CTCAE grade 2 or higher toxicity or needed hemodialysis.

Tumor motion tracking

Each patient got one gold fiducial implanted per lesion. Two patients had 2 and 3 gold fiducials for multiple lesions. There were no side effects with marker placement in the kidney or difficulties with marker migration observed. To position the patient as in planning CT, he was first aligned using the bony spine structures. Afterwards the position of the fiducial was tracked. The majority of the lesions (92.3%) were treated using MTS for motion compensation. The only robotic SABR done without tumor motion tracking was performed in a kidney transplant located in the left iliac fossa where no respiratory motion was suspected. For all patients, treatment was performed in "free-breathing", the largest respiratory-induced tumor motion was seen in superior-inferior direction with magnitudes between 3.0 mm and 24.7 mm. The left/right and anterior/posterior displacements of the tumor ranged from 0.7 to 10.6 mm, and 1.6 to 14.6 mm, respectively (Fig. 4). This motion was compensated by the CyberKnife with mean targeting errors over the complete treatment time of maximal 2.2 mm.

Discussion

In this retrospective study the efficacy of robotic SABR was assessed retrospectively in 10 patients with RCC and

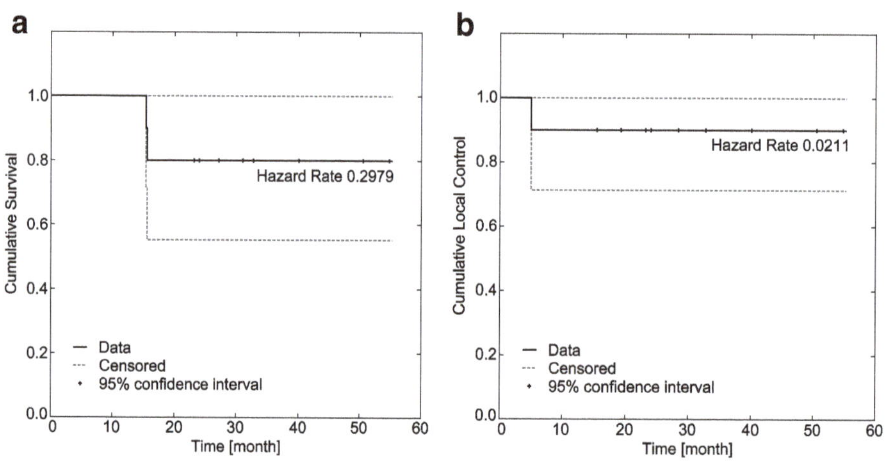

Fig. 2 Kaplan-Meier curves. **a** Shows overall survival and **b** local control for renal cell carcinoma patients after robotic stereotactic ablative radiotherapy

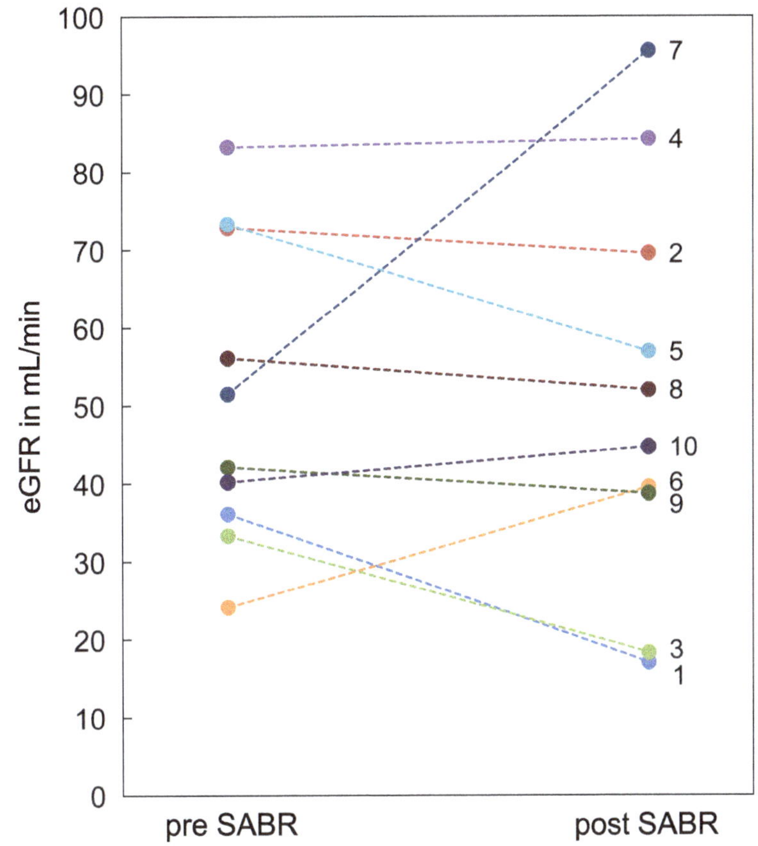

Fig. 3 Kidney function at baseline and follow-up. Estimated glomerular filtration rates (eGFR) before stereotactic ablative radiotherapy (pre SABR) and latest available follow-up (post SABR)

moderate to severe chronic kidney disease. Our study demonstrates that this minimal invasive and highly sophisticated treatment method provides good response rates and local control with negligible toxicity. SABR with motion compensation is a nephron-sparing treatment that perfectly adapts to patients with RCC and significant preexisting chronic renal failure.

Our results concerning local tumor control in 92.3% of all lesions and mild toxicity appear to be consistent with those available in the literature. A previous systematic review of 126 patients described a weighted local control rate of 94% and a grade 3 toxicity rate of 3.8% [10]. Since that study, 3 single-institution, prospective studies of 19 patients [11], 40 patients [2], and 33 patients [12] have reported similar findings, with local control rates ranging from 98 to 100% and grade $\geq$ 3 toxicity rates from 0 to 15.8%. Recently, 9 centers across Germany, Australia, the United States, Canada, and Japan formed an International Radiosurgery Oncology Consortium for Kidney and reported data of 223 patients [6]. The rates of LC, cancer-specific survival, and progression-free survival at 2 and 4 years were 97.8, 95.7, 77.4% and 97.8, 91.9, 65.4%, respectively. Multi-fraction SABR was associated with poorer progression-free survival and worse cancer-specific survival. Grade 1 and 2 toxicities were reported for 35.6% of patients whereas grade 3 and 4 toxicities were recorded in only 1.3% [6].

In patients with bilateral tumors or contralateral tumor recurrences after unilateral nephrectomy or partial resection treatment is especially challenging. The resection of the remaining kidney consecutively leads to the progression of chronic kidney disease including the need for hemodialysis treatment. In such cases, minimally invasive ablative techniques such as cryosurgery, radiofrequency ablation and SABR are possible alternatives to nephrectomy. A 2016 systematic review and meta-analysis reporting on survival across management strategies demonstrated a 95 to 100% cancer specific survival after nephrectomy and thermal ablation with a median follow-up period of 22 to 120 months. Whereas, for tumors more than 40 mm (T1b) survival rates decrease to around 90% and for tumors more than 70 mm (T2) between 82.5 and 86.7% [13]. A mostly retrospective data analysis by Kunkle and Uzzo [14] showed local tumor progression rates of 12.9% after RFA and 5.2% after renal cryoablation. In our series, tumor progression was

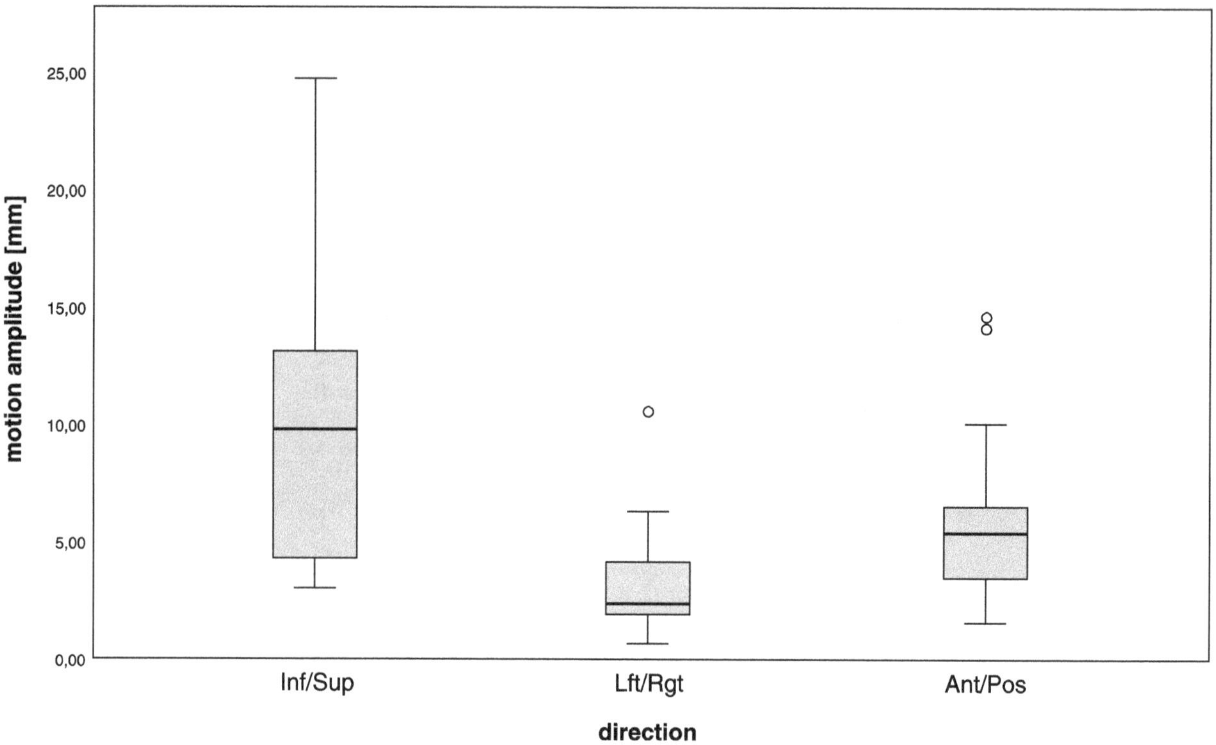

Fig. 4 A diagram of motion amplitudes. Maximal motion amplitudes of all treatment sessions in inferior/superior (Inf/Sup), left/right (Lft/Rgt) and anterior/posterior (Ant/Pos) direction in mm

recorded in 7.7% of all lesions, accordingly in one out of 10 patients (10%). In this case the tumor size was above the median, located close to renal pelvis and the PTV coverage was less than 90%.

Notably, renal function remained stable following treatment in all patients despite the high doses of radiation delivered to the kidney. This result raises two considerations. Firstly, preservation of renal function was assumed to be due to compensatory mechanisms of the contralateral kidney and the spared ipsilateral kidney volume described as renal functional reserve [15]. These results also suggest that it might be possible to rely on a compensatory capacity of the ipsilateral kidney in patients who already had contralateral nephrectomy and that, whenever oncologically suitable, a selective approach aimed to avoid post-treatment severe chronic kidney disease should be pursued. A second point concerns the radiation tolerance of the peritumoral kidney and the reliability of tumor tracking in robotic SABR. Cassady [16] proposed a threshold dose of 15 Gy for renal injury based on data of bilateral whole kidney irradiation in 3 fractions. Nevertheless, ours and other previous studies demonstrate a good tolerance to higher doses and stable kidney function. The prescribed dose (1 × 24–25 Gy or 3 × 12 Gy prescribed to the 70% isodose) was relatively high in order to overcome the radioresistance of RCC. The fraction number and prescribed dose of the two large studies from Staehler et al. [2] and Sun et al. [17] were similar to our dose concepts. Overall, they treated 80 patients with either 25 Gy in one fraction or 38 Gy in 3 fractions prescribed to the 70 or 80% isodose line. Both studies reported only grade 1 side effects with > 90% local control in a relatively short follow-up.

Svedman et al. [18] evaluated kidney injury following 3 fractions SABR in 7 patients with primary or metastatic renal disease with only one functioning kidney. In 5 patients, kidney function remained unaffected after SABR, with a kidney volume of 37.3% receiving 15 Gy (V15), whereas 2 patients exhibited modest changes in renal function without the requirement for medical intervention or hemodialysis. In SABR patients, a V15 limited to less than one third of the normal single remaining kidney could be an appropriate dose-volume constraint in patients with preexisting kidney disease. We therefore considered this dose constraint in our series for the three-fraction regiment.

Furthermore, the high doses used and the treatment result in terms of remission, local control and sparing of renal function, demonstrate that the robotic SABR is highly reliable in terms of targeting precision and dose delivery. According to our data, the median targeting accuracy was within 2.2 mm. This provided us an important information regarding the margins to be used. In fact, we believe that, unlike margins of up to 10 mm, as used in other studies, a moderate expansion of the tumor (i.e. 3.0 mm) is sufficient for the CyberKnife MTS. Since only one marker was implanted, rotations could neither be directly detected nor corrected. However, geometric calculations have shown that a 3.0 mm margin appears to be sufficient also if small rotations (< 5 °) occur.

Limitations

This study has several limitations. This is a retrospective series with a limited number of cases collected and a relatively short follow-up for renal function. Nevertheless, it should be considered as a proof-of-concept study for SABR on patients with impaired renal function gaining satisfactory results and providing a low risk for treatment-related side effects.

Conclusion

Robotic SABR is technically feasible for the treatment of early stage RCC in patients with preexisting kidney disease with good local control at short term follow-up. As an outpatient procedure, it may prevent (treatment related) loss of renal function with only mild side effects. Therefore robotic SABR with motion tracking represents a valid treatment option for these patients, who are at increased risk for progression to end-stage renal disease due to partial nephrectomy or other ablative techniques. Further studies are needed but warranted to determine long-term results of this treatment.

Abbreviations

CR: Complete remission; CT: Computed tomography; CTV: Clinical target volume; eGFR: Estimated glomerular filtration rate; GTV: Gross tumor volume; LC: Local control; MRI: Magnetic resonance images; MTS: Motion Tracking System; nCI: New conformity index; OAR: Organs at risk; OS: Overall survival; PD: Progressive disease; PR: Partial remission; PTV: Planning target volume; RCC: Renal cell carcinoma; RFA: Radiofrequency ablation; SABR: Stereotactic ablative radiotherapy; SD: Stable disease

Acknowledgments

Dr. Acker is participant of the BIH-Charité Clinician Scientist Program funded by the Charité – Universitätsmedizin Berlin and the Berlin Institute of Health.

Disclosure

Mathias Lukas is employed by Siemens Healthcare GmbH. The remaining authors report no conflict of interest concerning the materials or methods used in this study or the findings specified in this paper.

Authors' contributions

CS (Senger) acquired, analyzed and interpreted the patient data, drafted the manuscript. AC was a contributor in writing the manuscript. AK and DP provided technical support, preparation of figures and critical review of the manuscript. MK made substantial contributions to acquisition. ML conducted the statistical analysis. GA, AG, GK, JW and VB provided administrative support and critically revised the article. CS (Stromberger) participated in the design of the study, made substantial contributions to acquisition, analysis and interpretation of the data. CS (Senger) approved the final version of the manuscript on behalf of all authors. All authors read and approved the final manuscript.

Author details

[1]Department of Radiation Oncology, Charité - Universitätsmedizin Berlin, Augustenburger Platz 1, 13353 Berlin, Germany. [2]Charité CyberKnife Center, Charité - Universitätsmedizin Berlin, Augustenburger Platz 1, 13353 Berlin, Germany. [3]Department of Neurosurgery, University of Messina, Messina, Italy. [4]Department of Neurosurgery and Center for Stroke research Berlin (CSB), Charité - Universitätsmedizin Berlin, Charitéplatz 1, 10117 Berlin, Germany. [5]Berlin Institute of Health (BIH), Anna-Louisa-Karsch-Str. 2, 10178 Berlin, Germany. [6]Department of Nuclear Medicine, Charité - Universitätsmedizin Berlin, Charitéplatz 1, 10117 Berlin, Germany. [7]Department of Nephrology and Medical Intensive Care, Charité - Universitätsmedizin Berlin, Charitéplatz 1, 10117 Berlin, Germany.

References

1. Siegel R, Naishadham D, Jemal A. Cancer statistics, 2012. CA Cancer J Clin. 2012;62(1):10–29.
2. Staehler M, Bader M, Schlenker B, Casuscelli J, Karl A, Roosen A, et al. Single fraction radiosurgery for the treatment of renal tumors. J Urol. 2015;193(3): 771–5.
3. Guckenberger M, Andratschke N, Alheit H, Holy R, Moustakis C, Nestle U, et al. Definition of stereotactic body radiotherapy: principles and practice for the treatment of stage I non-small cell lung cancer. Strahlenther Onkol. 2014;190(1):26–33.
4. Schanne DH, Nestle U, Allgauer M, Andratschke N, Appold S, Dieckmann U, et al. Stereotactic body radiotherapy for centrally located stage I NSCLC: a multicenter analysis. Strahlenther Onkol. 2015;191(2):125–32.
5. Lo CH, Huang WY, Chao HL, Lin KT, Jen YM. Novel application of stereotactic ablative radiotherapy using CyberKnife((R)) for early-stage renal cell carcinoma in patients with pre-existing chronic kidney disease: initial clinical experiences. Oncol Lett. 2014;8(1):355–60.
6. Siva S, Louie AV, Warner A, Muacevic A, Gandhidasan S, Ponsky L, et al. Pooled analysis of stereotactic ablative radiotherapy for primary renal cell carcinoma: a report from the international radiosurgery oncology consortium for kidney (IROCK). Cancer. 2018;124(5):934–42.
7. Imura M, Yamazaki K, Shirato H, Onimaru R, Fujino M, Shimizu S, et al. Insertion and fixation of fiducial markers for setup and tracking of lung tumors in radiotherapy. Int J Radiat Oncol Biol Phys. 2005;63(5):1442–7.
8. Ning S, Trisler K, Wessels BW, Knox SJ. Radiobiologic studies of radioimmunotherapy and external beam radiotherapy in vitro and in vivo in human renal cell carcinoma xenografts. Cancer. 1997;80(12 Suppl):2519 28.
9. Emami B, Lyman J, Brown A, Coia L, Goitein M, Munzenrider JE, et al. Tolerance of normal tissue to therapeutic irradiation. Int J Radiat Oncol Biol Phys. 1991;21(1):109–22.
10. Siva S, Pham D, Gill S, Corcoran NM, Foroudi F. A systematic review of stereotactic radiotherapy ablation for primary renal cell carcinoma. BJU Int. 2012;110(11 Pt B):E737–43.
11. Ponsky L, Lo SS, Zhang Y, Schluchter M, Liu Y, Patel R, et al. Phase I dose-escalation study of stereotactic body radiotherapy (SBRT) for poor surgical candidates with localized renal cell carcinoma. Radiother Oncol. 2015;117(1):183–7.
12. Siva S, Pham D, Kron T, Bressel M, Lam J, Tan TH, et al. Stereotactic ablative body radiotherapy for inoperable primary kidney cancer: a prospective clinical trial. BJU Int. 2017;120(5):623–30.
13. Pierorazio PM, Johnson MH, Patel HD, Sozio SM, Sharma R, Iyoha E, et al. Management of Renal Masses and Localized Renal Cancer: systematic review and meta-analysis. J Urol. 2016;196(4):989–99.
14. Kunkle DA, Uzzo RG. Cryoablation or radiofrequency ablation of the small renal mass : a meta-analysis. Cancer. 2008;113(10):2671–80.
15. Thomas DM, Coles GA, Williams JD. What does the renal reserve mean? Kidney Int. 1994;45(2):411–6.
16. Cassady JR. Clinical radiation nephropathy. Int J Radiat Oncol Biol Phys. 1995;31(5):1249–56.
17. Sun MR, Brook A, Powell MF, Kaliannan K, Wagner AA, Kaplan ID, et al. Effect of stereotactic body radiotherapy on the growth kinetics and enhancement pattern of primary renal tumors. AJR Am J Roentgenol. 2016;206(3):544–53.
18. Svedman C, Karlsson K, Rutkowska E, Sandstrom P, Blomgren H, Lax I, et al. Stereotactic body radiotherapy of primary and metastatic renal lesions for patients with only one functioning kidney. Acta Oncol. 2008;47(8):1578–83.

21

Determinants of treatment in patients with stage IV renal cell carcinoma

Christopher S. Hollenbeak[1*], Eric W. Schaefer[2], Justin Doan[3] and Jay D. Raman[4]

Abstract

Background: Advances in systemic targeted therapies afford treatment opportunities in patients with metastatic renal cell carcinoma (RCC). Elderly patients with metastatic RCC present a subpopulation for consideration owing to competing causes of mortality and benefits seen with new therapeutic agents. We investigate treatment patterns for elderly patients with stage IV RCC and determine factors associated with not receiving treatment.

Methods: The Surveillance Epidemiology and End Results (SEER) Medicare linked data set contained 949 stage IV RCC patients over age 65 diagnosed between 2007 and 2011. Treatment approach was modeled using multinomial logistic regression. Landmark analysis at 6 months accounted for early death as a potential explanation for no treatment.

Results: Of the 949 patients with stage IV RCC, 26.2% received surgery and 34.1% received systemic therapy within 6 months of diagnosis. Among our entire cohort, over half (51.2%) had no evidence of receiving surgery or systemic therapy. Among the 447 patients who survived at least 6 months, 26.6% did not receive treatment during this time. Older patients and those with a higher Charlson Comorbidity Index (CCI) had lower odds of being treated with surgery, systemic therapy, or both. Conversely, married patients had higher odds of receiving these therapies. These associations were largely sustained in the 6-month landmark analyses.

Conclusions: Elderly patients with metastatic RCC present a unique subpopulation for consideration owing to competing causes of mortality. Many elderly patients with stage IV RCC did not receive surgery or systemic therapy up to 6 months from diagnosis. Several clinical and demographic factors were associated with this observation. Further investigation is needed to understand the rationale underlying the underutilization of systemic therapy in elderly patients.

Keywords: Renal cell carcinoma, Kidney cancer, Multinomial logistic regression, Systemic therapy, Landmark analysis

Background

The incidence of kidney cancer has continued to rise over the past three decades [1]. Much of this increase has been attributed to the diagnosis of incidental small kidney tumors detected on axial cross-sectional imaging [2]. Nonetheless, mortality from kidney cancer remains significant with an estimated 14,000 patients in the United States and over 125,000 worldwide dying from kidney cancer in 2017 [3].

The mainstay therapy of kidney cancer is surgical extirpation with resultant survival rates exceeding 90% for patients with localized disease [4]. Historically, however, the presence of regional and distant metastasis has been associated with a significantly poorer prognosis, with 5-year survival rates between 5 and 20% [5]. Cytokine-based therapies proved to carry significant patient toxicity with variable efficacy [6]. The discovery of VEGF inhibitors, mTOR inhibitors, and immunotherapy has changed the landscape for systemic treatment (ST) of metastatic kidney cancer [7]. Specifically, targeted anti-angiogenic therapies and immunotherapy through PDL-1 inhibition have become the foundation of metastatic RCC treatment, with improvements not only in progression-free survival but also overall survival compared with older therapies such as IL-2 and interferon [8]. Tolerability is generally superior compared to older agents, with side effects ranging from

* Correspondence: csh10@psu.edu
[1]Department of Health Policy and Administration, The Pennsylvania State University, 604E Donald H. Ford Building, University Park, State College, PA 16802, USA
Full list of author information is available at the end of the article

relatively mild (e.g. nausea, vomiting, fatigue) to less commonly severe sequelae (e.g. thrombolic events, bleeding).

Elderly patients with RCC present a unique population for treatment consideration. Population studies suggest that for localized renal tumors of any size, patients are more likely to die from other causes than from kidney cancer [9]. The scenario is different for metastatic stage IV disease where more biologically aggressive tumors have the potential for symptomatic metastasis. In theory, the availability of newer ST with improved tolerability profiles holds the promise of longer life and greater quality of life for many patients with metastatic RCC [10].

In this study, we explore the determinants of treatment for patients with stage IV renal cell carcinoma. We specifically focus on elderly patients, defined as Medicare beneficiaries, and explore factors associated with treatment selection. Most importantly, we determine the rates of no treatment in stage IV RCC and explore clinical and demographic factors that are associated with not receiving any form of treatment, including surgery and/or systemic therapy, or both surgery and systemic therapy.

Methods

Data

Data for this study came from the Surveillance Epidemiology and End Results (SEER)-Medicare linked database. The database includes patients in the SEER tumor registry who are covered by fee-for-service Medicare, along with all Medicare claims from the time of Medicare enrollment. We included all patients diagnosed between 2007 and 2011 with a first, single, stage IV cancer of the kidney, which we identified using an International Classification of Diseases for Oncology (ICD-O-3) code of C649 (kidney and renal pelvis).

We further included only patients with RCC by restricting cases to those with one of the following histologic types: clear cell adenocarcinoma; renal cell carcinoma; adenocarcinoma; adenocarcinoma with mixed subtype; papillary adenocarcinoma; cyst-associated renal cell carcinoma; renal cell carcinoma, chromophobe type; renal cell carcinoma, sarcomatoid; collecting duct carcinoma; granular cell carcinoma; and mucinous adenocarcinoma. In addition, we limited the sample to patients age 66 or older at the time of diagnosis, and we required that patients were continuously enrolled in fee-for-service Medicare (both Part A and Part B) from the time of diagnosis or until death or last follow-up. We also required patients to be covered by Medicare Part D in order to identify ST.

Variables

Analyses controlled for several demographic variables (age, sex, race/ethnicity, rurality, and marital status). An overall comorbidity score (or comorbidity weight) was computed from comorbidities identified using *International Classifications of Diseases, 9th Revision, Clinical Modification* (ICD-9) codes from inpatient and outpatient claims within one year of the date of diagnosis using the Deyo adaptation of the Charlson comorbidity index [11]. Procedure codes from the Romano adaptation were also included. Surgery (partial or total nephrectomy) was determined from claims using ICD-9 procedure codes (55.3x, 55.4, 55.5x) and Current Procedure Terminology (CPT) codes (50,220, 50,225, 50, 230, 50,240, 50,543, 50,545, 50,546, 50,548).

Systemic therapy

ST was determined from Medicare Parts A and B claims using Healthcare Common Procedure Coding System (HCPCS) level II codes for injection drugs, including temsirolimus (C9239, J9330), bevacizumab (C9257, J9035, Q2024), interferon-alfa (J9213, J9214), and interleukin-2 (J9015). In addition, Medicare Part D claims for prescription drugs were used to identify prescriptions that were filled for axitinitinib, bevacizumab, everolimus, pazopanib, sorafenib, sunitinib, and temsirolimus. Patients were classified as having received ST if a claim with one of these HCPCS codes or prescription drugs was found within 6 months of RCC diagnosis.

Statistical analysis

The objective was to investigate associations between patient factors and treatment choice among patients with stage IV kidney cancer, including no evidence of receiving treatment. We considered only surgery and ST to be primary treatments for kidney cancer. Although some RCC patients receive radiation therapy, it is not used as a primary treatment in kidney cancer but rather as palliative therapy for bone, brain, or other sites of metastases.

The primary outcome was treatment choice. To construct the primary outcome, patients were cross-classified by surgery and ST, resulting in four treatment groups: no treatment, surgery only, ST only, and both surgery and ST. Comparisons of demographic variables across treatment groups were made using analysis of variance (ANOVA) for continuous variables and chi-squared tests for categorical and binary variables.

We modeled treatment choice using multinomial logistic regression, an extension of logistic regression for outcomes with more than 2 categories. The log odds of receiving each treatment in comparison to the reference treatment were modeled as a function of covariates using a generalized logit link. Odds ratios (ORs) and their corresponding 95% confidence intervals (CIs) from the model were reported. By default, ORs were interpreted relative to the no treatment reference group.

However, ORs relative to other treatment groups can be calculated directly from model parameters and were therefore also reported. For the non-linear estimates of age, we reported ORs for 80 versus 70 years, or roughly the inter-quartile range. In addition, model results were reported graphically using the predicted probability of receiving treatment as a function of covariate values included in the model.

One final consideration is that treatment choice was necessarily unknown at the time of diagnosis; a patient must have lived long enough to receive any treatment. A patient classified as having no treatment within the first 6 months after diagnosis may have refused treatment, may have died before any planned treatment began, may have been observed clinically, or may have received no treatment for other reasons. As a way to control for this limitation, we used landmark analyses that fit the same multinomial logistic regression model but limited the sample to the subsets of patients who lived ≥6 months after diagnosis.

Results

The analysis sample contained 949 patients with Stage IV kidney cancer. Among these patients, 447 (47%) patients lived at least 6 months after diagnosis. Table 1 shows the distribution among treatment groups for all patients and for patients surviving ≥6 months. Most patients with Stage IV cancer did not receive surgery within 6 months ($n = 700$, 75%). A substantial number of patients received ST within 6 months ($n = 324$, 34%), but many did not.

Table 1 provides descriptive statistics for patient characteristics stratified by treatment group for the full patient sample. Significant differences in the distribution of patient characteristics were observed across the four treatment groups for all variables except for race and rurality. Unsurprisingly, patients who received both surgery and ST were younger on average than patients who received no treatment (mean age 72.2 vs. 78.7 years). Seventy percent (70.0%) of patients who received both surgery and ST were married, compared with 50.4% of patients receiving surgery alone and 51.9% of patients receiving ST alone. Among patients receiving no treatment, only 37.4% were married. Patients receiving no treatment had the highest mean CCI score (1.5) among all treatment groups.

Results of the multinomial logistic regression for all patients are presented in Table 2. Odds ratios from this model are interpreted in a similar fashion as for logistic regression models for each treatment relative to a given reference group. For example, patients who were married had 3.13 times greater odds than unmarried patients

Table 1 Characteristics of patients with Stage IV kidney cancer, stratified by treatment group

	All Patients[a]					Patients surviving ≥ 6 months				
	No treatment	Surgery only	ST only	Surgery + ST		No treatment	Surgery only	ST only	Surgery + ST	
Variable	($n = 486$)	($n = 139$)	($n = 214$)	($n = 110$)	*P*-value	($n = 237$)	($n = 146$)	($n = 164$)	($n = 71$)	*P*-value
Age at diagnosis					< 0.001					< 0.001
Mean (SD)	78.7 (7.43)	73.0 (5.39)	75.3 (5.67)	72.2 (5.26)		77.6 (7.39)	73.5 (5.31)	75.5 (5.6)	72.2 (5.19)	
Sex					0.017					0.121
Male	238 (49.0%)	70 (50.4%)	120 (56.1%)	71 (64.5%)		59 (49.6%)	50 (48.5%)	74 (56.9%)	60 (63.2%)	
Female	248 (51.0%)	69 (49.6%)	94 (43.9%)	39 (35.5%)		60 (50.4%)	53 (51.5%)	56 (43.1%)	35 (36.8%)	
Race					0.19					0.222
White	388 (79.8%)	119 (85.6%)	163 (76.2%)	89 (80.9%)		95 (79.8%)	89 (86.4%)	98 (75.4%)	76 (80%)	
Other	98 (20.2%)	20 (14.4%)	51 (23.8%)	21 (19.1%)		24 (20.2%)	14 (13.6%)	32 (24.6%)	19 (20%)	
Urban/rural code					0.424					0.119
Big metro	232 (47.7%)	61 (43.9%)	98 (45.8%)	62 (56.4%)		58 (48.7%)	46 (44.7%)	53 (40.8%)	54 (56.8%)	
Metro/urban	184 (37.9%)	53 (38.1%)	88 (41.1%)	35 (31.8%)		n/a	n/a	n/a	n/a	
Less urban/rural	70 (14.4%)	25 (18.0%)	28 (13.1%)	13 (11.8%)		n/a	n/a	n/a	n/a	
Other	n/a	n/a	n/a	n/a		61 (51.3%)	57 (55.3%)	77 (59.2%)	41 (43.2%)	
Marital status					< 0.001					< 0.001
Unmarried	304 (62.6%)	69 (49.6%)	103 (48.1%)	33 (30.0%)		65 (54.6%)	51 (49.5%)	67 (51.5%)	26 (27.4%)	
Married	182 (37.4%)	70 (50.4%)	111 (51.9%)	77 (70.0%)		54 (45.4%)	52 (50.5%)	63 (48.5%)	69 (72.6%)	
Charlson comorbidity index					< 0.001					0.056
Mean (SD)	1.5 (1.76)	0.9 (1.31)	1.1 (1.34)	1.0 (1.48)		1.2 (1.58)	0.9 (1.4)	1.2 (1.35)	1.0 (1.4)	

ST systemic therapy

[a]Subgroup for the landmark analysis at 6 months ($n = 447$): No treatment ($n = 119$); Surgery only ($n = 103$); ST only ($n = 130$); Surgery + ST ($n = 95$)

Table 2 Results of multinomial regression models for treatment approaches in patients with RCC. Two separate models are shown: one including all patients and the other including only the 6-month landmark analysis subgroup

	All patients w/ RCC				Patients w/ RCC in the 6-month landmark analysis			
	No treatment	Surgery only	ST only	Surgery + ST	No treatment	Surgery only	ST only	Surgery + ST
Variable	OR (95% CI)	OR (95% CI)	OR (95% CI)	OR (95% CI)	OR (95% CI)	OR (95% CI)	OR (95% CI)	OR (95% CI)
No Treatment as Reference								
Age (80 vs. 70)*	Reference	**0.46 (0.26–0.80)****	0.70 (0.46–1.07)	**0.39 (0.21–0.75)**	Reference	0.58 (0.26–1.32)	0.77 (0.37–1.61)	**0.40 (0.17–0.95)****
Sex (male vs. female)	Reference	0.71 (0.47–1.08)	0.99 (0.69–1.42)	1.01 (0.62–1.64)	Reference	0.74 (0.40–1.34)	1.27 (0.72–2.23)	1.00 (0.53–1.89)
Race (white vs. other)	Reference	1.23 (0.71–2.14)	0.75 (0.50–1.12)	0.94 (0.53–1.67)	Reference	1.20 (0.55–2.58)	0.70 (0.37–1.32)	0.80 (0.38–1.70)
Urban/rural code (ref: big metro)								
Metro/urban	Reference	0.89 (0.57–1.39)	1.03 (0.72–1.49)	**0.57 (0.35–0.94)**	Reference	0.97 (0.52–1.81)	1.61 (0.91–2.83)	0.68 (0.36–1.29)
Less urban/rural	Reference	1.09 (0.61–1.94)	0.84 (0.50–1.42)	0.54 (0.26–1.08)	Reference	1.32 (0.59–2.95)	1.04 (0.46–2.32)	0.51 (0.20–1.28)
Marital status (married vs. unmarried)	Reference	1.43 (0.94–2.18)	**1.48 (1.04–2.13)**	**3.13 (1.92–5.11)**	Reference	1.05 (0.58–1.91)	0.87 (0.50–1.53)	**2.51 (1.31–4.80)**
CCI (per 1-point increase)	Reference	**0.77 (0.66–0.89)**	**0.86 (0.77–0.96)**	**0.82 (0.70–0.96)**	Reference	0.89 (0.73–1.10)	1.04 (0.87–1.23)	0.92 (0.74–1.13)
Surgery only as Reference								
Age (80 vs. 70)*	**2.19 (1.25–3.82)**	Reference	1.54 (0.84–2.81)	0.86 (0.40–1.84)	1.72 (0.76–3.92)	Reference	1.32 (0.61–2.87)	0.58 (0.28–1.65)
Sex (male vs. female)	1.41 (0.92–2.15)	Reference	1.40 (0.88–2.22)	1.43 (0.83–2.46)	1.36 (0.75–2.48)	Reference	1.72 (0.97–3.05)	1.36 (0.73–2.53)
Race (white vs. other)	0.81 (0.47–1.41)	Reference	0.60 (0.34–1.08)	0.76 (0.38–1.53)	0.84 (0.39–1.81)	Reference	0.58 (0.28–1.19)	0.67 (0.30–1.49)
Urban/rural code (ref: big metro)								
Metro/urban	1.12 (0.72–1.75)	Reference	1.16 (0.72–1.87)	0.64 (0.37–1.13)	1.03 (0.55–1.92)	Reference	1.65 (0.92–3.00)	**0.70 (0.37–1.33)**
Less urban/rural	0.92 (0.51–1.63)	Reference	0.77 (0.41–1.46)	0.49 (0.23–1.06)	0.75 (0.34–1.68)	Reference	0.78 (0.36–1.70)	**0.38 (0.16–0.92)**
Marital status (married vs. unmarried)	0.70 (0.46–1.06)	Reference	1.04 (0.65–1.64)	**2.19 (1.26–3.80)**	0.95 (0.52–1.72)	Reference	0.83 (0.47–1.46)	**2.38 (1.26–4.50)**
CCI (per 1-point increase)	**1.30 (1.12–1.51)**	Reference	1.12 (0.95–1.32)	1.07 (0.88–1.30)	1.12 (0.91–1.37)	Reference	1.16 (0.95–1.41)	1.02 (0.82–1.28)
ST only as Reference								
Age (80 vs. 70)*	1.42 (0.93–2.17)	0.65 (0.36–1.19)	Reference	0.56 (0.28–1.10)	1.30 (0.62–2.73)	0.76 (0.35–1.64)	Reference	0.52 (0.23–1.18)
Sex (male vs. female)	1.01 (0.70–1.44)	0.72 (0.45–1.13)	Reference	1.02 (0.61–1.70)	0.79 (0.45–1.39)	0.58 (0.33–1.03)	Reference	0.79 (0.43–1.46)
Race (white vs. other)	1.34 (0.89–2.01)	1.66 (0.93–2.96)	Reference	1.27 (0.70–2.29)	1.44 (0.75–2.73)	1.72 (0.84–3.51)	Reference	1.15 (0.58–2.31)
Urban/rural code (ref: big metro)								
Metro/urban	0.97 (0.67–1.39)	0.86 (0.53–1.39)	Reference	**0.56 (0.33–0.94)**	0.62 (0.35–1.10)	0.60 (0.33–1.09)	Reference	**0.42 (0.23–0.78)**
Less urban/rural	1.19 (0.70–2.00)	1.30 (0.68–2.46)	Reference	0.64 (0.30–1.35)	0.96 (0.43–2.16)	1.28 (0.59–2.78)	Reference	0.49 (0.20–1.21)
Marital status (married vs. unmarried)	**0.67 (0.47–0.96)**	0.96 (0.61–1.52)	Reference	**2.11 (1.25–3.55)**	1.15 (0.65–2.02)	1.21 (0.69–2.14)	Reference	**2.88 (1.54–5.39)**
CCI (per 1-point increase)	**1.16 (1.04–1.30)**	0.89 (0.76–1.05)	Reference	0.96 (0.81–1.13)	0.96 (0.81–1.15)	0.86 (0.71–1.05)	Reference	0.88 (0.72–1.08)
Surgery + ST as Reference								

Table 2 Results of multinomial regression models for treatment approaches in patients with RCC. Two separate models are shown: one including all patients and the other including only the 6-month landmark analysis subgroup *(Continued)*

	All patients w/ RCC				Patients w/ RCC in the 6-month landmark analysis			
	No treatment	Surgery only	ST only	Surgery + ST	No treatment	Surgery only	ST only	Surgery + ST
Variable	OR (95% CI)	OR (95% CI)	OR (95% CI)	OR (95% CI)	OR (95% CI)	OR (95% CI)	OR (95% CI)	OR (95% CI)
Age (80 vs. 70) *	**2.55 (1.34–4.85)**	1.16 (0.54–2.50)	1.79 (0.91–3.53)	Reference	**2.52 (1.05–6.02)**	1.46 (0.61–3.53)	1.93 (0.85–4.40)	Reference
Sex (male vs. female)	0.99 (0.61–1.60)	0.70 (0.41–1.21)	0.98 (0.59–1.64)	Reference	1.00 (0.53–1.88)	0.74 (0.40–1.37)	1.26 (0.68–2.33)	Reference
Race (white vs. other)	1.06 (0.60–1.88)	1.31 (0.66–2.61)	0.79 (0.43–1.43)	Reference	1.24 (0.59–2.63)	1.49 (0.67–3.28)	0.87 (0.43–1.73)	Reference
Urban/rural code (ref: big metro)								
Metro/urban	**1.74 (1.06–2.86)**	1.55 (0.88–2.73)	**1.80 (1.07–3.04)**	Reference	1.47 (0.77–2.81)	1.43 (0.75–2.72)	**2.37 (1.28–4.38)**	Reference
Less urban/rural	1.87 (0.92–3.78)	2.04 (0.94–4.43)	1.57 (0.74–3.35)	Reference	1.98 (0.78–4.99)	**2.62 (1.09–6.30)**	2.05 (0.83–5.09)	Reference
Marital status (married vs. unmarried)	**0.32 (0.20–0.52)**	**0.46 (0.26–0.80)**	**0.47 (0.28–0.80)**	Reference	0.40 (0.21–0.76)	0.42 (0.22–0.79)	0.35 (0.19–0.65)	Reference
CCI (per 1-point increase)	**1.22 (1.04–1.42)**	0.94 (0.77–1.13)	1.05 (0.88–1.24)	Reference	1.09 (0.89–1.34)	0.98 (0.78–1.22)	1.13 (0.93–1.38)	Reference

*Odds ratio shown for 75th vs 25th percentile because age was modeled non-linearly
**Odds ratios and confidence intervals shown in bold are significant at the 5% level
RCC Renal Cell Carcinoma, *CCI* Charlson Comorbidity Index

(OR = 3.13, 95% CI 1.92–5.11) of having both surgery and ST within 6 months of diagnosis compared with patients who received no treatment, holding all other variables constant. Similarly, patients who were married had 0.67 times lower odds than unmarried patients (OR = 0.67, 95% CI 0.47–0.96) of having no treatment within 6 months compared with patients who received ST. The factors statistically significantly associated with treatment in the model (for any comparison) were age, marital status, and CCI. Older patients had lower odds of being treated with surgery, ST, or both compared to no treatment. Married patients had higher odds of being treated, and those with worse comorbidities had lower odds of being treated for all categories.

A more intuitive method of interpreting the fitted multinomial logistic regression model is examining predicted probabilities of each treatment group as a function of covariates in the model, which we present in Fig. 1. The probabilities for a given covariate were estimated after setting all other variables in the model to the median value (continuous variables) or most prevalent value (categorical variables). These values were age 76, male, white race, big metro, unmarried, and CCI = 1. In Fig. 1 we see the association between age and treatment group: the estimated probability of no treatment increases with age. Older patients (roughly ≥80 years) were more likely to receive no treatment than all other treatment groups combined. Similarly, patients with higher CCI (indicating more severe comorbidities) had increasing probabilities of receiving no treatment. Patients who were married had a higher probability of surgery and ST and a lower probability of no treatment, while the other treatment groups (surgery alone and chemo alone) stayed relatively constant for each marital status.

Similar patterns of patient characteristics were observed for the 6-month landmark analysis (Table 1). Whereas sex differences were statistically significant for all patients ($P = 0.017$), the differences were not significant for patients surviving ≥6 months ($P = 0.121$). However, this is largely due to the smaller sample size for the landmark analysis because the percentages of male and female were generally similar for each cohort.

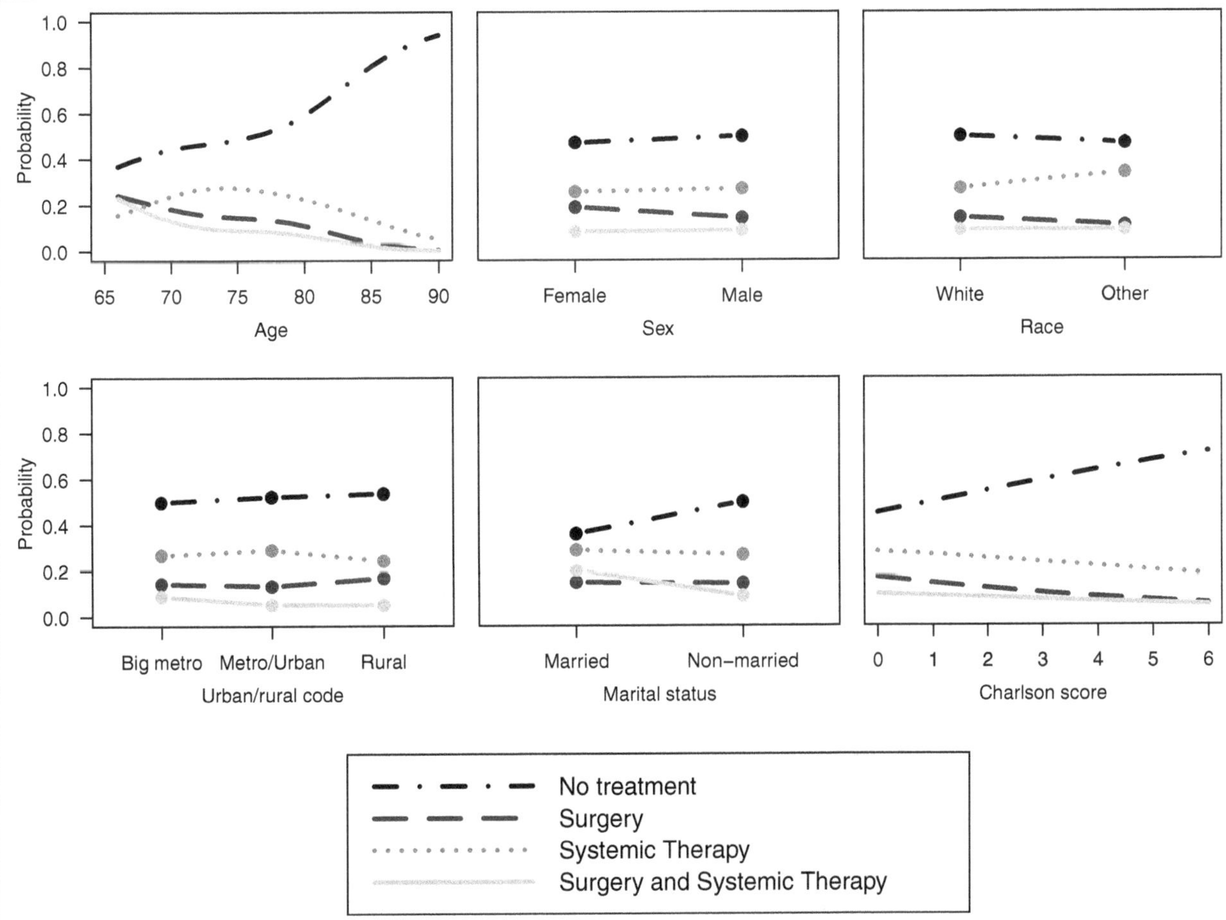

Fig. 1 Estimated probabilities from multinomial logistic regression model for each treatment group as a function of all variables in the model. For each plot, all other variables in the model were set to be the median (continuous variables) or most prevalent (categorical variables) value

Results of the multinomial logistic regression for patients surviving ≥6 months are presented in Table 2. Marital status, rurality, and age were the only significant predictors of treatment among this patient subgroup. Predicted probabilities of treatment from this model show that among patients who lived at least 6 months, the combination of surgery and systemic therapy was the highest probability treatment until age 80. For patients older then 80, no treatment was the highest probability treatment option (Fig. 2). Patients who were married had the highest probability of receiving both surgery and systemic therapy.

Discussion

In this study of almost 1000 Medicare beneficiaries with stage IV kidney cancer, we observed that over 50% did not receive any form of medical or surgical treatment. Even in our landmark analysis of patients who survived at least 6 months following diagnosis, 27% did not receive any therapy. Factors associated with patients not receiving treatment included clinical and sociodemographic factors such as older age, higher comorbidity burden, and unmarried status.

Cytoreductive nephrectomy is a potentially morbid operation with a risk of perioperative mortality (~ 3.2%) even in the most optimally selected patients [12]. This makes single or multi-agent systemic therapy a potentially attractive option in patients with impaired baseline renal function. Early experience with immune modulators, however, suggested treatment-related toxicity that significantly blunted therapeutic efficacy [13]. The introduction of tyrosine kinase inhibitors in the early 2000s heralded a new era in kidney cancer therapy with medications yielding significantly improved side effect profiles [14]. Subsequent investigations have identified a combination of agents with the capacity to target different components of the proliferative pathways [15, 16]. With both oral and parenteral routes of administration, options are available to a wide spectrum of patients, although treatment goals in this setting may be limited to partial response or stabilization of disease rather than complete remission. Additionally, the growth and expansion of

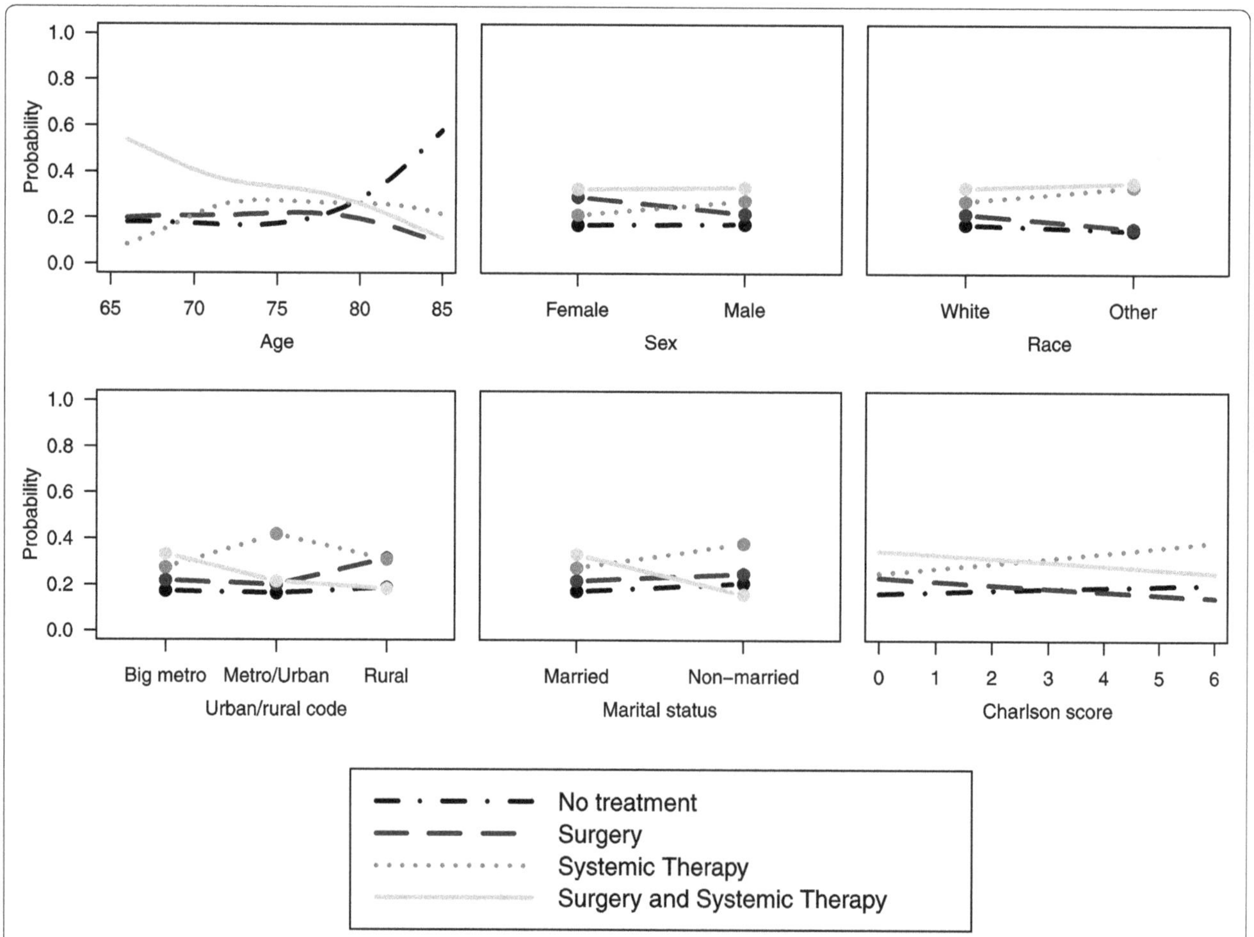

Fig. 2 Estimated probabilities from multinomial logistic regression model for each treatment group as a function of all variables in the model, for 6-month landmark. For each plot, all other variables in the model were set to be the median (continuous variables) or most prevalent (categorical variables) value

multiple agents in the second line setting, including nivolumab, cabozantinib, and combination lenvatinib and everolimus, show a survival advantage in this high-risk patient population [16]. In such settings, one must further consider potential advantages with regards to health-related quality of life (HRQoL) and time to onset of symptom improvement between agents [17]. Therefore, selection of subsequent therapy will depend on patient disease status, comorbidities, and resource availability [18]. Furthermore, other newer treatments may also provide treatments to patients who may otherwise have received little, including the robotic partial nephrectomy [19] and stereotactic ablative body radiotherapy [20].

One explanation for our finding that 27% of patients did not receive therapy is that the initial treatment strategy may have included active surveillance. A recent study by Rini et al. suggested that some patients with indolent growth of metastases could benefit from an initial active surveillance approach prior to administration of systemic targeted therapy [21]. Specifically, Rini found that among 48 patients the median time to surveillance interval was nearly 15 months; higher numbers of comorbidities and more metastatic disease sites were associated with shorter surveillance until initiation of systemic therapy or death [21]. While active surveillance may be an initial strategy for a select cohort of mRCC patients, the improved side effect profile of newer systemic therapies and their demonstrated effectiveness in elderly patients may obviate the need [22].

In our study, the negative association between age and CCI with receipt of therapy delivery was interesting and somewhat surprising. Clearly, the CCI is a measure of a patient's comorbidity complex, and therefore those who are ill are at risk for competing causes of mortality. In such patients, the costs of therapy must be balanced with expectations of prolonged life expectancy. The association with age, however, is more complex. In our cohort, the median age for the untreated group was 77, among which a percentage likely had an anticipated life expectancy of greater than 24–36 months post-diagnosis. The question remains whether such patients, particularly those untreated at 6-months after diagnosis, would have benefited from some therapy considering their low risk of imminent death.

Finally, the observation of marital status and receipt of treatment is not surprising. Previous research has found that factors beyond disease characteristics alone, including support- and infrastructure-related factors including marital status, socioeconomic status as determined by zip code, proximity to urban centers, as well as others being predictors not only for treatment but also survival in other cancers [23–27]. Such observations highlight potential opportunities for investment in a screening and survivorship initiative to bolster or ameliorate such factors.

We acknowledge several important limitations in this analysis, many of which are common in observational studies. First, as the information originated from an administrative dataset, we rely upon the coding in the part D component of Medicare to accurately assess delivery and type of treatment offered to patients, as well as comorbidities. Second, while the data allows evaluation of broad demographic and clinical factors, there is a lack of details regarding some of the specific factors that may have dictated the indication for treatment on an individual case basis. For example, Motzer et al. have shown that lab values and the Karnofsky score, measures not available in our data set, are predictive of risk [28, 29]. We were also unable to tell whether some patients received treatment as part of a clinical trial, nor were we able to distinguish between ST given as adjuvant therapy from neoadjuvant therapy among patients who received both surgery and ST. Finally, with the strict inclusion criteria utilized, the overall cohort of analysis was less than 1000 patients, thereby potentially limiting the applicability to a larger cohort with a broader age distribution. Nonetheless, these data are provocative and should prompt studies and discussions on the merits of intervention in patients particularly given those with anticipated life expectancy of greater than six months.

Conclusions

In this cohort of Medicare beneficiaries, many elderly patients with stage IV kidney cancer did not receive any form of therapy. Such observations persisted even among patients who survived at least six months after diagnosis. Given the increasing array of systemic targeted therapy with limited side effect profiles, the underlying reasons for such observations warrant further investigation as well as a consideration of the economic implications of therapy in this patient cohort.

Abbreviations

ANOVA: Analysis of variance; CCI: Charlson comorbidity index; CPT: Current procedural terminology; HCPCS: Healthcare common prodecure coding system; HRQoL: Health-related quality of life; ICD-9: International classification of diseases, ninth revision, clinical modification; ICD-O-3: International classification of diseases for oncology, 3rd edition; mRCC: Metastatic renal cell carcinoma; OR: Odds ratio; RCC: Renal cell carcinoma; SEER: Surveillane, Epidemiology and End Results; ST: Systemic therapy

Acknowledgements

Not applicable.

Authors' contributions
CH, JD, and ES conceived the study. JD and CH secured funding. ES and CH analyzed the data, while JD and JR interpreted the results. The manuscript was drafted by CH, ES, and JR, and JD provided critical review and revisions. All authors read and approved the final manuscript.
Table 1 Characteristics of patients with Stage IV kidney cancer, stratified by treatment group.

Author details
[1]Department of Health Policy and Administration, The Pennsylvania State University, 604E Donald H. Ford Building, University Park, State College, PA 16802, USA. [2]Department of Public Health Sciences, College of Medicine, The Pennsylvania State University, Hershey, PA, USA. [3]Bristol-Myers Squibb, Princeton, NJ, USA. [4]Department of Surgery, College of Medicine, The Pennsylvania State University, Hershey, PA, USA.

References

1. Smaldone MC, Egleston B, Hollingsworth JM, Hollenbeck BK, Miller DC, Morgan TM, Kim SP, Malhotra A, Handorf E, Wong YN, et al. Understanding treatment disconnect and mortality trends in renal cell carcinoma using tumor registry data. Med Care. 2017;55(4):398–404.
2. Hollingsworth JM, Miller DC, Daignault S, Hollenbeck BK. Rising incidence of small renal masses: a need to reassess treatment effect. J Natl Cancer Inst. 2006;98(18):1331–4.
3. Siegel RL, Miller KD, Jemal A. Cancer statistics, 2017. CA Cancer J Clin. 2017; 67(1):7–30.
4. Bazzi WM, Sjoberg DD, Feuerstein MA, Maschino A, Verma S, Bernstein M, O'Brien MF, Jang T, Lowrance W, Motzer RJ, et al. Long-term survival rates after resection for locally advanced kidney cancer: memorial Sloan Kettering Cancer center 1989 to 2012 experience. J Urol. 2015;193(6):1911–6.
5. Calvo E, Schmidinger M, Heng DY, Grunwald V, Escudier B. Improvement in survival end points of patients with metastatic renal cell carcinoma through sequential targeted therapy. Cancer Treat Rev. 2016;50:109–17.
6. Unverzagt S, Moldenhauer I, Nothacker M, Rossmeissl D, Hadjinicolaou AV, Peinemann F, Greco F, Seliger B. Immunotherapy for metastatic renal cell carcinoma. Cochrane Database Syst Rev. 2017;5:Cd011673.
7. Bedke J, Gauler T, Grunwald V, Hegele A, Herrmann E, Hinz S, Janssen J, Schmitz S, Schostak M, Tesch H, et al. Systemic therapy in metastatic renal cell carcinoma. World J Urol. 2017;35(2):179–88.
8. Kumbla RA, Figlin RA, Posadas EM. Recent advances in the medical treatment of recurrent or metastatic renal cell Cancer. Drugs. 2017;77(1): 17–28.
9. Hollingsworth JM, Miller DC, Daignault S, Hollenbeck BK. Five-year survival after surgical treatment for kidney cancer: a population-based competing risk analysis. Cancer. 2007;109(9):1763–8.
10. Randrup Hansen C, Grimm D, Bauer J, Wehland M, Magnusson NE. Effects and side effects of using sorafenib and sunitinib in the treatment of metastatic renal cell carcinoma. Int J Mol Sci. 2017;18(2):E461.
11. Deyo RA, Cherkin DC, Ciol MA. Adapting a clinical comorbidity index for use with ICD-9-CM administrative databases. J Clin Epidemiol. 1992;45(6):613–9.
12. Wallis CJ, Bjarnason G, Byrne J, Cheung DC, Hoffman A, Kulkarni GS, Nathens AB, Nam RK, Satkunasivam R. Morbidity and mortality of radical nephrectomy for patients with disseminated Cancer: an analysis of the National Surgical Quality Improvement Program Database. Urology. 2016;95:95–102.
13. Pham A, Ye DW, Pal S. Overview and management of toxicities associated with systemic therapies for advanced renal cell carcinoma. Urol Oncol. 2015; 33(12):517–27.
14. Kuenen BC, Tabernero J, Baselga J, Cavalli F, Pfanner E, Conte PF, Seeber S, Madhusudan S, Deplanque G, Huisman H, et al. Efficacy and toxicity of the angiogenesis inhibitor SU5416 as a single agent in patients with advanced renal cell carcinoma, melanoma, and soft tissue sarcoma. Clin Cancer Res. 2003;9(5):1648–55.
15. Merza H, Bilusic M. Current management strategy for metastatic renal cell carcinoma and future directions. Curr Oncol Rep. 2017;19(4):27.
16. Jonasch E. Incorporating new systemic therapies in kidney Cancer treatment. J Natl Compr Cancer Netw. 2017;15(5S):703–5.
17. Grimm MO, Grunwald V. Health-related quality of life as a prognostic measure of clinical outcomes in renal cell carcinoma: a review of the CheckMate 025 trial. Oncol Ther. 2017;5(1):75–8.
18. Fernandez-Pello S, Hofmann F, Tahbaz R, Marconi L, Lam TB, Albiges L, Bensalah K, Canfield SE, Dabestani S, Giles RH, et al. A systematic review and meta-analysis comparing the effectiveness and adverse effects of different systemic treatments for non-clear cell renal cell carcinoma. Eur Urol. 2017; 71(3):426–36.
19. Hennessey DB, Wei G, Moon D, Kinnear N, Bolton DM, Lawrentschuk N, Chan YK. Strategies for success: a multi-institutional study on robot-assisted partial nephrectomy for complex renal lesions. BJU Int. 2018;121(Suppl 3):40–7.
20. Siva S, Pham D, Kron T, Bressel M, Lam J, Tan TH, Chesson B, Shaw M, Chander S, Gill S, et al. Stereotactic ablative body radiotherapy for inoperable primary kidney cancer: a prospective clinical trial. BJU Int. 2017; 120(5):623–30.
21. Rini BI, Dorff TB, Elson P, Rodriguez CS, Shepard D, Wood L, Humbert J, Pyle L, Wong YN, Finke JH, et al. Active surveillance in metastatic renal-cell carcinoma: a prospective, phase 2 trial. Lancet Oncol. 2016;17(9):1317–24.
22. Vitale MG, Scagliarini S, Galli L, Pignata S, Lo Re G, Berruti A, Defferrari C, Spada M, Masini C, Santini D, et al. Efficacy and safety data in elderly patients with metastatic renal cell carcinoma included in the nivolumab expanded access program (EAP) in Italy. PLoS One. 2018;13(7):e0199642.
23. Schaefer EW, Wilson MZ, Goldenberg D, Mackley H, Koch W, Hollenbeak CS. Effect of marriage on outcomes for elderly patients with head and neck cancer. Head Neck. 2015;37(5):735–42.
24. Wang L, Wilson SE, Stewart DB, Hollenbeak CS, Schaefer EW, Wilson MZ, Goldenberg D, Mackley H, Koch W, Hollenbeak CS. Marital status and colon cancer outcomes in US surveillance, epidemiology and end results registries: does marriage affect cancer survival by gender and stage? Effect of marriage on outcomes for elderly patients with head and neck cancer. Cancer Epidemiol. 2011;35(5):417–22.
25. Megwalu UC. Impact of county-level socioeconomic status on Oropharyngeal Cancer survival in the United States. Otolaryngol Head Neck Surg. 2017;156(4):665–70.
26. Hinyard L, Wirth LS, Clancy JM, Schwartz T. The effect of marital status on breast cancer-related outcomes in women under 65: a SEER database analysis. Breast. 2017;32:13–7.
27. Vetterlein MW, Meyer CP, Leyh-Bannurah SR, Mayr R, Gierth M, Fritsche HM, Burger M, Keck B, Wullich B, Martini T, et al. Effect of hospital and surgeon case volume on perioperative quality of care and short-term outcomes after radical cystectomy for muscle-invasive bladder Cancer: results from a European tertiary care center cohort. Clin Genitourin Cancer. 2017;15(5):e809–17.
28. Motzer RJ, Bacik J, Mazumdar M. Prognostic factors for survival of patients with stage IV renal cell carcinoma: memorial sloan-kettering cancer center experience. Clin Cancer Res. 2004;10(18 Pt 2):6302s–3s.
29. Mekhail TM, Abou-Jawde RM, Boumerhi G, Malhi S, Wood L, Elson P, Bukowski R. Validation and extension of the memorial Sloan-Kettering prognostic factors model for survival in patients with previously untreated metastatic renal cell carcinoma. J Clin Oncol. 2005;23(4):832–41.

22

Optical puncture combined with balloon dilation PCNL vs. conventional puncture dilation PCNL for kidney stones without hydronephrosis

Mi Zhou, Xiang He, Yuelong Zhang and Weiwen Yu*

Abstract

Background: Accurate puncture and dilation of the target kidney calices for percutaneous nephrolithotomy (PCNL) can be difficult. This study aimed to investigate the advantages of PCNL using optical puncture (i.e. the puncture is visualized on a screen as seen through the needle) combined with balloon dilation vs. conventional puncture methods.

Methods: This was a retrospective study of 58 consecutive patients with kidney stones without hydronephrosis and treated at the Minimally Invasive Urology Center of Zhejiang Provincial People's Hospital between 10/2016 and 12/2017. Twenty-one patients underwent optical puncture combined with balloon dilation PCNL. Thirty-seven patients underwent conventional puncture instrument dilation PCNL (controls). Success rate, tubeless rate, blood loss, pain, and complications were compared between the two groups.

Results: The one-time puncture success rate (95.2% [20/21] vs. 67.6% [25/37], $P = 0.02$) and the postoperative tubeless rate (81.0% [17/21] vs. 54.1% [20/37], $P = 0.04$) were higher in the optical puncture group compared with controls. The average postoperative hemoglobin reduction was smaller (1.13 ± 0.63 vs. 1.56 ± 0.59 g/dL, $P = 0.01$), the postoperative VAS score was lower (1.6 ± 0.9 vs. 2.5 ± 1.2, $P = 0.004$), the rate of postoperative analgesic use was lower (14.3% [3/21] vs. 40.5% [15/37], $P = 0.04$), and the postoperative mean hospitalization days was shorter (3.7 ± 0.9 vs. 4.4 ± 0.8, $P = 0.005$) in the optical puncture group vs. controls. There was no case of urinary sepsis, blood transfusion, perirenal hematoma, pleural injury, and visceral organ damage.

Conclusions: Optical puncture combined with balloon dilation PCNL could be associated with good therapeutic effect and low frequency of complications for the treatment of kidney stones without hydronephrosis.

Keywords: Optical puncture, Balloon dilation, Percutaneous nephrolithotomy, Kidney stones without hydronephrosis

Background

Most kidney stones do not lead to significant symptoms, but partial, intermittent, or complete urinary tract obstruction will result in pain [1]. The reported lifetime incidence of kidney stone is 1–15%, depending on countries and lifestyle habits [2, 3], and the incidence is high in Western countries and in children [4, 5]. In China, the prevalence of kidney stones is around 7.5% and shows a rising trend [6].

Percutaneous nephrolithotomy (PCNL) is the main minimally invasive surgical method for the treatment of large or complex stones [7]. The successful establishment of the percutaneous renal channel is the basis for PCNL. Accurate puncture and dilation of the target kidney calices are keys to establish the percutaneous renal channel. The renal cortex in patients with kidney stones without hydronephrosis is relatively thick, the space in the target kidney calices is limited, and routine PCNL puncture and dilation are associated with risks of hemorrhage and channel loss [8]. Therefore, the selection of the best PCNL approach for the treatment of

* Correspondence: hfhyww@163.com
Department of Urology, Zhejiang Provincial People's Hospital/People's Hospital of Hangzhou Medical College, Hangzhou, China

kidney stones without hydronephrosis is still a challenge for urologists.

Optical puncture technology can be used to confirm whether the puncture site is reliable and reasonable [9, 10]. The application of balloon dilation can reduce the damage to the renal parenchyma [11–13]. The combination of the two could decrease the risk of complications of kidney stones without hydronephrosis and improve the postoperative stone clearance rate.

Therefore, this study was designed to investigate the advantages of optical puncture combined with balloon dilation PCNL. Although observational, this study could provide some basis for the selection of the best PCNL approach and for an eventual randomized controlled trial.

Methods

Study design and patients

This was a retrospective analysis of 58 consecutive patients with kidney stones without hydronephrosis and treated at the Minimally Invasive Urology Center of Zhejiang Provincial People's Hospital between October 1, 2016 and December 31, 2017. The study was approved by the ethics committee of Zhejiang Provincial People's Hospital. The need for individual consent was waived by the committee because of the retrospective nature of the study.

The inclusion criteria were: 1) kidney stones maximum diameter of > 2 cm; and 2) no hydronephrosis or mild hydronephrosis (level 1 or 2 in Grignon's grading) by IVP/CTU examination [14]. The exclusion criteria were: 1) distal stone obstruction; 2) severe heart or lung disease; 3) diseases with hemorrhagic tendency; 4) ASA grade III or above; 5) solitary kidney or functional solitary kidney; 6) abnormal renal function; or 7) upper urinary tract infection with unsatisfying preoperative control.

Preoperative examinations

All patients completed the preoperative examinations including blood routine, blood type, urine routine, urine culture, stool routine, occult blood, biochemical tests (liver and kidney function, fasting blood glucose, lipids, and electrolytes), coagulation function, thyroid function, parathyroid function, tests for infectious diseases (hepatitis B, hepatitis C, syphilis, and AIDS, as per Chinese guidelines for PCNL), electrocardiogram, chest X-ray, abdominal ultrasound, urinary B ultrasound, and IVP/CTU.

Surgical methods

All procedures were conducted by three senior physicians (> 20 years of experience and completed more than 500 PCNL procedures) under general anesthesia. After effective anesthesia, a F6 ureteral catheter was implanted into the ureters in the lithotomy position (to prevent the stone fragment moving to the distal ureter during operation). A 16F Foley urethral catheter was implanted into the bladder. Then, the patient was converted to the prone position. Puncture was performed under ultrasound positioning. The puncture site was between the scapular line and the posterior axillary line under the 11th or 12th rib. The puncture entered into the renal calyx at the fornix.

For optical puncture combined with balloon dilation PCNL, a 16 G (1.5 mm) Kangge puncture needle (Shanghai Shangyi Kangge Medical Equipment Co., Ltd., China) was used for puncture after B-mode ultrasound (BK Ultrasound Machines, Denmark) positioning. Two optical methods were used during the study period. The UMP nephroscope (F3, Schoelly, Germany) was used to monitor the whole puncture process through the lumen of the puncture needle by the visualization platform; or the process was observed with a Poly optical puncture nephroscope (F4.8, Poly, Germany) until the puncture needle entered the target renal calyx and the stones were seen. The visualization approach, the type of puncture instrument, the type of guide wire, and the brand of the dilation balloon were selected according to the physicians' experience.

A Bard (Bard Biopsy Systems, Tempe, AZ, USA)/Cook (Cook Medical, Bloomington, IN, USA) super smooth guide wire was placed through a puncture needle and a Bard (Bard, USA)/Cook (Cook, USA) nephroscope dilation balloon catheter was placed along the guide wire. B-mode ultrasound positioning was used to confirm that the balloon was in the target renal calyx. Saline was injected into the balloon and the water pressure was set to 20–25 atm for coaxial radial expansion and maintained for 3–5 min. A 24 Fr outer sheath was placed along the balloon catheter into the target renal calyx. The balloon catheter was withdrawn. A 18 Fr Wolf nephroscope (Richard-wolf, Germany) was used to start the lithotripsy procedure. The perfusion pump was used to infuse physiological saline into the collecting system during lithotripsy and flow rate was kept at 350–400 ml per minute. Ultrasound combined with a pneumatic ballistic suction system (EMS, Switzerland) was used for lithotripsy and clearing the stones. After lithotripsy, the collecting system was carefully examined for each renal calyx and the junctions of the renal pelvis and ureter. B-mode ultrasound was used for confirmation of no apparent residual stones left. A super smooth guide wire was placed into the collecting system. The F6 ureteral catheter was removed and a 6 Fr DJ stent was indwelled into the ureter along the guide wire. The puncture channel and renal parenchyma were observed for bleeding. A 20 Fr nephrostomy tube was indwelled. The 24 Fr outer sheath was gradually withdrawn. Dressing was directly applied on the skin incision.

If hemorrhage was found at the end of operation, a bipolar columnar electrocoagulation rod/Nd laser was used to stop the hemorrhage along the channel. If there were no injury to the collecting system, no severe hydronephrosis, no intrarenal infection, and no residual stone > 4 mm, the nephrostomy tube was not indwelled (postoperative tubeless). If there were no visible bleeding and residual stones after surgery, the DJ stent was not indwelled (completely postoperative tubeless).

In the control group, the conventional punctures were performed using the Create puncture instrument (Dalian Create Medical Products Co., Ltd., China) or the UROVISION puncture instrument (LAKH, Inc., Germany). Puncture needles (18G) were used to puncture the target renal calyx under ultrasound guidance. After successful puncture, a Bard (Bard, USA)/Cook (Cook, USA) super smooth guide wire was implanted. After the skin was incised, the percutaneous renal passage was dilated to 24 Fr using a fascial dilator and another sheath was indwelled. The remaining operations were similar to the operations of optical puncture combined with balloon dilation PCNL, as above.

Postoperative management

Blood routine, CRP, PCT, and coagulation function examinations were completed on the day of surgery and the following day. Postoperative blood loss, inflammatory responses, and stability of the internal environment were evaluated. Antibiotics were routinely used for 3–5 days after surgery. The patients' vital signs, urine color, and urine volume were observed. CT plain scan of the urinary system was repeated 1–3 days after surgery to assess whether there were any perinephric effusion and hematocele after surgery, complications, residual stones, and whether the nephrostomy tube should be removed. All patients were given non-steroidal anti-inflammatory drugs on the day of surgery. Postoperative pain was evaluated by visual analogue scale (VAS) on the following day. If VAS was ≥3, the patients continued to use analgesics. The patient was required to stand and be active 1–3 days after surgery and adjust the amount of activity according to the change of urine color. Normal diet was given after postoperative defecation. If there was obviously active hematuria after surgery, digital subtraction angiography (DSA) hemostasis was completed as soon as possible. The urethral catheters and nephrostomy tubes were removed 2–7 days after surgery (for patients with nephrostomy tube) and the patients were discharged. Stone specimens were physicochemically analyzed by infrared spectroscopy. DJ stents were removed at the outpatient clinic one month after surgery (for patients with DJ stents). CT plain scan of the urinary system was performed to evaluate the stone-free rate (SFR), defined as no residual stones or residual stones with a maximum diameter ≤ 4 mm and no clinical symptoms [15]. If the stone-free state was not achieved, CT plain scan of the urinary system was performed again 3 months after surgery to assess the SFR.

Follow-up

Since this study aimed to observe the surgical complications and the postoperative SFR, only 3 months of follow-up after surgery was considered.

Statistical analysis

SPSS 19.0 (IBM, Armonk, NY, USA) was used for statistical analysis. Continuous data were tested for normal distribution using the Kolmogorov-Smirnov test. All data were found to be normally distributed, presented as means ± standard deviation, and analyzed using the Student t test. Categorical data were presented as frequencies and analyzed using the Fisher's exact test. Two-sided P values ≤0.05 were considered statistically significant.

Results

Characteristics of the patients

General clinical data and postoperative analysis of stone composition in the 21 patients in the optical puncture group and the 37 patients in the control group are shown in Table 1. There were 35 males and 23 females. They were 21–77 years of age (mean of 45.2 ± 13.4 years). The mean maximum diameter of the stones was 3.9 ± 1.2 cm. There were 16 patients with single stones and 42 with multiple stones (25 patients with stag horns). The kidney stones were on the left side in 22 patients and on the right side in 36. The ASA scores were I in 34 patients and II in 24. Thirteen patients had diabetes mellitus, 19 had hypertension, and three had coronary heart disease. There were no significant differences in sex, age, ASA score, stone size, location, number of stones, and stone composition between the two groups.

Surgery and therapeutic effect

Surgical characteristics and therapeutic effects are shown in Table 2. The first-time puncture success rate (95.2% vs. 67.6%, $P = 0.02$) and the postoperative tubeless rate (81.0% vs. 54.1%, $P = 0.04$) were higher in the optical puncture group compared with controls. Postoperative hemoglobin reduction was lower (1.13 ± 0.63 vs. 1.56 ± 0.59 g/dL, $P = 0.01$), postoperative VAS score was lower (1.6 ± 0.9 vs. 2.5 ± 1.2, $P = 0.004$), rate of postoperative analgesic use was lower (14.3% vs. 40.5%, P = 0.04), and mean postoperative hospitalization days was shorter (3.7 ± 0.9 vs. 4.4 ± 0.8, $P = 0.005$) in the optical puncture group compared with controls. There were no significant differences in the mean operation time and completely

Table 1 Characteristics of the patients and stones

	Optical puncture group (*n* = 21)	Control group (*n* = 37)	P
Sex, n (%)			0.710
Male	12 (57.1)	23 (62.2)	
Female	9 (42.9)	14 (37.8)	
Mean age (years)	46.8 ± 12.4	44.2 ± 14.0	0.483
Maximum stone diameter (mm)	4.0 ± 1.0	3.9 ± 1.3	0.666
Number of stones, n (%)			0.900
Single	6 (28.6)	10 (27.0)	
Multiple	15 (71.4)	27 (73.0)	
Stone position, n (%)			0.985
Left side	8 (38.1)	14 (37.8)	
Right side	13 (61.9)	23 (62.2)	
ASA score, n (%)			0.431
I	12 (57.1)	25 (67.6)	
II	9 (42.9)	12 (32.4)	
Stone composition, n (%)			0.822
Calcium oxalate	3 (14.3)	5 (13.5)	
Calcium phosphate	2 (9.5)	6 (16.2)	
Magnesium phosphate	3 (14.3)	4 (10.8)	
Uric acid	1 (4.8)	1 (2.7)	
Mixed	12 (57.1)	21 (56.8)	

Table 2 Surgical data and therapeutic effect

	Optical puncture group (*n* = 21)	Control group (*n* = 37)	P
Mean operation time (min)	57 ± 8	53 ± 7	0.058
One-time success rate of puncture, n (%)	20 (95.2)	25 (67.6)	0.016
Hemorrhage			
Mean reduction of postoperative Hb (g/dL)	1.13 ± 0.63	1.56 ± 0.59	0.012
Postoperative DSA rate, n (%)	1 (4.8)	2 (5.4)	0.916
Infection, n (%)			
Postoperative fever rate	2 (9.5)	4 (10.8)	0.878
Incidence of urinary sepsis	0	0	1
Pain situation			
Postoperative VAS score	1.6 ± 0.9	2.5 ± 1.2	0.004
Postoperative analgesic usage, n (%)	3 (14.3)	15 (40.5)	0.039
Average postoperative hospitalization days	3.7 ± 0.9	4.4 ± 0.8	0.005
Postoperative tubeless rate, n (%)	17 (81.0)	20 (54.1)	0.042
Postoperative completely tubeless rate	23.8%(5)	18.9%(7)	0.661
Stone-free rate after 1 month of operation, n (%)	16 (76.2)	29 (78.3)	0.849
Stone-free rate after 3 month of operation, n (%)	20 (95.2)	35 (94.6)	0.916

postoperative tubeless rate. Urethral catheters and nephrostomy tubes (for patients with nephrostomy tubes) were successfully removed for all patients before discharge. The DJ stents were removed one month after surgery (for patients with DJ stents).

Complications

There were two and four patients with postoperative fever in the optical puncture and control groups, respectively. All of them were transient fever, without clinical manifestations of urinary sepsis. Fresh gross hematuria was observed in two and five patients, respectively. Among them, one and two patients, respectively, had DSA embolization for hemostasis. No patients required blood transfusion. The postoperative CT examination showed no significant perirenal hematoma, no pleural injury, or visceral organ damage.

Residual stones

In the optical puncture group, residual stones were found in five patients who underwent CT scan reexamination at 1 month after surgery. There was still one patient with residual stones at 3 months after surgery, which was treated with extracorporeal lithotripsy. In the control group, residual stones were found in eight patients who underwent CT scan reexamination at 1 month after surgery. There were still two patients with residual stones at 3 months after surgery. One patient underwent extracorporeal lithotripsy and the other one underwent ureteroscopic lithotripsy. All remaining patients achieved SFR on CT scan at 3 months after surgery.

Discussion

PCNL is difficult because the space of the target calyces is small. Therefore, this study was designed to investigate the advantages of optical puncture combined with balloon dilation PCNL. The results suggest that optical puncture combined with balloon dilation PCNL could be associated with good therapeutic effect and small frequency complications for the treatment of kidney stones without hydronephrosis.

In 1976, Fernström et al. [16] first reported the PCNL minimally invasive method for the treatment of urolithiasis. At present, PCNL is still the first choice for the treatment of kidney stones and upper ureteral stone of

> 2 cm or > 500 mm^2 [17, 18]. According to the size of the channel, percutaneous nephroscopes can be divided into standard-channel (24F–30F) or conventional-channel (>22F), mini-channel (14-22F), ultra/super-mini-channel (12F–14F), mini-micro-channel (8F), and micro-channel (<5F) [19–22]. The preferred channel for treating stag horn stone is still standard-channel PCNL [23]. In the treatment of large stones, negative pressure suction combined with standard-channel puncture and using ultrasound and pneumatic lithotripsy could effectively shorten the operation time, reduce intrarenal perfusion pressure during surgery, increase stone clearance rate, and reduce complications during and after the operation, especially the occurrence of urinary sepsis [24, 25]. Nevertheless, surgery with standard channel may increase the risk of bleeding. It requires accurate puncture techniques and effective channel establishment. In cases of kidney stone without hydronephrosis, the ultrasound localization of kidney stone is limited, and it is easy to lose the channel when the channel is established because the effective space of the renal calyces is small, increasing the difficulty of operation.

In 1997, Bellman et al. [26] selected 50 patients who underwent tubeless PCNL surgery and retained only DJ stent after operation, and compared them with 50 cases of conventional catheterization. They found that the tubeless treatment group had a lower use of analgesics, shorter hospitalization, and reduced treatment costs compared with the traditional catheterization group. In a prospective trial, Aghamir et al. [27] randomized 70 patients to a completely tubeless technique (no retention of nephrostomy tube and DJ stent) and a traditional catheterization group, and the outcomes were similar (i.e. there were no significant differences in postoperative bleeding, postoperative complications, secondary operation rate, and stone removal rate). The premise of tubeless PCNL is that kidney bleeding is controlled at the end of the operation and kidney drainage is unobstructed after operation. Therefore, the tubeless PCNL requires more precise surgical techniques, but there should be no bleeding, no iatrogenic injury, and no residual stone at the end of operation.

In patients with kidney stone without hydronephrosis, the traditional method aims to establish artificial hydronephrosis in order to increase the success rate of targeted calyceal puncture [28]. A ureteral catheter placed on the affected side prior to puncture, and the assistant pushes saline into the targeted renal calyx, which increases the success rate of puncture. But sometimes water injection will increase the intrarenal pressure of the renal pelvis and renal calyx, and it may increase the risk of septicemia. Recently, studies reported an improved success rate of renal puncture using GPS ultrasound positioning systems [29, 30]. Indeed, the GPS ultrasound positioning system can be used to adjust the angle and direction of the puncture needle in real time, and guide the depth of puncture. It could reduce the difficulty of puncture to a certain extent. It is still based on ultrasound and had no advantage to determine the calyceal fornix without hydronephrosis. In addition, its real-time location depended on the magnetic field sensing system, and errors may occur. Jie et al. [31] used B-mode ultrasound combined with X-ray to guide the puncture, and reported improved accuracy of puncture by using the two methods. Nevertheless, this combined method requires the repeated use of B-mode ultrasound and C-arm X-ray, which lengthen the operation time. In addition, the repeated use of the C-arm X-ray machine increases radiation exposure of patients and medical personnel.

In the present study, the optical puncture technique was used to improve the success rate of the puncture of kidney without hydronephrosis. X-ray is not required in this method. The optical puncture technique was first reported by Bader et al. [9]. Using this method, the whole puncture process is completed under direct vision for entering into the target renal calyx. Desai et al. [10] and Hanqing et al. [10, 32] used the optical puncture system to perform ultra-microchannel lithotripsy to treat kidney stones < 2 cm, and achieved good surgical results. In the present study, seven patients were treated with a 16G (1.5 mm) Kangge puncture needle combined with UMP nephroscope (F3) under a needle sheath, and 14 patients were treated with a Poly optical puncture nephroscope (F4.8). In the direct vision puncture process, the puncture is first completed with B-mode ultrasound localization. The needle tip position is observed by intrathecal endoscopy and the depth of the needle tip in the targeted renal calyx is adjusted properly to ensure that the guide wire in the narrow space of the renal calyx is placed exactly. During the process of localization observation, because of its rigid characteristics, the puncture nephroscope can pass staghorn calculi without hydronephrosis, and is successful regarding the insertion of the guide wire into the renal pelvis and keeping it in the space of UPJ. The puncture needle has a water injection channel to achieve a clear view. Using direct vision, the accuracy of puncture position is determined by the optical puncture technique. When the stone is not observed during the puncture process, the puncture angle can be adjusted. The needle tip position can be observed by intrathecal endoscopy and the depth of needle in the targeted renal calyx can be adjusted properly to ensure that the guide wire in the narrow space of the renal calyx is placed exactly. In addition, B-mode ultrasound localization and optical puncture can be performed simultaneously without increasing the number of punctures. In the 21 patients, the success rate of the first puncture was 95.2% (20/21). Postoperative routine CT examinations of the urinary system can help rule out complications, display residual stones, and help decide whether the nephrostomy tube should be removed. Previous studies suggest that some inconclusive results are to be expected when evaluating a patient using ultrasound, and imaging with a low-dose CT in these circumstances is reasonable [33–35]. Therefore, in the present study, a CT scan was performed 1–3 days after the operation.

Another difficulty in the operation of kidney stones without hydronephrosis is channel establishment. The space of the targeted renal calyx is occupied by stones. After puncture needle enters the targeted renal calyx, the guide wire can easily become curled in the renal calyx or be blocked by the stone in calyceal fornix, and cannot enter the renal pelvis and ureter. In this case, the guide wire can easily slide out of the kidney calyx when the channel is expanded step by step, leading to loss of channel and injury to the renal parenchyma. In order to reduce channel loss, the "two-step method" or the "improved one-step method" is generally used [36, 37]. Although this method can reduce the probability of channel loss to some extent, it still damages the renal parenchyma due to the shearing force of axial expansion. If the puncture needle is not fully perpendicular to the fornix of calix at the time of puncture, it might damage the interlobar artery and cause bleeding during dilation. We selected the method of balloon expansion when we established the channel. In this method, the balloon catheter is pushed along the guide wire under real-time B-mode ultrasound guidance after the guide wire is confirmed to be into the collection system. The puncture channel is expanded by water injection. This is a "coaxial radial one-step dilatation" method for the establishment of skin-kidney channel. It converts the axial shearing force of the traditional fascial dilators into a radial compression force, reducing the cutting damage to the renal tissue and performing some kind of compression hemostasis when expanding.

A number of studies demonstrated that balloon dilation has more advantages than traditional fascial dilators in establishing channels, especially in patients with kidney stone without hydronephrosis [13, 23, 38]. Balloon dilation can significantly increase the success rate of first dilation and reduce the surgical risks. On the other hand, some studies suggested that there is no significant difference in the effects of balloon dilators and Amplaz fascial dilators and metal sleeve dilators during PCNL surgery [11, 12]. It is worth noting that these negative studies were not performed in patients with kidney stones without hydronephrosis.

In our study, PCNL was performed in 21 patients with kidney stone without hydronephrosis, of which 17 patients underwent tubeless treatment without retention of nephrostomy tube, and 5 patients underwent completely tubeless treatment. None of the 17 cases had delayed hemorrhage, sepsis, or perirenal effusion/hematoma after surgery. In a previous study [39], we summarized the surgical experience of tubeless PCNL with common puncture dilation standard channel. The criteria for the selection of tubeless treatment are: 1) no active bleeding or hemorrhage spot, or the hemorrhage of small blood vessels was stopped by bipolar columnar electrocoagulation rod/Nd laser; 2) no injury to the collecting system; 3) no severe hydronephrosis and intrarenal infection; 4) no obvious residual stone; and 5) 11 intercostals or 12 subcostal single channel. We hypothesize that optical puncture combined with balloon dilation standard-channel PCNL lithotripsy can increase the accuracy of puncture and reduce the skin-kidney channel loss, leading to smaller rates of repeated puncture. Thus, it can decrease blood loss and increase the tubeless rate, which may relieve postoperative pain. It can also reduce the length of hospital stay. Nevertheless, we should pay attention on the additional expense of this technique. Both the additionally needed scope and balloon add to the total cost.

This study has limitations. It was not a prospective study and there was probably an inherent selection bias. The sample size was small. There were some subjective judgments on the determination of tubeless treatment selection. The effectiveness still needs to be confirmed by multicenter, large-sample studies.

Conclusions

Our study suggests that optical puncture combined with balloon dilatation standard channel PCNL lithotripsy in patients with kidney stone > 2 cm without hydronephrosis can increase the accuracy of puncture and success rate of the skin-kidney channel establishment, ensure the stone removal rate, and increase the postoperative tubeless rate. As a result, it can also reduce the length of hospital stay and postoperative pain, and promote rapid recovery after PCNL.

Abbreviations

PCNL: percutaneous nephrolithotomy; VAS: visual analogue scale

Acknowledgements

Not applicable.

Authors' contributions

MZ designed and coordinated the study, designed, performed and analyzed the experiments, and wrote the paper. XH, YLZ, and WWY carried out data collection, data analysis, and revised the paper. All authors reviewed the results and approved the final version of the manuscript.

References

1. Pietrow PK, Karellas ME. Medical management of common urinary calculi. Am Fam Physician. 2006;74:86–94.

2. Scales CD Jr, Smith AC, Hanley JM, Saigal CS, Urologic Diseases in America P. Prevalence of kidney stones in the United States. Eur Urol. 2012;62:160–5.
3. Morgan MS, Pearle MS. Medical management of renal stones. BMJ. 2016; 352:i52.
4. Sas DJ, Hulsey TC, Shatat IF, Orak JK. Increasing incidence of kidney stones in children evaluated in the emergency department. J Pediatr. 2010;157:132–7.
5. Turney BW, Reynard JM, Noble JG, Keoghane SR. Trends in urological stone disease. BJU Int. 2012;109:1082–7.
6. Wang W, Fan J, Huang G, Li J, Zhu X, Tian Y, et al. Prevalence of kidney stones in mainland China: a systematic review. Sci Rep. 2017;7:41630.
7. Ganpule AP, Vijayakumar M, Malpani A, Desai MR. Percutaneous nephrolithotomy (PCNL) a critical review. Int J Surg. 2016;36:660–4.
8. Ying H, Hui W, Zhigang C. Application of ureteral balloon dilation catheter in treatment of renal calculi without hydronephrosis. Chin J Endourol. 2013;7:21–3.
9. Bader MJ, Gratzke C, Seitz M, Sharma R, Stief CG, Desai M. The "all-seeing needle": initial results of an optical puncture system confirming access in percutaneous nephrolithotomy. Eur Urol. 2011;59:1054–9.
10. Desai MR, Sharma R, Mishra S, Sabnis RB, Stief C, Bader M. Single-step percutaneous nephrolithotomy (microperc): the initial clinical report. J Urol. 2011;186:140–5.
11. El-Shazly M, Salem S, Allam A, Hathout B. Balloon dilator versus telescopic metal dilators for tract dilatation during percutaneous nephrolithotomy for staghorn stones and calyceal stones. Arab J Urol. 2015;13:80–3.
12. Ozcift B, Bal K, Dincel C. A comparison of balloon and amplatz dilators in percutaneous nephrolithotomy: a retrospective evaluation. Turk J Urol. 2013; 39:226–31.
13. Ren M, Zhang C, Fu W, Fu Y, Ma L, Zhao W, et al. Balloon dilation versus Amplatz dilation during ultrasound-guided percutaneous nephrolithotomy for staghorn stones. Chin Med J. 2014;127:1057–61.
14. Grignon A, Filion R, Filiatrault D, Robitaille P, Homsy Y, Boutin H, et al. Urinary tract dilatation in utero: classification and clinical applications. Radiology. 1986;160:645–7.
15. Somani BK, Desai M, Traxer O, Lahme S. Stone-free rate (SFR): a new proposal for defining levels of SFR. Urolithiasis. 2014;42:95.
16. Fernstrom I, Johansson B. Percutaneous pyelolithotomy. A new extraction technique. Scand J Urol Nephrol. 1976;10:257–9.
17. Lingeman JE, Newman D, Mertz JH, Mosbaugh PG, Steele RE, Kahnoski RJ, et al. Extracorporeal shock wave lithotripsy: the Methodist Hospital of Indiana experience. J Urol. 1986;135:1134–7.
18. Lam HS, Lingeman JE, Barron M, Newman DM, Mosbaugh PG, Steele RE, et al. Staghorn calculi: analysis of treatment results between initial percutaneous nephrostolithotomy and extracorporeal shock wave lithotripsy monotherapy with reference to surface area. J Urol. 1992;147: 1219–25.
19. Zeng G, Zhu W, Lam W. Miniaturised percutaneous nephrolithotomy: its role in the treatment of urolithiasis and our experience. Asian J Urol. 2018;5: 295–302.
20. Mishra S, Sharma R, Garg C, Kurien A, Sabnis R, Desai M. Prospective comparative study of miniperc and standard PNL for treatment of 1 to 2 cm size renal stone. BJU Int. 2011;108:896–9 discussion 9-900.
21. Schilling D, Husch T, Bader M, Herrmann TR, Nagele U. Training, et al. nomenclature in PCNL or the tower of babel: a proposal for a uniform terminology. World J Urol. 2015;33:1905–7.
22. Rassweiler J, Rassweiler MC, Klein J. New technology in ureteroscopy and percutaneous nephrolithotomy. Curr Opin Urol. 2016;26:95–106.
23. Tiejun P, Xumin X, HGongcheng L. Clinical study of balloon dilation in percutaneous nephrolithotomy for staghorn stones. Chin J Urol. 2014; 35:881–4.
24. De S, Sarkissian C, Marchinni G, Monga M. Concurrent stone stabilization improves ultrasonic and pneumatic efficacy during cystolithopaxy: an in vitro analysis. Int Braz J Urol. 2015;41:134–8.
25. Pugh JW, Canales BK. New instrumentation in percutaneous nephrolithotomy. Indian J Urol. 2010;26:389–94.
26. Bellman GC, Davidoff R, Candela J, Gerspach J, Kurtz S, Stout L. Tubeless percutaneous renal surgery. J Urol. 1997;157:1578–82.
27. Aghamir SM, Modaresi SS, Aloosh M, Tajik A. Totally tubeless percutaneous nephrolithotomy for upper pole renal stone using subcostal access. J Endourol. 2011;25:583–6.
28. Huan W, Xingqiu F, Changhui W. Percutaneous nephrolithotomy for treatment of renal stone in non-dilated collecting system. Guide Chin Med. 2016;14:21–2.
29. Zhihua Z, Jian L, Qiqing F. Application of percutaneous nephrolithotomy with GPS-ultrasound guidance. J Minimally Invasive Urol. 2016;5:16–8.
30. Shan R, Renjing P, Dejun Z. Application of SonixGPS system in percutaneous nephrostomy. Chin Pract Med. 2014;5:45–6.
31. Jie C, Moing L, Youbin P. Application experience of type-B ultrasonic joint x-ray in percutaneous nephroscope treatment of complicated kidney stones. Chin Med Innov. 2013;13:44–6.
32. Hanqing X, Qi C, Hai Z. Ultra-mini percutaneous nephrolithotomy for the treatment of renal or upper ureteral stones (report of 32 cases). Chin J Urol. 2016;37:427–30.
33. Weinrich JM, Bannas P, Regier M, Keller S, Kluth L, Adam G, et al. Low-dose CT for evaluation of suspected Urolithiasis: diagnostic yield for assessment of alternative diagnoses. AJR Am J Roentgenol. 2018;210:557–63.
34. Brisbane W, Bailey MR, Sorensen MD. An overview of kidney stone imaging techniques. Nat Rev Urol. 2016;13:654–62.
35. Moore CL, Daniels B, Singh D, Luty S, Gunabushanam G, Ghita M, et al. Ureteral stones: implementation of a reduced-dose CT protocol in patients in the emergency department with moderate to high likelihood of calculi on the basis of STONE score. Radiology. 2016;280:743–51.
36. Bo Y, Jianxing L, Weiguo H. Two-step method to establish standard channel percutaneous nephrolithotomy: 3052 cases of clinical reports. J Peking Univ (Med Sci). 2010;42:447–50.
37. Yihua Z, Xumin J, Wei H. Application of establish standard percutaneous renal access by ultrasound-guided "improved one-step method" in percutaneous nephrolithotomy. J Wenzhou Med Univ. 2014;44:913–6.
38. Pengtao W, Qi L, Zingtao H. Comparison of balloon dilator and amplatz dilator in establishing percutaneous nephrolithotomy access (136 cases). Chin J Endosc. 2014;20:1145–8.
39. Weiwen Y, Xiang H, Yuelong Z. Tubeless standerd tract PCNL in the treatment of upper urinary tract calculi (report of 67cases). Chin J Laparosc Surg. 2013;6:11–4.

23

Supernumerary kidneys: A clinical and radiological analysis of nine cases

Peter Rehder[1†], Rafael Rehwald[2,3†], Julia M. Böhm[4], Astrid E. Grams[5], Alexander Loizides[4], Marco Pedrini[1], Jannik Stühmeier[1] and Bernhard Glodny[4*]

Abstract

Background: A supernumerary kidney (SK) is an additional kidney with its own capsule and blood supply that is not fused with the ipsilateral kidney (IK). Because individual case reports indicate a high morbidity rate, the aim of this retrospective study was a detailed analysis of this rare anatomical variant.

Methods: Our systematic imaging-based search for SKs, conducted in the period from 2000 and to 2017, yielded 9 cases in total (5 men, 4 women; mean age: 51.8 ± 22.8 years).

Results: The SKs were observed on the right in six and on the left side in three cases. In six subjects (66%) they were located caudal and in three cases (33%) cranial to the ipsilateral kidney. Calculi were found in three (33%) of the renal collecting systems. Five (56%) of the SKs had hydronephrosis grade IV and one SK had recurrent pyelonephritis (11%). Two of the ureters opened into the ipsilateral seminal vesicle (22%). Two (22%) SKs were functional but atrophic. Clinically relevant findings were made in 33% of the IKs: atrophy (n = 2), calculi (n = 1), and reflux with recurrent pyelonephritis (n = 1); another 33% had anatomical anomalies without functional impairment. The correct diagnosis of a SK is possible using CT imaging in all subjects. The prevalence of SK based on CT imaging can be estimated to be 1:26750.

Conclusions: CT is the method of choice for visualizing SKs. The correct diagnosis is crucial in preventing dispensable surgical procedures and for providing optimal patient treatment and outcome.

Keywords: Supernumerary kidneys, Computed tomography, Renal variants, Diagnostic imaging, Duplex kidneys, Ureter fissus

Background

Supernumerary kidneys (SKs) are usually one [1], rarely two [2–5] additional kidneys, distinguished from the significantly more common duplex kidneys by the fact that they are not fused with the other kidney and have their own capsule and blood supply [1]. Most SKs are smaller than normal kidneys [6], but they can also be larger [1, 6, 7]. SKs are usually located caudal, less frequently cranial to the ipsilateral kidney [1]. While there is as yet no comprehensive description of the blood supply of SKs because of its high variability [1], the ureters of a SK tend to join with those of the ipsilateral kidney (IK) [1]. However, completely separate ureters draining into the bladder [1, 8], the vagina [9], the vulva [10], the prostatic urethra, or into vesical or vaginal pouches [1] have also been described.

Supernumerary kidneys have no inherent clinical relevance [1]. They are– however– often accompanied by urolithiasis, pyonephrosis, infections or hydronephrosis [1, 6, 11]. Individual cases have also been reported in which an associated adenocarcinoma [12], a Wilms tumor [13] or a cyst [7] were observed. Furthermore, SKs can be subject to traumatic injuries [14].

Formerly, most cases of SKs were detected during surgery or autopsy [6, 15]. Diagnostic methods such as retrograde pyelography [16], urography [12, 17–19], or angiography [12, 18–20] were less likely to lead to such a finding. Today, supernumerary kidneys are more frequently diagnosed using computed tomography (CT) [21], ultrasound, Tc-99^{m} MAG3 scintigraphy [22], Tc-

* Correspondence: bernhard.glodny@i-med.ac.at
†Peter Rehder and Rafael Rehwald contributed equally to this work.
4Department of Radiology, Medical University of Innsbruck, Anichstraße 35, 6020 Innsbruck, Austria
Full list of author information is available at the end of the article

99^m DTPA scintigraphy [23] or magnetic resonance imaging (MRI) [24].

One notable reason for the increased morbidity appears to arise from misinterpretations in the assessment of diagnostic procedures, in which SKs are not recognized as such. There may be no consequences [25], but this can at worst also lead to unnecessary interventions, such as biopsies [26] or surgery [27], including the risk of further complications [28].

The prevalence of SKs is unknown. There are only case reports of incidental findings of supernumerary kidneys, with a few exceptions of reports including two [1] or three cases [29, 30].

This study represents the yet largest case series, describing nine patients with supernumerary kidneys–the result of a systematic imaging-based assessment between 2000 and 2017. The aim of the present study was to estimate the frequency of SKs and to precisely describe and summarize both the anatomy and the clinical features of these patients for the first time.

Methods

A SK was defined as organ with a typically asymmetric collecting system to which a ureter is connected, having its own capsule and blood supply and not being fused with the other ipsilateral kidney, distinguishing it from duplex kidneys [1]. The ureter of the SK may not open into the vagina in order to rule out confusion with Gartner's duct cysts [31, 32], and no ureter may open into the presumed supernumerary kidney [32, 33]. The SK must be connected to the lower urinary tract [32, 34] and it must not be filled with blood or mucus at the onset of puberty [32, 35].

A total of 461,500 radiological examinations of the abdomen (without duplicate examinations), performed between 2000 and 2017 at our institution were systematically reviewed for anomalies of the kidneys: 214,000 contrast-enhanced CT scans acquired on spiral CT machines from different vendors (Genesis HiSpeed RP, QXi LightSpeed 4 Slice, LightSpeed 16, LightSpeed VCT 64, General Electric, W.I., USA; Somatom Sensation 4, 16 and 64 series, Somatom Definition Flash, Siemens AG, Erlangen, Germany), 31,500 MRI scans, performed on various systems (1.5 T Sonata, Symphony and Avanto, 3 T Magnetom Skyra, Siemens AG, Erlangen, Germany), 208,000 abdominal ultrasound examinations (HDI 5000, iU22, CX50 and EPIQ 7 ultrasound systems, Koninklijke Philips N.V., Best, the Netherlands; Xario 200, Aplio a550 and i800 series, Canon Medical Europe B.V., Zoetermeer, the Netherlands), as well as 8000 angiographies and urographies (Integris angiography unit, Koninklijke Philips N.V., Best, the Netherlands).

Most CT scans in patients with supernumerary kidneys were acquired after the intravenous application of iodinated contrast medium during a parenchymatous phase in 5 mm slice-thickness, while a urographic phase was almost always missing. All MRI examinations in which a supernumerary kidney was identified consisted of at least a T_2-weighted sequence.

A significant part of the abdominal CT and MRI examinations was evaluated in the context of daily clinical routine. Additionally, the radiological reports of all included modalities were systematically screened for incidental findings of the urogenital tract, and the respectively identified imaging material carefully assessed. In a second step, every detected anomaly was independently re-evaluated and classified by both a senior board-certified radiologist (BG) and urologist (PR), resulting in nine cases of a SK beeing identified based on the inclusion criteria described (an organ with an asymmetric renal collecting system with an arising ureter, own capsule and blood supply and without fusion with the other kidney). A histopathological examination of the SK was available for four cases.

The renal anatomy of each identified SK has been comprehensively illustrated based on the imaging material available (Fig. 1), and additional coronal and sagittal CT and MRI reconstructions are presented for some patients in Fig. 2a-c, as these planes are considered particularly well suited to demonstrate supernumerary kidneys [36].

Descriptive statistics were performed using IBM SPSS Statistics for Windows, version 21 (IBM Corp., Armonk, N.Y., USA), with mean values and standard deviations given. For the statistical analysis, Fisher's exact test was used for categorical and the Mann–Whitney U test for continuous variables. The sensitivity of the modalities was estimated under the assumption that kidneys can be reliably diagnosed using computed tomography [37]. The prevalence was determined based on the total number of patients examined between 2000 and 2017 with each imaging modality, respectively. A $p < 0.05$ was considered to be statistically significant.

Results

Nine patients with a SK were identified; five men and four women (mean age 51.8 ± 22.8 years). The SKs were identified on the right in six cases and on the left in three cases ($p = 0.132$, Fisher's exact test), caudal to the IK in six cases (cases 1, 4, 5, 6, 7, and 9) and cranial in three cases (cases 2, 3, and 8). The supernumerary kidneys are illustrated in Fig. 1a-I. Figure 2a-c shows sectional images, as well as ostensive images of selected cases.

Three out of nine patients (cases 4, 6, and 9; 33%) were clinically symptomatic due to the SK (infection and pain in case 4, pain in cases 6 and 9). The other cases were incidental findings (66%). None of the patients had initially had a urological examination; in three cases,

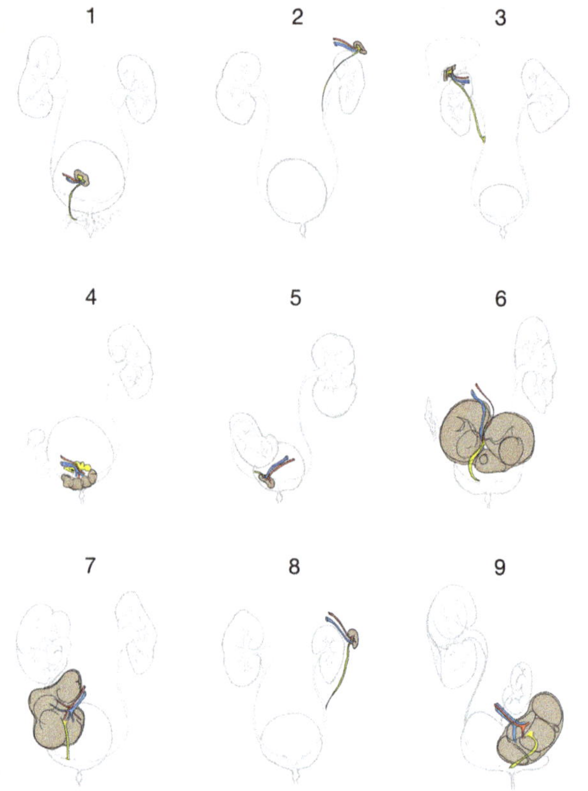

Fig. 1 Illustration of the renal anatomy of the nine cases of supernumerary kidneys, derived from the abdominal imaging available for each individual patient. SK posterior to the bladder (Case 1; **a**); SK anterior to the upper pole of the ipsilateral kidney, sharing a common ureter (Case 2; **b**). SK cranial and lateral to the right kidney (Case 3; **c**; Fig. 2a and b). SK located posterior to the bladder (Case 4; **d**). SK cranial to the right seminal vesicle (Case 5; **e**). SK located posterior and cranial to the bladder, as an inferior crossed ectopia from left to right (Case 6; **f**). SK located caudal to the right kidney, sharing a ureter fissus (Case 7; **g**). SK was cranial to the left kidney, with a ureter fissus to the hydronephrotic IK (Case 8; **h**). SK located cranial and posterior to the bladder (Case 9; **i**)

urology was consulted later. The working diagnoses for the referral to imaging are listed in Table 1.

In two patients, the diagnosis had initially been made based on imaging (cases 1 and 6), in two other patients, the SKs were only described without further interpretation (cases 2 and 8). The other cases were misdiagnosed as a mesenteric cyst (case 7), a metastasis (case 3), an abscess (case 4), a megaureter (case 9) or a unknown tumor (case 5) (Table 2). Thus, the correct diagnosis had initially been made in only 22% of the cases, no diagnosis in 22% and an incorrect diagnosis in 66% of the cases.

The initial imaging modality was CT in seven subjects (78%) and ultrasound in the other two cases (cases 6 and 9; 22%). A total of 28 CT scans (8 patients; range: 1–8), 16 sonographies (6 patients; range 0–5), 12 MRI scans (5 patients; range 0–6), 4 voiding cystourethrograms (3 patients; range 1–2), 2 PET-CT scans (2 patients; range 0–1), 1 urography and one angiography (range 0–1) has been performed. Retrospectively, all initially acquired CT scans (100%), both PET-CT scans (100%), three of five initial MRIs (60%), and one of three voiding cystourethrographies (VCUG, 33%) were sufficient to establish the correct diagnosis. A sensitivity of 100% was achieved with CT and PET-CT, 60% with MRI and VCUG and 0% with angiography and sonography. Specificity estimates as well as positive and negative predictive values could not reliably be obtained, as discussed below.

Due to the number of individual examinations performed between 2000 and 2017, the period prevalence rates of SKs were estimated to be 1:26750 based on the CT scans and 1:31500 based on MR imaging. All other examinations were either performed for diagnostic purposes or were follow-up examinations after the initial CT scans.

None of the SKs were normal. The two (22%) still functional SKs (cases 3 and 5) were shrunken. Three of the collecting systems had calculi (cases 1, 2, and 8; 33%). Five SKs had hydronephrosis grade IV (cases 4, 6, 7, 8, and 9; 56%), and one of these suffered from recurrent pyelonephritis (case 4; 11%). Two ureters opened into the ipsilateral seminal vesicle (cases 1 and 5; 22%). The SK's were with 5.7 ± 3.6 cm versus 9.2 ± 1.7 cm smaller than the IKs ($p < 0.05$).

Five patients underwent medical procedures related to their SK. One non-functioning SK with calculi which has been observed for 12 years was finally removed during a prostatectomy (case 1). In case 4, the patient presented externally with lower abdominal pain and fever. A hydronephrotic, orthotopic IK had been removed previously and the pyelonephritic SK in the small pelvis was misinterpreted to be an abscess. A vesicorectal fistula developed as a complication after the surgery. In case 5, imaging follow-up of the SK was planned, as a tumor was previously reported. The abdominal pain of patients 6 and 9 could be cured by surgical removal of their SKs.

Four out of the nine IKs were normal (cases 1, 2, 3, and 7; 44%). Three were ectopic and located caudally in the pelvis (cases 5, 6, and 9; 33%), one had calculi (case 8) and one had been removed because of recurrent pyelonephritis and vesicoureteral reflux (case 4). Four out of nine ipsilateral kidneys had a ureter fissus that branched to the SK (cases 2, 3, 7, and 8; 44%). Two of the kidneys were atrophic (cases 6 and 8, 22%). All contralateral kidneys were normal.

Three patients (33%) presented with a spina bifida occulta of the 5th (cases 6 and 9) or 6th lumbar vertebral arch (case 5). No other deformities were found.

Discussion

The prevalence of supernumerary kidneys can be estimated to be 1:26750 with CT imaging. Supernumerary kidneys have been found more frequently located caudal than cranial to the ipsilateral kidney, and more often on

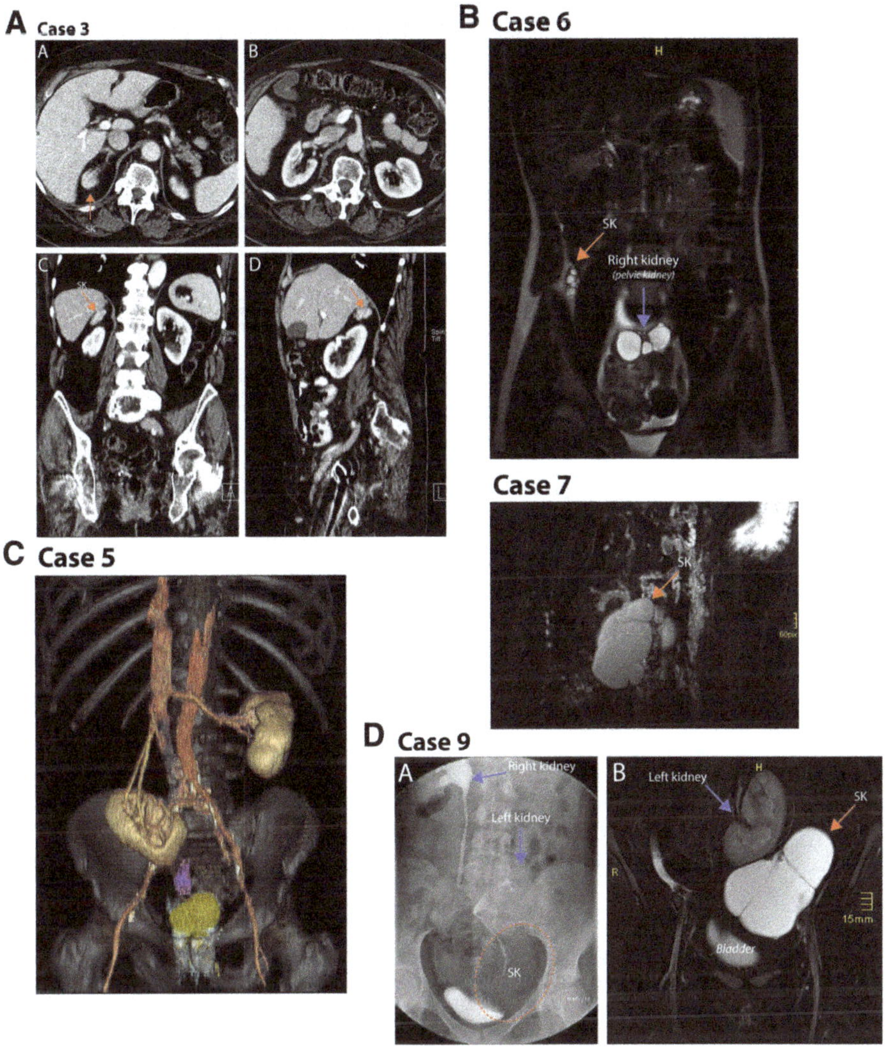

Fig. 2 Case 3: (**a**) Transversal contrast-enhanced CT of a supernumerary kidney (SK) on the right, located dorso-lateral and at the same level as the ipsilateral adrenal gland. The SK presents with the same attenuation as the contralateral kidney. **b** Transversal contrast-enhanced CT of the normal kidneys bilaterally. **c** Sagittal CT-reconstruction. SK located cranial to the normal kidney. **d** Coronal CT-reconstruction with SK located cranial to the normal kidney. **Case 5:** Coronal 3D volume rendering reconstruction of a contrast-enhanced CT, SK in violet, bladder in yellow. **Case 6:** T_2-weighted coronal image of the abdomen, showing the supernumerary kidney and the hydronephrotic right kidney (pelvic kidney). **Case 7:** T_2-weighted thick-slab semi-coronal image of the supernumerary kidney and the normal kidney. **Case 9:** (**a**) T_2-weighted coronal slice of the left kidney, the SK and bladder. (B) Intravenous pyelogram (15 min after i.v. contrast administration) depicting the right and left kidney as well as the supernumerary kidney as a mass and bladder

the right than on the left side. All SKs were either hydronephrotic, atrophic, or had calculi while only two were still functional (22%). Three of the IKs (33%) were atrophic, hydronephrotic, or had calculi. However, only one third of the patients suffered from clinical symptoms; they all had pain that was cured after successful nephrectomy. The other cases can be considered as incidental radiological findings. Based on the criteria of a retroperitoneal organ with its own blood supply and capsule and an asymmetrical collecting system [1], all SKs could be identified as such using computed tomography as the imaging modality of choice.

This study has some limitations to consider. A histological examination of the SK was only available for four of the nine cases (cases 1, 4, 6, and 9). Furthermore, while the CT scans were of generally high quality, they were not specifically modified for optimal visualization of the kidneys. The retrospective estimate of the total number of examinations evaluated is also subject to a certain degree of uncertainty. One argument for the reliability is the good agreement of the prevalence of 1: 27000 estimated based on CT and of 1:31500 based on MR imaging. The validity of the data regarding the accuracy of the presented diagnostic measures is however

Table 1 Clinical details of the 9 patients with supernumerary kidneys

No.	Age group	Initial reason for radiological examination	Referred to radiology by?	Initial modality	Additional modalities	Correctly diagnosed	Initial diagnosis reported	Initial diagnosis to surgery	Patient management
1	Adult	Pneumonia and gastrointestinal bleeding	Pulmonology	CT	2 CT scans 1 Cystography	Yes	SK; diagnosis rejected 12 years later. DD: *"tumor"*	12 years	Watch-and-wait surgery 12 years later together with prostatectomy
2	Adult	Liver cirrhosis	Gastroenterology	CT	7 CT scans 1 MR scan	No	Described, but without diagnosis or interpretation	–	No consequence
3	Adult	Uterine Carcinoma	Gynecology	CT	3 CT scans 6 US exams	No	Metastasis of the adrenal gland	–	No consequence
4	Adult	Urinary tract infections	Surgery	CT	5 CT scans 4 US exam 2 Cystographies 3 MR scans	No	Abscess	2 days	Series of operations. Complications: urinary leakage; fistula to rectum and urine bladder
5	Adult	Lumbalgia	GP	CT	–	No	Recurrence of a presumably resected tumor	–	Watch-and-wait
6	Child	Lower abdominal pain	Pediatrics	US	1 CT 2 US exam 1 MR scan	Yes	SK	11 years	Resection of the hydronephrotic SK and ureter; shrunken IK remained in situ
7	Adult	Tumor palpated	Gastroenterology	CT	6 MR scans	No	Mesenterial cyst or lymphocele	–	No consequence
8	Adult	Aortic dissection	Surgery	CT	2 CT scans 1 US exam	No	Described, but without diagnosis or interpretation	–	No consequence
9	Adolescent	Inguinal hernia and pain	Surgery	US	2 US exams 1 Cystography 1 Urography 1 MR scan	No	Megaureter or cyst	17 years	Resection

Abbreviations: *DD* Differential diagnosis, *IK* Ipsilateral kidney, *SK* Supernumerary kidney, *UF* Ureter fissus, *US* Ultrasound

limited. Whereas the sensitivity of the different imaging modalities (100% for CT and PET-CT, 60% for MRI and VCUG, and 0% for angiography and sonography) can be considered reliable for at least in their magnitude, other markers of diagnostic accuracy–such as specificity, positive and negative predictive values as indicators of diagnostic effectiveness [38]–could not be obtained due to an unknown rate of true negative cases. Moreover, it has to be acknowledged that some of the STARD criteria have not been met by the present study [39]. The MRI and CT cohorts, for example, do at least partly differ and do not fully comprise of the same patients, whilst the readers of one modality were not blinded to the results and reports from other modalities. Finally, the number of patients is too limited to calculate confidence intervals.

While it was possible to make the diagnosis retrospectively in all of the CT scans, no supernumerary kidney was clearly identified by ultrasound, although the SKs were sonographically visualized in cases 6 and 9 and abdominal ultrasounds were available for 55% of the patients. Sonography thus appears to be not suitable for the reliable detection of SKs. In two cases in which MRI had been performed, the SK was not completely within the field of view. When fully scanned, it was possible to make the correct diagnosis. Only the PET-CT scan appears to allow the diagnosis to be made as reliably as CT imaging. It appears, that the main reason for an initially incorrect diagnosis in 78% of the cases is the relatively unknown nature of a SK which is not even considered as a differential diagnosis and that patients with

Table 2 Anatomical details of the 9 pat ents with supernumerary kidneys

No.	Supernumerary kidney			Contralateral kidney	Ipsilateral kidney	Artery	Vein	Ureter	Complications		
	Side	*Size (cm)*	*Localization*						*Urologic*	*Genital*	*Other*
1	right	3.0 × 2.1 × 1.9	Dorsal of the bladder	Left, normal	Right, normal	Internal Iliac	Internal Iliac	Seminal vesicle	Concrements in SK without function	–	–
2	left	1.7 × 1.5 × 1.2	Ventral of the upper pole of the left kidney	Right, normal	Left, normal *(Ureter fissus)*	Aorta	Caval vein	Orifice in ureter of normal IK *(Ureter fissus)*	Concrements in SK	–	–
3	right	3.7 × 3.2 × 1.5	Cranial of the right kidney	Right, normal	Right, normal	Aorta	Caval vein	Orifice in ureter of normal IK *(Ureter fissus)*		–	–
4	right	8.5 × 8.1 × 6.5	Dorsal of the bladder, median and paramedian	Left, normal	Right; reflux; pyelonephritis; removed	Internal Iliac	Internal iliac	Bladder	Hydronephrosis IV in SK; Pyelonephritis in SK and IK	–	–
5	right	2.9 × 2.0 × 2.0	Dorsal of the bladder; cranial of the seminal vesicle	Left, normal	Right; pelvic kidney	Internal Iliac	Internal iliac	Seminal vesicle		–	6 lumbar vertebrae; Cleft of 6th vertebrate body arc
6	right	9.4 × 7.6 × 7.5	Dorsal and cranial of the bladder, median and paramedian	Left, normal	Right; pelvic kidney; cirrhosis of the kidney	Internal Iliac	Internal iliac	Bladder	Hydronephrosis IV in SK; cirrhosis of IK	–	Cleft of 5th vertebrate body arc
7	right	9.3 × 6.6 × 4.2	Caudal of the right kidney	Left, normal	Right, normal	Aorta	Caval vein	Orifice in ureter of IK *(Ureter fissus)*	Hydronephrosis IV in SK	–	–
8	left	6.7 × 5.2 × 6.2	Cranial of the left kidney	Right, normal	Cirrhosis of the kidney; kidney stones	Aorta	Caval vein	Orifice in ureter of IK *(Ureter fissus)*	Hydronephrosis IV in SK; cirrhosis of IK; kidney stones in common stem of ureter fissus	–	–
9	left	12.2 × 8.8 × 8.9	Caudal and lateral of the left kidney	Right, normal	Left; pelvic kidney	Internal Iliac	Internal Iliac	Bladder *(caudal)*	Hydronephrosis IV in SK; ipsilateral indirect inguinal hernia	–	Cleft of 5th vertebrate body arc

Abbreviations: *DD* Differential diagnosis, *IK* Ipsilateral kidney unclear retroperitoneal masses are generally rarely referred to urology.

It can therefore be argued that there is currently no universally established diagnostic approach to reliably diagnose supernumerary kidneys. Performing an intravenous pyelogram or CT urography (CTU) assumes an intention to diagnose, something that has been missing in most, if not all, cases presented in this work. Furthermore, such a radiological approach would still most likely not solely be expedient to secure a definitive diagnosis, as no urinary excretion was observed from most of the SKs. A MRI scan of the kidneys acquired on an up-to-date system and utilizing a heavily T_2-weighted sequence would allow for a higher detection rate and a more precise diagnosis. However, a justified suspicion before referring a patient to MRI is nevertheless both from a clinical and economic perspective advantageous. Additionally, the appropriate area of interest in which the kidney is suspected should be carefully selected, as even in modern scanners the field of view (FOV) is often highly focused.

In all cases, the renal artery and the renal vein could be clearly identified, likewise the ureter, and the abdominal organs were separate from the IK in all cases, so that the criteria of Geisinger [1] were fulfilled. Therefore, a differential diagnosis of a Gartner's duct cyst combined with a Müllerian duct obstruction and ipsilateral renal dysgenesis [32] was not considered in any of the four female patients with SKs while, however, three such cases were identified but excluded.

While two of the SKs (cases 6 and 9) were larger than the other kidneys due to hydronephrosis grade IV, the other seven SKs were considerably smaller than regular kidneys. Only in cases 3 and 5 there no apparent cause other than atrophy as defined by Geisinger [1] is likely. Although the smallest supernumerary kidney was only 1.7 × 1.5 × 1.2 cm (case 2), it was not a so-called *"Beiniere"*, a term first introduced by Neckarsulmer [40] in 1914 to describe a kidney that was attached to the upper pole of the adjacent kidney like a hood [1]. We found no case of such a non-functional *"Beiniere"* [1] without an excretory duct [41] or with a rudimentary collecting system, but non-functioning parenchyma [40] that was connected with the IK [1]. Instead, in case 2, a narrow bridge to the adjacent IK was observed, as described by Geisinger [1] in his second case, but with the difference that the third kidney was located lateral, not medial to the upper pole of the IK. A functional SK of normal size thus likely to be rare.

While all patients had a normal contralateral kidney, four on the right and five on the left side, 66% of the IKs were conspicuous. An ureter fissus (cases 2, 3, 7, and 8), or caudal ectopia (cases 5, 6, and 9) are not clinically relevant. However, two IKs were shrunken, one of them with calculi, and a third had to be surgically removed because of recurrent pyelonephritis. Therefore, and as suggested by Rubin [42], special attention needs to be given also to the normal ipsilateral kidney.

Concomitant deformities occurred in 33% of the patients, consisting of fusion defects in the lumbosacral junctions which were clinically irrelevant and no further deformities were observed in other organ systems.

Detecting and correctly interpreting a supernumerary kidney by imaging is important for several reasons. Unnecessary procedures, as in case 1, could be prevented, and even more importantly complications of dispensable surgical procedures, such as in case 4, could be avoided, as the kidney should have been surgically removed *in toto*. The correct diagnosis is possible with a CT scan, and elaborate follow-ups would not be required. If there is no UF, the diagnosis can be confirmed by cystoscopy and verifying the presence of the ureter ostium. An accurate diagnosis is essential for providing an effective and successful therapy, which should ultimately consist of uretro-nephrectomy. This radical therapeutic approach is, however, only indicated if the kidney is clinically symptomatic. In conclusion, for the purpose of the most effective therapy, no generally valid treatment recommendations can be offered, except that each therapeutic decision should be tailored to the individual circumstances.

Conclusion

In summary, our results show that SKs occur with a prevalence of 1:26750. None of the SKs were normal, however only one third of the patients had clinical manifestations. Surgery is rarely indicated, but can cure the pain that is sometimes present. Supernumerary kidneys can be identified by CT using Geisinger's [1] criteria: a retroperitoneal organ with its own blood supply and own capsule and an asymmetric collecting system. In order to avoid unnecessary operations and the concomitant risk of complications, the correct diagnosis is of utmost importance for the individual patients.

Abbreviations

CT: Computed tomography; CTU: Computed tomography urography; FOV: Field of view; IK: Ipsilateral kidney; MRI: Magnetic resonance imaging; PET: Positron emmision tomography; SK: Supernumerary kidney; UF: Ureter fissus; US: Ultrasound; VCUG: Voiding cystourethrography

Acknowledgements

N/A

Authors' contributions

PR, RR and GB were the chief investigators of this study. PR, RR, JMB, AEG and GB conducted, designed and managed this study, acquired, analysed and interpreted the data, performed the literature search, wrote the final version of the manuscript and revised it critically. AL, MP and JS analysed and interpreted the data, contributed to the literature search and the final version of the manuscript and revised it critically. All authors reviewed and approved the final version of the manuscript.

Author details
[1]University Hospital for Urology, Department of Surgery, Medical University of Innsbruck, Innsbruck, Austria. [2]Department of Radiology, University of Cambridge, Cambridge, UK. [3]Queen Square Institute of Neurology, University College London, London, UK. [4]Department of Radiology, Medical University of Innsbruck, Anichstraße 35, 6020 Innsbruck, Austria. [5]Department of Neuroradiology, Medical University of Innsbruck, Innsbruck, Austria.

References

1. Geisinger JF. Supernumerary kidney. J Urol. 1939;38(4):331–56.
2. Pintér AB, Schäfer J, Varró J. Two supernumerary kidneys with ureteral atresia. J Urol. 1982;127(1):119–20.
3. Shane JH. Supernumerary kidney with vaginal ureteral orifice. J Urol. 1942;47:344.
4. Saccone AH, H. B. Supernumerary kidney: report of a case and review of the literature. J Urol. 1934;31:711–20.
5. Budniok R, Suchowsky G. A case of bilateral supernumerary kidney and bilateral supernumerary ureter with extravesicular orifices a contribution on anomalies of the urinary tract. Z Urol. 1951;44(7):453–63.
6. Carlson HE. Supernumerary kidney: a summary of 51 reported cases. J Urol. 1950;64(2):224–9.
7. Wulfekuhler WV, Dube VE. Free supernumerary kidney: report of a case. J Urol. 1971;106(6):802–4.
8. Fischer K, Rosenloecher K. Über einen Fall von dritter Niere mit selbstständigem Harnleiter. Zeitschrift für Urologische Chirurgie. 1925;17:61–6.
9. Headings DM, Palmer RE. Supernumerary kidney with ureter opening into vagina. Am J Surg. 1946;71:370–3.
10. Van den Bulcke C, Keutgen JM, Van Hees JN. Apropos of a case of supernumerary kidney with megaureter leading into the vulva. Acta Urol Belg. 1966;34(3):282–6.
11. Costantino L. The supernumerary kidney. On a case Minerva Chirurgica. 1974;29(21):1132–5.
12. Fratkin LB, Johnson HW, Moscovich BB. Adenocarcinoma in supernumerary kidney. Can J Surg. 1963;6:195–8.
13. Wu JP, Garcia J. Supernumerary kidney with Wilms' tumor. Wis Med J. 1971; 70(10):211–6.
14. Ogreid PI, Bo O, Loovas J. Traumatic haematuria in supernumerary hydronephrotic kidney. A case report. Scand J Urol Nephrol. 1979;13(1):127–30.
15. Burgess SB. Supernumerary kidney: report of a case. Arch Pathol. 1960;69:154–7.
16. Stewart CM. True right supernumerary kidney diagnosed preoperatively. J Urol. 1949;61(2):327–32.
17. Jensenius H, Munck T. Supernumerary kidney with megalo-ureter; report of a case. Acta Chir Scand. 1955;109(1):20–5.
18. Hvezdoslav S. Eine klinisch diagnostizierte überzählige Niere. Zeitschrift für Urologie. 1956;49:343–9.
19. Browne MK, Glashan RW. Multiple pathology in a unilateral supernumerary kidney. Br J Surg. 1971;58(1):73–6.
20. Sasidharan K, Babu AS, Rao MM, Bhat HS. Free supernumerary kidney. Br J Urol. 1976;48(5):388.
21. Khalda E, Singh GN, Mandal AK, Kumar R. Unilateral supernumerary kidney with contra lateral hydronephrosis-a rare case report. Australas Med J. 2014; 7(5):213–7.
22. Kim N, Yung E, Katz DS. Supernumerary left kidney. Clin Nucl Med. 2004; 29(12):852–3.
23. Sy WM, Seo IS, Sze PC, Kimmel MA, Homs CJ, McBride JG, et al. A patient with three kidneys: a correlative imaging case report. Clin Nucl Med. 1999; 24(4):264–6.
24. Moses KA, Kirsch AJ, Heiss EA, Gow KW. Supernumerary kidney in a term infant with VATER association. Am Surg. 2008;74(9):874–6.
25. Nouira K, Menif E, Nouira Y, Baccar S, Salem A, Horchani A, et al. Supernumerary kidney: a case report. Tunis Med. 2002;80(3):152–4.
26. Bernik TR, Ravnic DJ, Bernik SF, Wallack MK. Ectopic supernumerary kidney, a cause of Para-aortic mass: case report and review. Am Surg. 2001;67(7):657–9.
27. Truc E, Grasset D, Balmes M. Giant hydronephrosis in a supernumerary kidney. J Urol Nephrol (Paris). 1962;68:356–8.
28. Yousef AK, Abu Khadra AL, Dajani AM. A pitfall in the diagnosis of supernumerary kidney. Br J Urol. 1991;67(1):100.
29. Macpherson RI. Supernumerary kidney: typical and atypical features. Can Assoc Radiol J. 1987;38(2):116–9.
30. Campbell MF. Anomalies of the kidney. In: Campbell MF, Harrison JH, editors. Urology. 2. 3rd ed. Philadelphia: W. B. Saunders Co.; 1970.
31. Gotoh T, Koyanagi T. Clinicopathological and embryological considerations of single ectopic ureters opening into Gartner's duct cyst: a unique subtype of single vaginal ectopia. J Urol. 1987;137(5):969–72.
32. Sheih CP, Liao YJ, Hung CS, Huang TS, Li YW. Duplex kidney, Gartner's duct cyst and ipsilateral Mullerian duct obstruction. J Urol. 1998;159(6):2120–1.
33. Gotoh T, Morita H, Tokunaka S, Koyanagi T, Tsuji I. Single ectopic ureter. J Urol. 1983;129(2):271–4.
34. Sheih CP, Hung CS, Wei CF, Lin CY. Cystic dilatations within the pelvis in patients with ipsilateral renal agenesis or dysplasia. J Urol. 1990;144(2 Pt 1):324–7.
35. Sheih CP, Li YW, Chen WL, Chang CH, Hung CS. Unilateral occlusion of duplicated mullerian ducts associated with ipsilateral Gartner's duct cyst: report of 3 cases. J Urol. 1993;149(3):543–5.
36. Chien JC-W, Chan WP. Bilateral Supernumerary Kidney. J Korean Med Sci. 2016;31(5):822–3.
37. Schlunt LB, Harper JD, Broome DR, Baron PW, Watkins GE, Ojogho ON, et al. Improved detection of renal vascular anatomy using multidetector CT angiography: is 100% detection possible? J Endourol. 2007;21(1):12–7.
38. Simundic AM. Measures of diagnostic accuracy: basic definitions. EJIFCC. 2009;19(4):203–11.
39. Ames A 3rd. CNS energy metabolism as related to function. Brain Res Brain Res Rev. 2000;34(1–2):42–68.
40. Neckarsulmer K. Über Beinieren. Berliner klinische Wochenschrift. 1914;61: 1641–3.
41. Cobb F, Giddings HG. VII. Supernumerary kidney subject of Cystadenoma: report of a case verified by operation. Ann Surg. 1911;53(3):367–72.
42. Rubin JS. Supernumerary kidney with aberrant ureter terminating externally. J Urol. 1948;60(3):405–8.

24

Intrarenal arteriovenous malformation following flexible ureterorenoscopy and holmium laser stone fragmentation

Abdelrahman Bashar[1] and Fayez T. Hammad[2*]

Abstract

Background: Flexible ureterorenoscopy (FURS) and holmium laser lithotripsy is currently considered as one of the treatment options for large renal calculi. It has been shown to be safer than percutaneous nephrolithotomy. The latter can sometimes be complicated by the formation of intrarenal arteriovenous malformation (AVM). AVM is extremely rare following FURS and laser lithotripsy. Indeed only one case has been reported on reviewing the literature up to June 2018. We report on the second case illustrating the possibility of developing this major complication following this procedure.

Case presentation: A 79 years old diabetic and hypertensive male with stage-4 chronic kidney disease who previously had left extracorporeal shockwave lithotripsy and FURS with Holmium laser lithotripsy, presented with bilateral large renal calculi. He underwent simultaneous bilateral FURS and Holmium laser lithotripsy and was discharged home the following day with almost clear urine. Four days post-discharge, he presented with gross hematuria for which he required hospitalization and blood transfusion. CT scan demonstrated left subcapsular, perinephric and retroperitoneal hematoma. Angiography showed contrast extravasation from pseudoaneurysms in two small branches of left renal artery. Both were selectively embolized with micro-coils and this led to the cessation of the hematuria.

Conclusions: Despite the relative safety of FURS and Holmium laser lithotripsy, it can be associated with major complications like intrarenal AVM. This can probably be prevented by careful and judicious use of laser energy in patients with large stone burden and premorbid conditions.

Keywords: Arteriovenous malformation, Flexible ureterorenoscopy, Holmium laser

Background

The recent and on-going advances in flexible instrumentation and laser technology have expanded the indications of retrograde intrarenal surgery. As per many guidelines, flexible ureterorenoscopy (FURS) and holmium laser lithotripsy is currently considered as one of the treatment options for renal stones larger than 2 cm in diameter. It has less complication rate compared to the more invasive procedures such as percutaneous nephrolithotomy [1, 2]. Following percutaneous nephrolithotomy, the formation of intrarenal arteriovenous malformations (AVM) in the form of arteriovenous fistulae or pseudoaneurysms, although rare with an incidence of around 1.4%, is a well-known complication [3, 4]. However, this complication is extremely rare following FURS and holmium laser lithotripsy. To our knowledge, and by reviewing the English literature in the Medline up to June 2018, there was only one case of reported AVM following this procedure [5]. Herein, we report on the second case of AVM following FURS and holmium laser lithotripsy, which presented with delayed hematuria and required angio-embolisation.

* Correspondence: fayezhammad@hotmail.com
[2]Department of Surgery, College of Medicine and Health Sciences, United Arab Emirates University, Po Box 17666, Al Ain, UAE
Full list of author information is available at the end of the article

Case report

A 79 years old male with multiple comorbidities including hypertension, valvular heart disease, diabetes mellitus and stage 4 chronic kidney disease with a baseline creatinine of more than 300 μmol/L presented with bilateral symptomatic large renal stones for which he underwent staged stone treatment. Prior to presentation to our hospital, he had bilateral double J stent (DJS) insertion and left extracorporeal shockwave lithotripsy followed by FURS and laser stone fragmentation of the left renal stones. Subsequently, he sought medical advice in our facility. Non-contrast CT scan showed multiple bilateral renal stones. In the left kidney, there were 3 stones distributed to middle and lower pole calyces with a stone burden of approximately 3.0 cm as measured using the CT scan. In the right kidney there were also three stones, two in middle calyces and one in the pelvis with a total stone burden of 3.2 cm. After stopping the aspirin for seven days, he underwent simultaneous bilateral FURS and holmium laser lithotripsy and insertion of bilateral DJS under general anesthesia with endotracheal intubation. The surgical procedure took 125 min (65 min for the left side followed by 60 min for the right one) and the procedure was similar in both sides. Following insertion of a hydrophilic tip guidewire (Sensor, 0.038 in), a ureteral access sheath (Inner diameter: 12 Fr, Length: 55 cm) was inserted and the tip was located approximated at the level of ureteropelvic junction. Karl Storz flexible ureterorenoscope (8.5 Fr) was used. During the procedure the normal saline was allowed to run from the bag (approximately 80 cm above the level of the patient pelvis without a pump) and the outflow of saline from around the scope was observed throughout the procedure. Laser energy between 1.0–1.2 joules with a frequency ranging between 8 and 12 Hz (short pulses) were used in both sides. 4200 and 4066 pulses were used in the left and right sides respectively. He was discharged home in a good condition the next day with almost clear urine. Four days later, he reported back to the emergency department with severe suprapubic pain and gross hematuria which required continuous bladder irrigation with a three-way catheter. His hemoglobin dropped dramatically from 121 to 84 g/dl requiring an initial transfusion of two units of packed red blood cells. CT scan showed left-sided subcapsular, perinephric and retroperitoneal hematoma (Fig. 1), bladder clots and complete dislodgement of the left DJS. Cystoscopy revealed bleeding from the left ureteric orifice. Evacuation of clots and change of the DJS were performed. Postoperatively, he continued to have hematuria which was initially treated conservatively with bladder irrigation. His Hb dropped again from 113 to 85 g/dl and in view of the ongoing hematuria he required an additional five units of packed red blood cells. In view of the impaired renal functions, the patient was initially reluctant to have angiogram but ultimately it was performed and showed pseudoaneurysms in two small branches of the left main renal artery with extravasation of the contrast outside the renal parenchyma (Fig. 2). Both branches were then selectively embolized using 3x2mm microcoils. As results, the hematuria ceased and he was discharged home two days later. On follow-up, his creatinine remained similar to the pre-operative values and in view of the patient comorbidities and of what happened during this procedure; he decided not to go for another procedures for the residual stones.

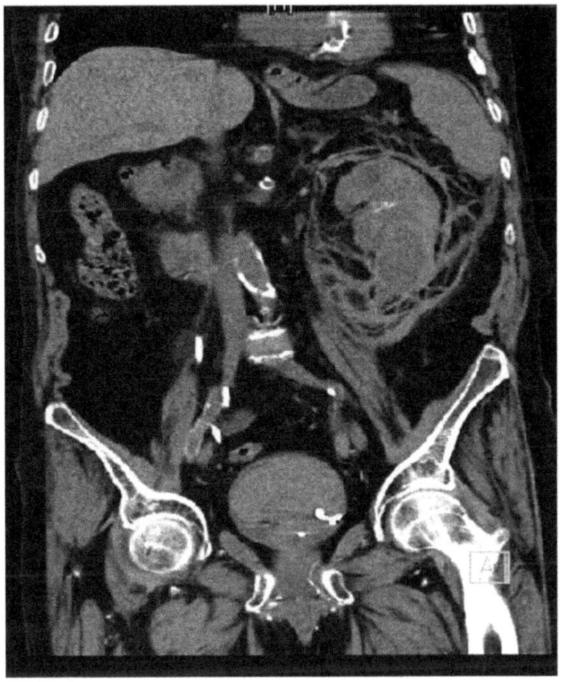

Fig. 1 Coronal view of the non-contrast CT scan showing severe left-sided perinephric and retroperitoneal hematoma. It also demonstrates the intra-vesical part of the dislodged double coil stent. Minimal stone fragments are left over

Discussion and conclusions

Like all other types of surgery, the use of FURS and holmium laser lithotripsy is not without complications. These complications, although relatively rare, include urosepsis, mucosal injury and bleeding [6, 7]. Unlike percutaneous renal stone surgery [3, 4], the formation of AVM malformation is extremely rare following FURS and holmium laser lithotripsy. To our knowledge, only one case of AVM was reported following this procedure [5]. Our case is another evidence of the possible occurrence of AVM following the use of FURS and holmium laser lithotripsy.

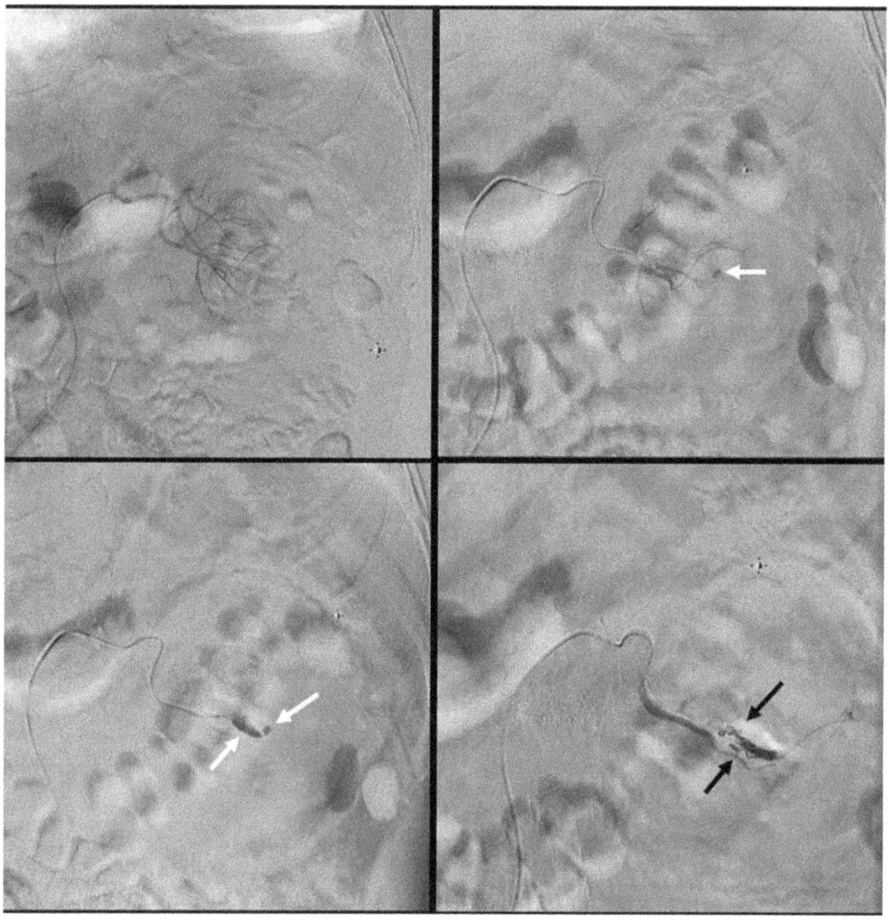

Fig. 2 Lower pole selective angiogram showing two small pseudo aneurysms with extravasation of contrast material outside the renal parenchyma (light arrows). Selective embolisation of both branches using microcoils (dark arrows)

The exact etiology for the formation of AVM in our case is difficult to ascertain and could be multifactorial. Theoretically, the AVM could have formed as a result of the possible mechanical trauma to the renal tissues by the laser probe or guidewire during the initial manipulation. The fact that there was no significant bleeding soon after the procedure and the fact that the hematuria was delayed till the fourth post-operative day refute this possibility. A more likely possibility would be the thermal injury caused by laser lithotripsy during stone fragmentation as suggested by Tiplitsky et al. [5]. Additional contributing factors in our case could be the previous treatment with FURS and laser stone fragmentation and extracorporeal shock wave lithotripsy which could have affected the renal vessels making them more liable for the laser-induced trauma [8, 9]. Further, and despite the observation of free outflow of saline from the access sheath around the scope during the procedure a high intrarenal pressure could have been reached leading to renal dilation and further thinning of the parenchyma during the procedure and hence exacerbated the injury of blood vessels. Moreover, the cardiovascular disease and renal impairment and the associated effect on renal vasculature in this patient could have also exacerbated the laser effect [10]. Collectively, it is more likely that the formation of AVM was due to the use of laser lithotripsy rather than the use of FURS per se. With this regard, other lithotripsy modalities such as electrohydraulic lithotripsy was also shown to result in intra-renal AVM although extremely rare and indeed only one case was reported following the use of FURS and electrohydraulic lithotripsy [10].

Regardless of the exact cause of the AVM post-FURS and laser lithotripsy, a high index of suspension is required to diagnose these cases when such patients present with delayed hematuria. Moreover, every effort should be made to decrease the laser-induced trauma to renal tissues. This could be achieved by careful use of guidewires and laser probes and keeping them away from the urothelium as much as possible and by using the minimum energy required to fragment the stone especially in patients with underlying morbidities which affect the integrity of renal vasculature. Every effort should be made to insure a clear vision and low intrarenal pressure and certainly multi-stage procedures should be performed instead of one long-procedure especially when there is poor visibility and large stones. Further, despite the rarity of this complication, it might need to be discussed during pre-operative counselling of high risk patients.

Abbreviations

AVM: arteriovenous malformation; DJS: double J stent; FURS: flexible ureterorenoscopy

Acknowledgements

None.

Author details

[1]Urology Division, Tawam Hospital in affiliation with Johns Hopkins Medicine, Al Ain, UAE. [2]Department of Surgery, College of Medicine and Health Sciences, United Arab Emirates University, Po Box 17666, Al Ain, UAE.

References

1. Aboumarzouk OM, Somani BK, Monga M. Flexible ureteroscopy and holmium: YAG laser lithotripsy for stone disease in patients with bleeding diathesis: a systematic review of the literature. Int Braz J Urol. 2012;38(3): 298–305; discussion 306.
2. Elbir F, et al. Flexible ureterorenoscopy results: analysis of 279 cases. Turk J Urol. 2015;41(3):113–8.
3. Srivastava A, et al. Vascular complications after percutaneous nephrolithotomy: are there any predictive factors? Urology. 2005;66(1):38–40.
4. Kallidonis P, et al. Complications of percutaneous nephrolithotomy: classification, management, and prevention. Curr Opin Urol. 2016;26(1):88–94.
5. Tiplitsky SI, et al. Case report: intrarenal arteriovenous fistula after ureteroscopic stone extraction with holmium laser lithotripsy. J Endourol. 2007;21(5):530–2.
6. Cindolo L, et al. Mortality and flexible ureteroscopy: analysis of six cases. World J Urol. 2016;34(3):305–10.
7. Bas O, et al. Factors affecting complication rates of retrograde flexible ureterorenoscopy: analysis of 1571 procedures-a single-center experience. World J Urol. 2017;35(5):819–26.
8. Delius M, et al. Biological effects of shock waves: kidney damage by shock waves in dogs--dose dependence. Ultrasound Med Biol. 1988;14(2):117–22.
9. Jaeger. P., et al., *[Do shock waves damage the kidney? Morphologic and functional changes of the kidney following exposure to shock waves]*. Schweiz Med Wochenschr. 1989;119(26):944–9.
10. Aston W, et al. Pseudoaneurysm formation after flexible ureterorenoscopy and electrohydraulic lithotripsy. Int J Clin Pract. 2004;58(3):310–1.

25

Which is the best treatment of pediatric upper urinary tract stones among extracorporeal shockwave lithotripsy, percutaneous nephrolithotomy and retrograde intrarenal surgery

Qing He†, Kaiwen Xiao†, Yuntian Chen, Banghua Liao, Hong Li and Kunjie Wang*

Abstract

Background: Although the indications of minimally invasive treatments for pediatric urolithiasis are similar to those in adults, it is still crucial to make the right treatment decision due to the special considerations of children. This review aims to evaluate the efficacy and safety of extracorporeal shockwave lithotripsy (SWL), percutaneous nephrolithotomy (PCNL), and retrograde intrarenal surgery (RIRS) in the management of pediatric upper urinary tract stones.

Methods: EMBASE, PubMed, and the Cochrane Library were searched from their first available date to March 2018. The studies that meet the inclusive criteria were included. The efficacy and safety of the treatments were assessed by means of meta-analysis of the stone free rate (SFR), complication rate, effectiveness quotient (EQ) and secondary outcome indicators.

Results: A total of 13 comparative studies were identified for data analysis. PCNL presented a significantly higher SFR compared with SWL. Similarly, the single-session SFR of RIRS was significantly higher than SWL. However, no significant difference was found between RIRS and SWL in the overall SFR. There was no significant difference between PCNL and RIRS in the SFR. Furthermore, no significant differences in complication rates were found among the three therapies. Compared with the other two treatments, PCNL had a longer operative time, fluoroscopy time and hospital stay. SWL had a shorter hospital stay, higher retreatment rate and auxiliary rate in comparison with the other two treatments. The present data also showed that PCNL presented a higher EQ than the other two treatments, and RIRS had a lower efficiency than SWL and PCNL. In the subgroup analysis of pediatric patients with stone ≤20 mm, the comparative results were similar to those described above, except for the higher complication rate of PCNL than SWL.

(Continued on next page)

* Correspondence: wangkj@scu.edu.cn
†Qing He and Kaiwen Xiao contributed equally to this work.
Department of Urology, Institute of Urology (Laboratory of Reconstructive Urology), West China Hospital, Sichuan University, No. 37 Guo Xue Xiang, Chengdu, Sichuan 610041, People's Republic of China

(Continued from previous page)

Conclusions: Although SWL as an outpatient procedure provides shorter hospital stay and reduces operative time, it has a lower SFR and higher retreatment rate than the other two treatments. PCNL exhibits a higher SFR and EQ than SWL; nevertheless, it has a longer operative time and fluoroscopy time than the other two procedures. RIRS offers a similar SFR as PCNL but a lower efficiency than PCNL.

Keywords: Extracorporeal shockwave lithotripsy, Pediatric, Percutaneous nephrolithotomy, Retrograde intrarenal surgery, upper urinary tract stone

Background

Pediatric urolithiasis is an important global medical issue, particularly in regards to the selection of different treatments by care providers. The primary risk factors of forming stones among children include geographical conditions, climates, and diet customs. Additionally, the morbidity is opposite to the level of economic development; the morbidity is 1 to 5% in developed nations and 5 to 15% in developing nations [1]. Nevertheless, rates of pediatric urolithiasis have increased in developed countries. Extracorporeal shockwave lithotripsy (SWL) has long been considered as the first-line therapy for pediatric urolithiasis less than 20 mm [2]. There is a growing trend in the management of pediatric urolithiasis with endourologic procedures due to the technological advances and miniaturization of instruments. SWL, percutaneous nephrolithotomy (PCNL), and retrograde intrarenal surgery (RIRS) have become standard therapeutic options for adult urinary stones and can be extended to pediatric stones.

SWL is still the first choice for pediatric renal stones since it is the least-invasive approach for managing pediatric urolithiasis. The indications of SWL for pediatric urolithiasis are similar to those of adults, according to the European Association of Urology (EAU) guideline, and the stone fragments are more easily passed by pediatric patients than adult patients [3]. Similarly, the American Urological Association (AUA) guideline recommends that clinicians offer SWL or RIRS as first-line therapy for pediatric patient with a total renal stone burden under 20 mm [4]. However, the high retreatment rates and the potential biological effects on the immature kidneys and adjacent tissues may limit the range of application of SWL.

Age is not a limiting factor, since there are appropriately sized PCNL instruments for children, and this approach has even been reported in a 5-month-old infant [5, 6]. In children, PCNL is recommended to manage renal stones larger than 20 mm [3, 4], especially multiple renal stones. The most common complications are fever and bleeding with some serious cases requiring blood transfusions to prevent ischaemia. The necessary radiation exposure and its effects on pediatric renal function remain controversial [7].RIRS is considered as an ideal choice for medium and large-sized pediatric renal or ureteric stones. With their smaller diameter, excellent optical properties, relatively wider range of motion, and the multiple secure and effective lithotripsy techniques available, increasing numbers of urologists prefer to treat pediatric upper urinary tract stones using ureteroscopy [8, 9]. Nevertheless, ureteroscopy, especially flexible ureteroscopy, is quite a challenge for clinicians who lack the necessary training. In addition, the high purchase and maintenance costs of RIRS result in this technique not being available in every medical centre.

In adults, any of the above three procedures could be recommended to patients with stones smaller than 20 mm located in the renal pelvis and upper or middle calices [3]. Although the indications for treatment in pediatric urolithiasis are similar to those of adults, the unique considerations, such as a smaller anatomical structure and immature kidneys, make it vital to identify the most effective and safest procedure for children. To evaluate the efficacy and safety of SWL, PCNL, and RIRS in the management of pediatric upper urinary tract stones, we performed a systematic review, synthesizing the available high-level studies.

Methods

Study identification

Literature databases including EMBASE, PubMed, and the Cochrane Library, were searched from their first available date to March 2018. The first search procedure was performed to identify all relevant trials retrieved using the following search terms: (extracorporeal shock wave lithotripsy/ESWL/SWL or percutaneous nephrolithotomy/percutaneous lithotripsy/PCNL or Retrograde intrarenal surgery/RIRS/flexible ureterorenoscopy/flexible ureteroscopy/URS/FURS) and (Pediatric/pediatrics/child/children). The language was restricted to English. Scanning the reference lists of the selected articles to identify additional articles was also conducted.

Inclusion and exclusion criteria

The inclusion criteria were: 1) comparative studies evaluating the efficacy of SWL versus PCNL, SWL versus RIRS, PCNL versus RIRS, or SWL versus PCNL versus RIRS in the treatment of pediatric renal or upper ureteral calculi; and 2) the stone-free status was evaluated postoperatively by KUB film and/or ultrasonography. In addition, for the exclusion criteria were: 1) abstracts, comments, reviews, conference papers, or systematic reviews; and 2) inclusion of children with distal ureteral stones, uncontrolled coagulation disorders, active urinary tract infections, obstructive urinary tract anomalies, severe hydronephrosis or kidney failure (GFR < 15 mL/min). Duplicated studies were included in our research, however, only the latest data were assessed in our review.

Data extraction and outcome measurement

Two investigators reviewed the titles and abstracts identified by the search strategies. The following data were extracted from each study if available by using a Microsoft Excel worksheet: first author's name, year of publication, mean age of the patients, type of stones, stone sizes, stone free rate (SFR), complications, operative time, length of hospital stay, need for auxiliary procedures, and retreatments. We graded the complications according to the Clavien-Dindo classification of surgical complications [10]. To increase the comparability among these treatment modalities, the effectiveness quotients (EQs) were calculated according to the equation reported by Clayman and colleagues [11]. Dichotomous data were classified into two-by-two tables. For continuous data, available summary estimates per group (mean, changes in means) and measures of variability (standard deviation [SD], 95% confidence interval [CI]) were extracted.

Evaluation of study quality

The levels of evidence (LE) of all included studies were assessed by the Oxford Centre for Evidence Based Medicine-Levels of Evidence [12]. The methodological quality of the studies was evaluated according to the Modified Jadad Scale for randomized controlled trials (RCTs) [13] and the Newcastle-Ottawa Scale (NOS) for nonrandomized controlled trials [14].

Statistical analysis

The efficacy and safety of SWL, PCNL, and RIRS in the treatment of pediatric renal or ureteral calculi was accessed by the OR and mean difference with corresponding 95% CI under the paired comparisons among the three treatment techniques. The OR value was calculated by using the Z test. In addition, if $p < 0.05$, the difference was considered as statistically significant. When comparing the risk of continuous variables, the mean values and SDs are necessary for the pooled data. The random-effects model was used to generate the most conservative estimate. The chi-squared-based Q test was used to assess the heterogeneity with the significance level set to $p < 0.10$. Subgroup analysis was conducted according to stone size ≤20 mm to increase the comparability of these procedures and reduce the heterogeneity of results. All of the statistical analyses were performed using the RevMan5.3 software.

Results

Study identification and characteristics

The process of the selection of studies included in this review is summarized in Fig. 1. In total, 13 articles were included in this quantitative synthesis [15–27]. There were 3 randomized controlled trials [17, 21, 24] (RCTs) (LE: 2b), 1 prospective case controlled study [16] (LE: 3b) and 9 retrospective case controlled studies [15, 18–20, 22, 23, 25–27] (LE: 3b) (Table 1). Seven nonrandomized studies were relatively high (NOS: 6 of 9 points) and 3 nonrandomized studies were medium (NOS: 5 of 9 points) in methodological quality. The methodological quality of the 3 RCTs were relatively low (Modified Jadad Scale: 2 of 3 points and 1 of 2 points) due to a lack allocation concealment and a lack blinding methods.

A total of 529 SWL cases (50.38%), 241 PCNL cases (22.95%), and 280 RIRS cases (26.67%) were included. The baseline characteristics of the children are summarized in Table 2.

Meta-analysis outcomes

Overall SFR and single-session SFR

All the included studies defined stone free as no residual fragments except one study [22] that defined stone free as fragments no larger than 4 mm. PCNL presented a significantly higher overall SFR (OR 2.69, 95% CI 1.48 to 4.91, $p = 0.001$) and single-session SFR (OR 4.67, 95% CI 1.68 to 12.98, $p = 0.003$) than SWL. Similarly, the single-session SFR of RIRS was significantly higher than SWL (OR 2.34, 95% CI 1.21 to 4.54, $p = 0.01$), but there was no significant difference in the overall SFR between RIRS and SWL (OR 2.12, 95% CI 1.00 to 4.48, $p = 0.05$). Furthermore, PCNL had similar effects in the overall SFR and single-session SFR in comparison with RIRS (OR 1.42, 95% CI 0.70 to 2.88, $p = 0.33$; OR 1.28, 95% CI 0.71 to 2.32, $p = 0.41$). (Fig. 2).

Complication rate, minor (Clavien-Dindo I–II) complication rate and major (Clavien-Dindo III–IV) complication rate

Intriguingly, no significant difference in the complication rate was found among the three procedures (SWL vs PCNL OR 0.85, 95% CI 0.25 to 2.89, $p = 0.79$; SWL vs RIRS OR 0.69, 95% CI 0.28 to 1.66, $p = 0.40$; and RIRS vs PCNL OR 0.65, 95% CI 0.32 to 1.30, $p = 0.22$). Furthermore, we analysed the postoperative complications according to grade. The results showed, similar to the overall complication rates, the minor (Clavien-Dindo I–II) complication rates (SWL vs PCNL OR 0.57, 95% CI 0.20 to 1.57, $p = 0.27$;

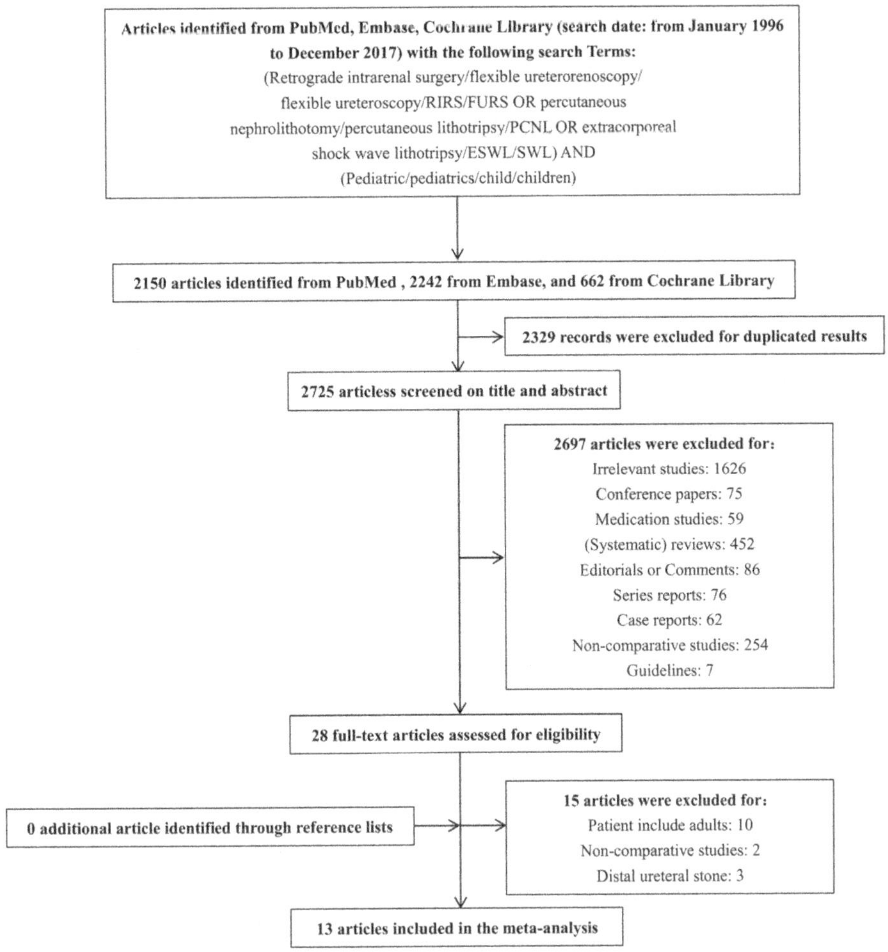

Fig. 1 PRISMA flow diagram of study selection

Table 1 Summary of publications included in the meta-analysis

Study	Study period	Country	Study design	Cases, n			LE	Study quality
				SWL	PCNL	RIRS		
Zeng et al [15]	2005–2011	China	RCCS	22	24	–	3b	6[b]
Wadhwa et al [16]	2005–2005	India	PCCS	8	6	–	3b	5[b]
Kumar et al [17]	2012–2013	India	RCT	106	106	–	2b	3[a]
Hatipoglu et al [18]	2010–2012	Turkey	RCCS	108	37	–	3b	6[b]
Shokeir et al [19]	1995–2004	Egypt	RCCS	91	75	–	3b	6[b]
ElSheemy et al [20]	2010–2014	Egypt	RCCS	64	54	–	3b	6[b]
Mokhless et al [21]	3 months follow-up	Egypt	RCT	30	–	30	2b	3[a]
Freton et al [22]	2000–2014	France	RCCS	100	–	46	3b	5[b]
Resorlu et al [23]	2008–2011	Turkey	MRCCS	–	106	95	3b	6[b]
Saad et al [24]	2011–2014	Egypt	RCT	–	20	18	2b	2[a]
Bas et al [25]	2011–2015	Turkey	RCCS	–	45	36	3b	6[b]
Sen et al [26]	2015–2016	Turkey	RCCS	–	25	23	3b	5[b]
Pelit et al [27]	2013–2016	Turkey	RCCS	–	45	32	3b	6[b]

a.Modified Jadad scale (score from 0 to 7); b. Newcastle-Ottawa scale (score from 0 to 9). *SWL* Extracorporeal shockwave lithotripsy, *PCNL* Percutaneous nephrolithotomy, *RIRS* Retrograde intrarenal surgery, *LE* Level of evidence, *RCCS* Retrospective case control study, *PCCS* Prospective case control study, *RCT* Randomized control trail, *MRCCS* Multicenter retrospective case control study

Table 2 Summary of pediatric patients' baseline of included studies

Author	Treatment	Age, years	Sex		Stone location, n (units)					Side		Stone size, mm
					Pelvis	Caliceal	Pelvis + caliceal	Staghorn stone				
		(Mean ± SD)	Male	Female				Partial	Complete	Unilateral	Bilateral	(Mean ± SD)
Zeng et al [15]	SWL	1.96 ± 0.55	17	5	5(5)	0(0)	2(2)	15(15)	0(0)	22	0	21.7 ± 1.7
	PCNL	1.92 ± 0.8	15	9	6(7)	0(0)	3(4)	12(12)	3(3)	24	1	21.4 ± 3.5
Wadhwa et al [16]	SWL	3~12	11	3	8(9)	0(0)	0(0)	0(0)	0(0)	NA		220.4[a]
	PCNL	5.9			NA(4)	0(0)	NA(4)	1(1)	0(0)			1393.4[a]
Kumar et al [17]	SWL	10.7 ± 1.3	52	54	NA					106	0	12.9 ± 1.3
	PCNL	10.3 ± 1.2	51	55						106	0	12.7 ± 1.2
Hatipoglu et al [18]	SWL	5.91 ± 4.03	61	47	50	58	0(0)	0(0)	0(0)	108	0	11.32 ± 2.84
	PCNL	8.43 ± 4.84	15	22	10	27	0(0)	0(0)	0(0)	37	0	14.78 ± 5.39
Shokeir et al [19]	SWL	6.4 ± 1.4	50	41	NA(70)	NA(11)	NA(12)	0(0)	0(0)	89	2	13.9 ± 4.2
	PCNL	6.6 ± 1.2	45	30	NA(52)	NA(14)	NA(16)	0(0)	0(0)	68	7	14.4 ± 3.1
ElSheemy et al [20]	SWL	4.06 ± 0.96	44	20	52	12	0(0)	0(0)	0(0)	64	0	14.87 ± 4.05
	PCNL	3.84 ± 1.44	33	21	39	15	0(0)	0(0)	0(0)	54	0	15.98 ± 4.31
Mokhless et al [21]	SWL	1~6	40	20	15(NA)	5(NA)	10(NA)	0(0)	0(0)	60	0	10–20
	RIRS	2.4 ± 1.3			17(NA)	7(NA)	6(NA)	0(0)	0(0)			10–20
Freton et al [22]	SWL	6.7 ± 0.6	NA		Upper tract urinary stones (upper ureter or kidney)					NA		19.5 ± 1.5
	RIRS	9.1 ± 0.9										21.6 ± 2.0
Resorlu et al [23]	PCNL	9.6 ± 4.9	56	50	36(NA)	70(NA)	0(0)	0(0)	0(0)			23.7 ± 4.42
	RIRS	9.3 ± 5.2	53	42	29(NA)	66(NA)	0(0)	0(0)	0(0)			14.3 ± 3.81
Saad et al [24]	PCNL	6.93 ± 3.55	14	8	2(2)[b]		17(17)[c]	3(3)		22	0	>20
	RIRS	6.44 ± 4.84	14	7	5(5)[b]		11(11)[c]	5(5)		21	0	>20
Bas et al [25]	PCNL	5.62 ± 4.50	23	22	27	18	0(0)	0(0)	0(0)	45	0	13.97 ± 3.46
	RIRS	8.39 ± 4.72	15	21	14	22	0(0)	0(0)	0(0)	36	0	12.80 ± 3.03
Sen et al [26]	PCNL	4 ± 2.3	NA		1	24	0(0)	0(0)	0(0)	NA		12.2 ± 2.8
	RIRS	10.9 ± 3			0	23	0(0)	0(0)	0(0)			13.7 ± 3.5
Pelit et al [27]	PCNL	3.71 ± 1.89	24	21	Renal stones					NA		21.06 ± 5.61
	RIRS	3.65 ± 1.95	17	15								19.30 ± 4.21

a. mm2, b. single stone, c. multiple stones. *SWL* Extracorporeal shockwave lithotripsy, *PCNL* Percutaneous nephrolithotomy, *RIRS* Retrograde intrarenal surgery, *NA* Not available

SWL vs RIRS OR 0.98, 95% CI 0.37 to 2.60, $p = 0.97$; and RIRS vs PCNL OR 0.69, 95% CI 0.39 to 1.22, $p = 0.20$) and the major (Clavien-Dindo III–IV) complication rates (SWL vs PCNL OR 1.45, 95% CI 0.49 to 4.31, $p = 0.28$; SWL vs RIRS OR 0.14, 95% CI 0.01 to 1.43, $p = 0.10$; and RIRS vs PCNL OR 0.92, 95% CI 0.17 to 5.00, $p = 0.92$) were not significantly different among these three procedures (Fig. 3). The detailed complications reported by the included studies are summarized in Table 3.

Operative time, fluoroscopy time and hospital stay

Compared with the other two procedures, PCNL had a longer operative time, fluoroscopy time and hospital stay than SWL and RIRS (Fig. 4). In addition, SWL had a significantly shorter operative time (weighted mean difference [WMD] − 12.10, 95% CI − 15.16 to − 9.04, $p < 0.00001$) and hospital stay (WMD − 0.38, 95% CI − 0.63 to − 0.14, $p = 0.002$) than RIRS. There was no significant difference in fluoroscopy time between SWL and RIRS (WMD 10.00, 95% CI − 9.56 to 29.56, $p = 0.32$). (Fig. 4).

Retreatment rate and auxiliary procedure rate

SWL exhibited a significantly higher retreatment rate than PCNL (OR 14.41, 95% CI 8.41 to 24.71, $p < 0.00001$) and RIRS (OR 26.95, 95% CI 1.49 to 488.33, $p = 0.03$), while the retreatment rate between PCNL and RIRS (OR 0.55, 95% CI 0.18 to 1.71, $p = 0.30$) did not show any significant difference. The auxiliary procedure rate of RIRS had no significant difference compared with the other two treatments. Furthermore, SWL had a significantly higher auxiliary procedure rate compared with PCNL (OR 2.78, 95% CI 1.39 to 5.55, $p = 0.004$) (Fig. 5).

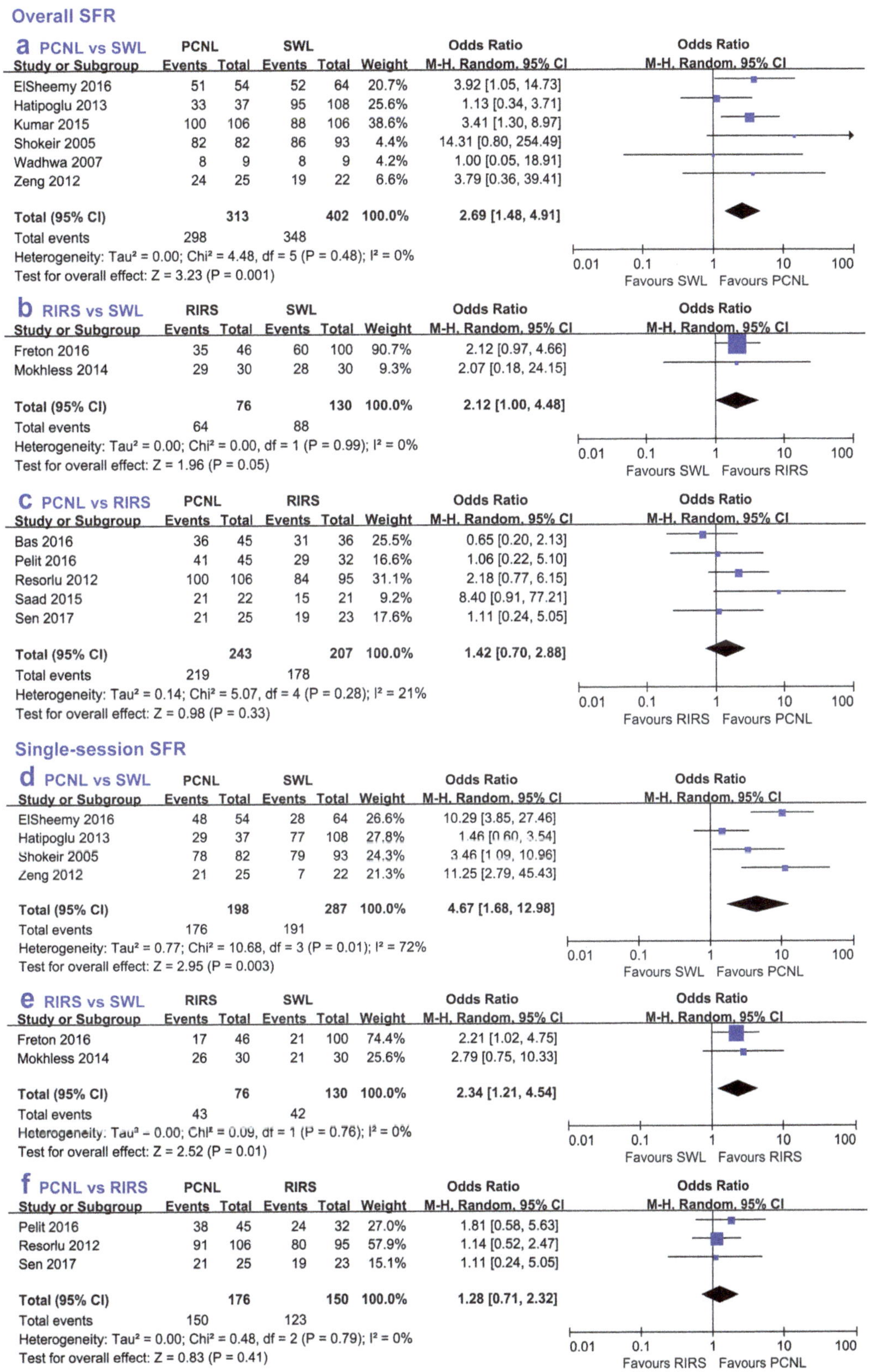

Fig. 2 Forest plot comparing overall SFR between (**a**) PCNL and SWL, **b** RIRS and SWL, **c** PCNL and RIRS, and single-session SFR between (**d**) PCNL and SWL, **e** RIRS and SWL, **f** PCNL and RIRS

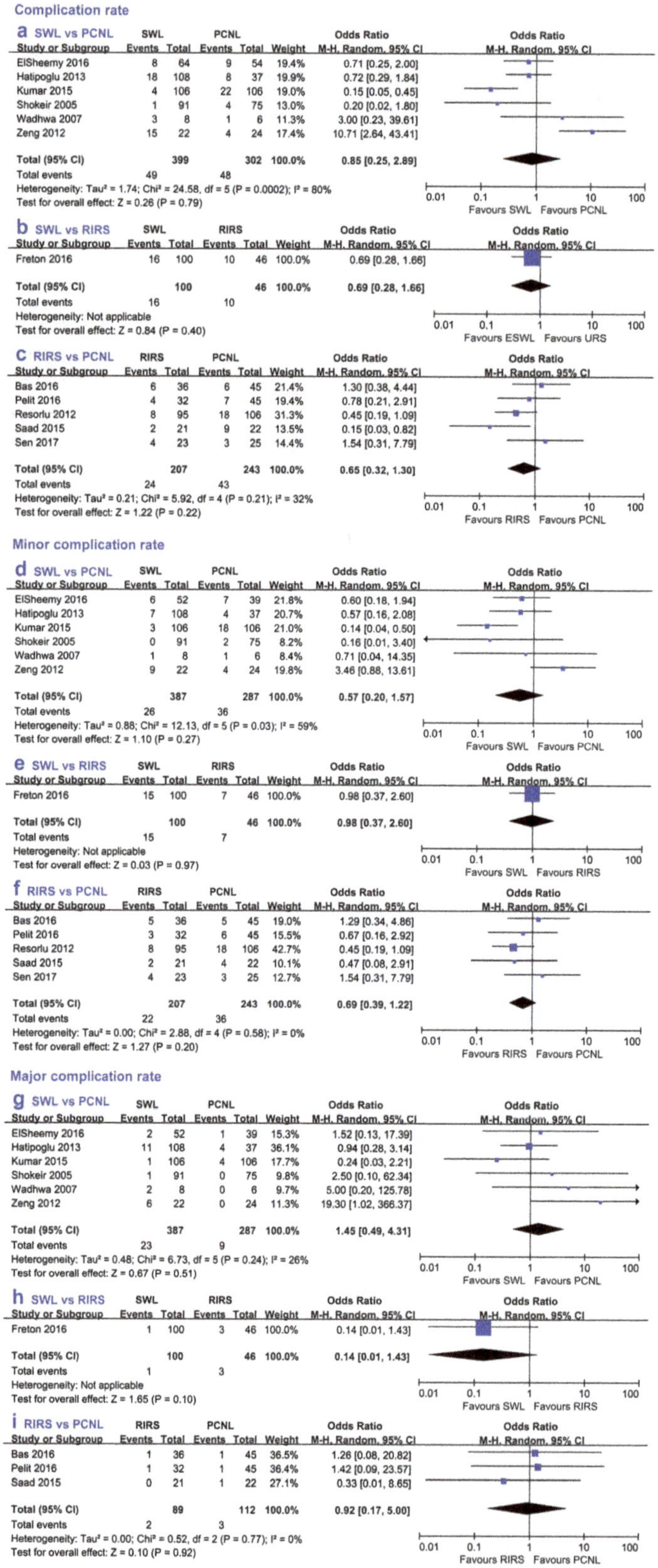

Fig. 3 Forest plot comparing complication rate between (**a**) SWL and PCNL, **b** SWL and RIRS, **c** RIRS and PCNL, minor complication rate between (**d**) SWL and PCNL, **e** SWL and RIRS, **f** RIRS and PCNL, and major complication rate between (**g**) SWL and PCNL, **h** SWL and RIRS, **i** RIRS and PCNL

Table 3 Summary of detailed complications of included studies

Author	Treatment	Complications, n(%)										
		Total	Renal colic	Fever	Urinary infection	Hematuria	Uroepsis	Steinstrasse	Blood transfusion	Ureteral injury	Perforation	Others
Zeng et al [15]	SWL	15(68.19)	5(22.73)	4(18.19)	–	1(4.55)	–	4(18.19)	–	–	–	1(4.55)
	PCNL	4(16)	–	4(16)	–	–	–	–	–	–	–	–
Wadhwa et al [16]	SWL	3(37.5)	–	1(12.5)	–	–	–	2(25)	–	–	–	–
	PCNL	1(16.7)	–	1(16.7)	–	–	–	–	–	–	–	–
Kumar et al [17]	SWL	4(3.7)	2(1.85)	–	1(0.93)	1(0.93)	–	–	–	–	–	–
	PCNL	22(20.75)	5(4.72)	–	9(8.49)	8(7.55)	–	–	–	–	–	–
Hatipoglu et al [18]	SWL	18(16.67)	7(6.6)	–	–	–	–	11(10.38)	–	–	–	–
	PCNL	8(21.62)	4(10.81)	–	–	–	–	1(2.70)	–	–	–	3(8.11)
Shokeir et al [19]	SWL	1(1.1)	–	–	–	–	–	1(1.1)	–	–	–	–
	PCNL	4(5.41)	–	2(2.7)	–	–	–	–	1(1.35)	–	1(1.35)	–
ElSheemy et al [20]	SWL	8(15.4)	–	4(7.7)	4(7.7)	–	–	4(7.7)	–	–	–	–
	PCNL	8(20.5)	–	7(17.94)	2(5.1)	–	–	–	–	–	1(2.6)	2(5.1)
Mokhless et al [21]	SWL	NA[a]	–	–	–	–	–	–	–	–	–	–
	RIRS	NA[a]	–	–	–	–	–	–	–	–	–	–
Freton et al [22]	SWL	16(16)	11(11)	1(1)	2(2)	–	–	–	–	–	–	2(2)
	RIRS	10(21.7)	–	–	3(6.5)	1(2.2)	–	1(2.2)	–	–	–	5(10.9)
Resorlu et al [23]	PCNL	18(17)[b]	–	–	–	–	–	–	–	–	–	–
	RIRS	8(8.4)[b]	–	–	–	–	–	–	–	–	–	–
Saad et al [24]	PCNL	9(40.9)	–	4(18.2)	–	–	–	–	3(13.6)	–	–	2(9.1)
	RIRS	2(9.5)	–	2(9.5)	–	–	–	–	–	–	–	–
Bas et al [25]	PCNL	6(13.3)	4(8.9)	1(2.2)	1(2.2)	–	–	–	–	–	–	–
	RIRS	6(16.7)	2(5.6)	2(5.6)	2(5.6)	–	–	–	–	–	–	–
Sen et al [26]	PCNL	3(12)	3(12)	2(8)	–	–	–	–	–	–	–	–
	RIRS	4(17.3)	4(17.3)	4(17.3)	–	–	1(4.3)	–	–	–	–	–
Pelit et al [27]	PCNL	7(15.5)	–	–	2(4.4)	–	–	–	3(6.7)	–	1(2.2)	1(2.2)
	RIRS	4(12.5)	–	–	3(9.4)	–	–	–	–	1(3.1)	–	–

a. No major complications; b. No detailed complications. *SWL* Extracorporeal shockwave lithotripsy, *PCNL* Percutaneous nephrolithotomy, *RIRS* Retrograde intrarenal surgery

EQ

According to the calculated EQs (Fig. 6), PCNL had a higher efficiency than SWL (OR 5.49, 95% CI 3.73 to 8.06, $p < 0.00001$) and RIRS (OR 8.14, 95% CI 4.75 to 13.98, $p < 0.00001$). Only one study [20], which compared RIRS to SWL, provided enough data to identify a lower EQ of RIRS than SWL (OR 0.32, 95% CI 0.11 to 0.94, $p = 0.04$).

Subgroup analyses

PCNL and SWL

Obviously, PCNL still presented a significantly higher overall SFR (OR 3.94, 95% CI 1.58 to 9.86, $p = 0.003$) and single-session SFR (OR 5.46, 95% CI 2.34 to 12.73, $p < 0.0001$) than SWL in the treatment of pediatric patients with upper urinary tract stone of ≤20 mm (Fig. 7). Except for the approximate major complication rate (OR 1.74, 95% CI 0.19 to 15.80, $p = 0.62$), PCNL had both a significantly higher complication rate (OR 6.32, 95% CI 2.35 to 16.98, $p = 0.0003$) and a higher minor complication rate (OR 6.90, 95% CI 2.16 to 22.03, $p = 0.001$) (Fig. 7). However, pediatric patients with a stone size ≤20 mm who were treated with SWL were more likely to have multiple operations (PCNL vs SWL: OR 0.07, 95% CI 0.04 to 0.13, $p < 0.00001$) and additional procedures (PCNL vs SWL: OR 0.43, 95% CI 0.20 to 0.92, $p = 0.03$) (Fig. 7).

RIRS and SWL

RIRS had a significantly higher single-session SFR than SWL (OR 3.16, 95% CI 1.21 to 8.28, $p = 0.02$) (Fig. 8). Although SWL was always conducted as an outpatient procedure, the results of the subgroup analyses did not show statistically significant differences of hospital stay

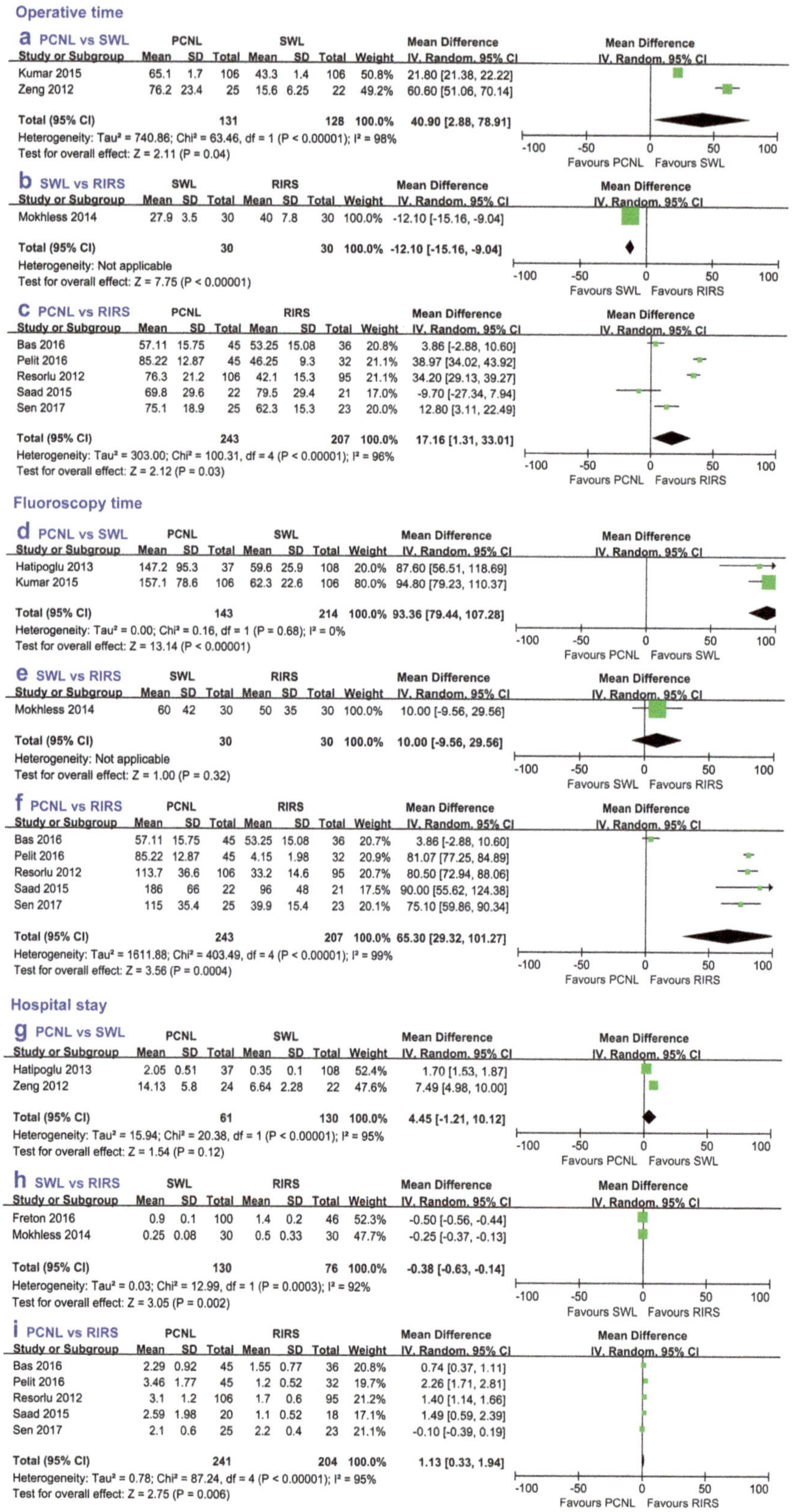

Fig. 4 Forest plot comparing operative time between (**a**) PCNL and SWL, **b** SWL and RIRS, **c** PCNL and RIRS, fluoroscopy time between (**d**) PCNL and SWL, **e** SWL and RIRS, **f** PCNL and RIRS, and hospital stay between (**g**) PCNL and SWL, **h** SWL and RIRS, **i** PCNL and RIRS

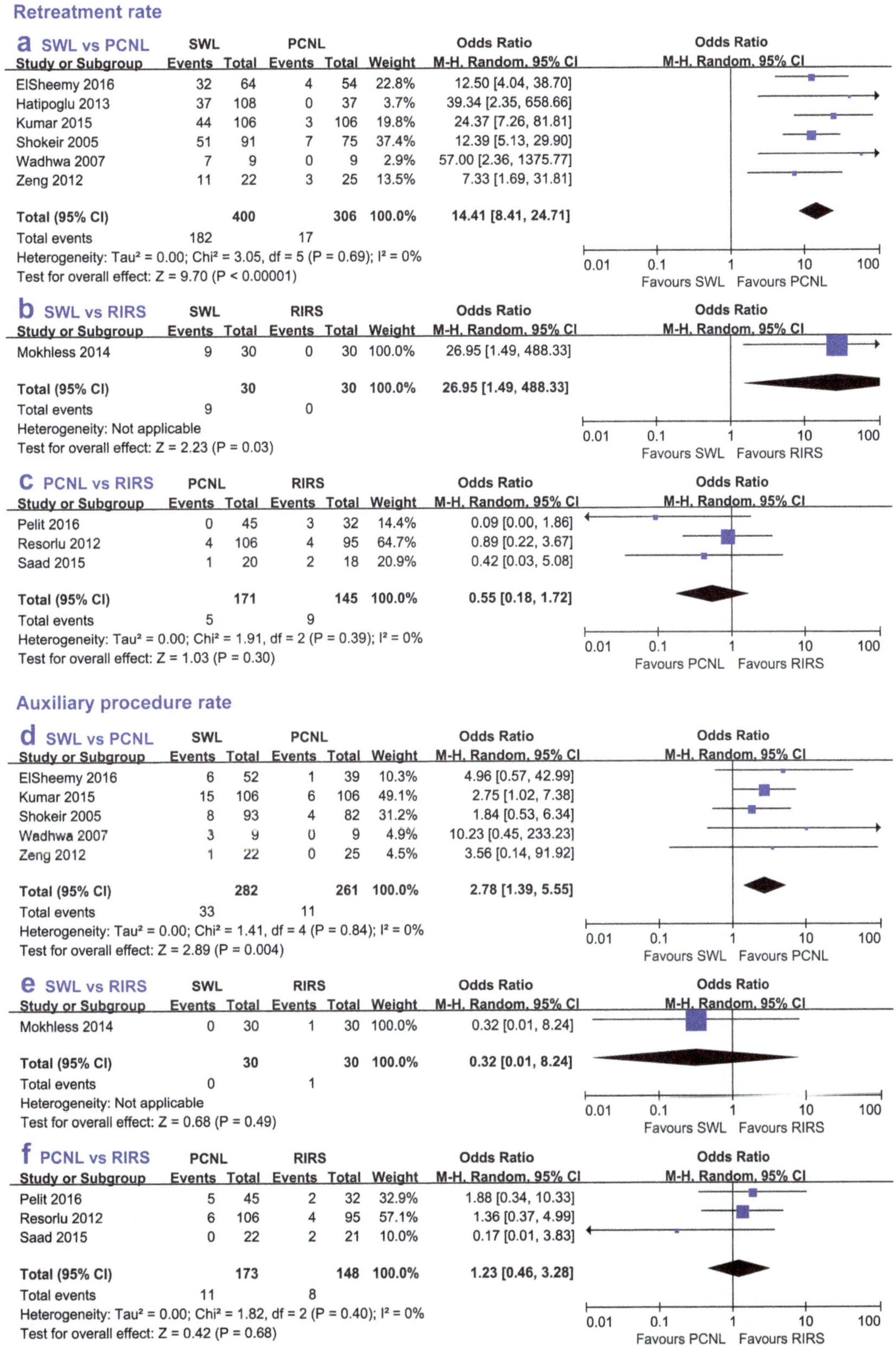

Fig. 5 Forest plot comparing retreatment rate between (**a**) SWL and PCNL, **b** SWL and RIRS, **c** RIRS and PCNL, and auxiliary procedure rate between (d) SWL and PCNL, **e** SWL and RIRS, **f** RIRS and PCNL

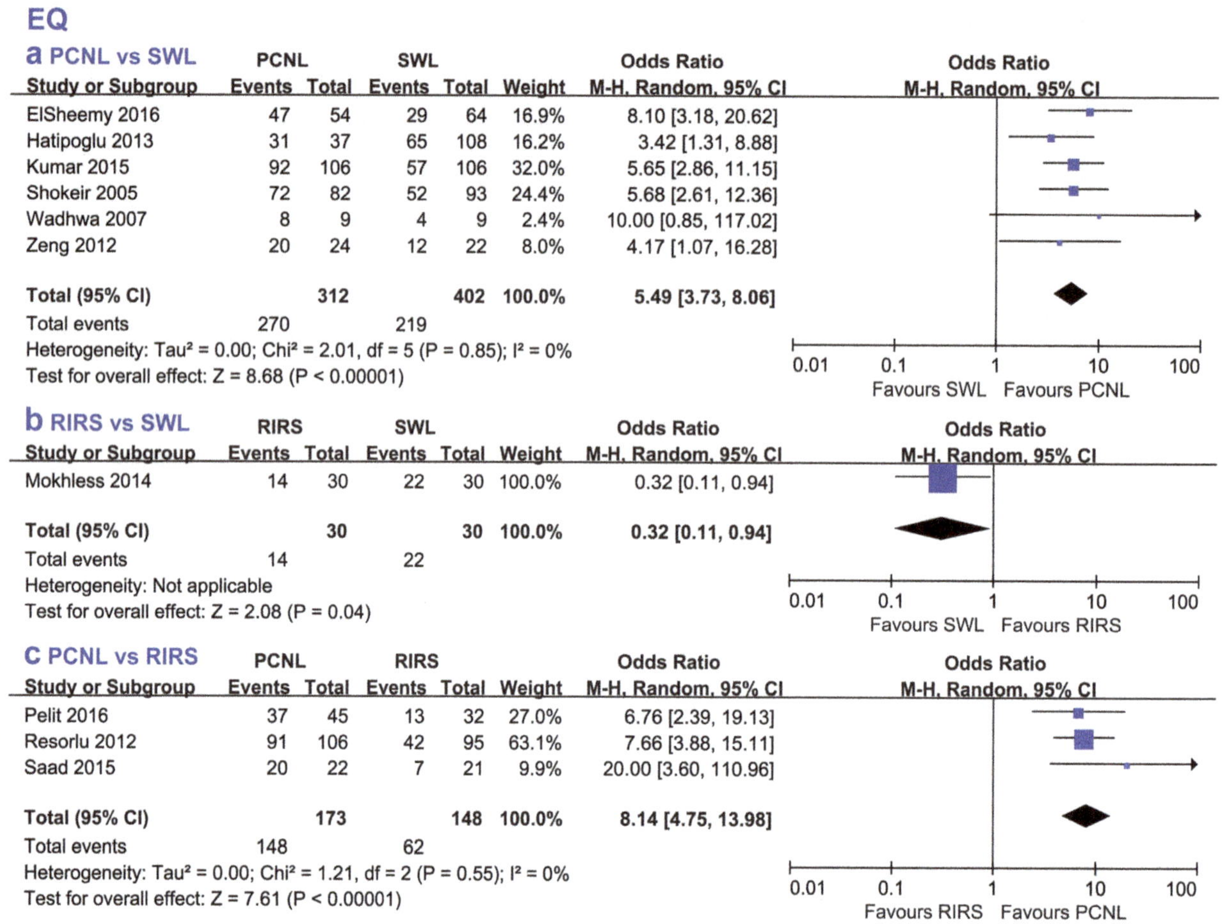

Fig. 6 Forest plot comparing effectiveness quotient (EQ) between (**a**) PCNL and SWL, **b** RIRS and SWL, **c** PCNL and RIRS

between RIRS and SWL (WMD 0.57, 95% CI − 0.06 to 1.21, $p = 0.08$) (Fig. 8).

PCNL and RIRS

Overall SFR, single-session SFR, complication rate, minor complication rate, operative time, fluoroscopy time and hospital stay were all not significantly different between PCNL and RIRS (Fig. 9).

Discussion

Pediatric urolithiasis, which has a high risk of a relapse, can currently be managed by SWL, PCNL, RIRS, and laparoscopic or open surgery. Regardless of the selection of treatment modalities, the final objective is to render the pediatric patient stone free and to reduce the recurrence risk to a minimum. The results from this systematic review illustrated that PCNL presented a significantly higher overall SFR (OR 2.69, 95% CI 1.48 to 4.91, $p = 0.001$), higher single-session SFR (OR 4.67, 95% CI 1.68 to 12.98, $p = 0.003$), and higher EQ. (OR 5.49, 95% CI 3.73 to 8.06, $p < 0.00001$) compared with SWL. The RCT of SWL vs PCNL conducted by Kumar A, et al. [17] proved that PCNL was more efficient for stone sizes of 10–20 mm than SWL (EQ: 86.96% vs 53.33%), and the identical conclusion was also reached by the retrospective case controlled studies. Although the pooled results demonstrated the overall SFR and single-session SFR of PCNL were both significantly higher than SWL, there was no significant difference in several studies in terms of the overall SFR (PCNL vs SWL: 96% vs 86.3%; 88% vs 88%; 89.2% vs 88%; 94.9% vs 84.6%) [15, 16, 18, 20]. Considering the lower retreatment rate and auxiliary procedure rate, these studies claimed that PCNL is a feasible and more efficient treatment for pediatric renal stones.

The pooled results revealed there was no significant difference in the SFR between PCNL and RIRS regardless of the stone size of the pediatric patients. Although Resorlu B, et al. [23] also reported that no significant difference of the SFR was found between PCNL and RIRS (94.3% vs 92.6%), if dividing patients into subgroups according to stone size, PCNL was apparently superior to RIRS (> 20 mm: 83.9% vs 50%; < 20 mm: 100% vs 87.3%). Nevertheless, the length of hospital stay was significantly shorter in RIRS pediatric patients in comparison with

PCNL vs SWL

Overall SFR

Study or Subgroup	PCNL Events	PCNL Total	SWL Events	SWL Total	Weight	Odds Ratio M-H, Random, 95% CI
Kumar 2015	100	106	88	106	89.9%	3.41 [1.30, 8.97]
Shokeir 2005	82	82	86	93	10.1%	14.31 [0.80, 254.49]
Total (95% CI)		**188**		**199**	**100.0%**	**3.94 [1.58, 9.86]**
Total events	182		174			

Heterogeneity: Tau² = 0.00; Chi² = 0.91, df = 1 (P = 0.34); I² = 0%
Test for overall effect: Z = 2.93 (P = 0.003)

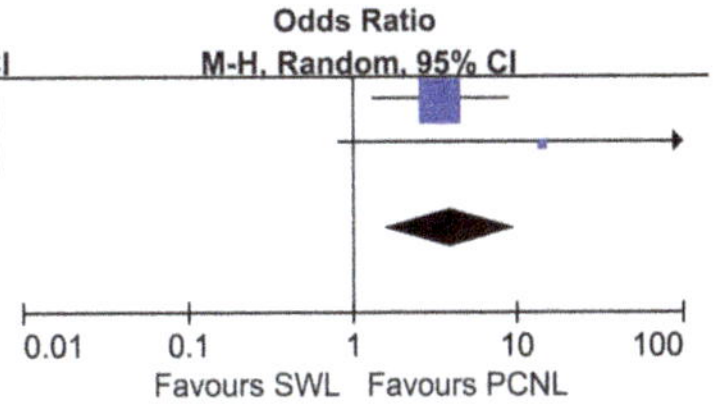

Single-session SFR

Study or Subgroup	PCNL Events	PCNL Total	SWL Events	SWL Total	Weight	Odds Ratio M-H, Random, 95% CI
ElSheemy 2016	38	43	25	52	52.9%	8.21 [2.79, 24.16]
Shokeir 2005	78	82	79	93	47.1%	3.46 [1.09, 10.96]
Total (95% CI)		**125**		**145**	**100.0%**	**5.46 [2.34, 12.73]**
Total events	116		104			

Heterogeneity: Tau² = 0.05; Chi² = 1.15, df = 1 (P = 0.28); I² = 13%
Test for overall effect: Z = 3.93 (P < 0.0001)

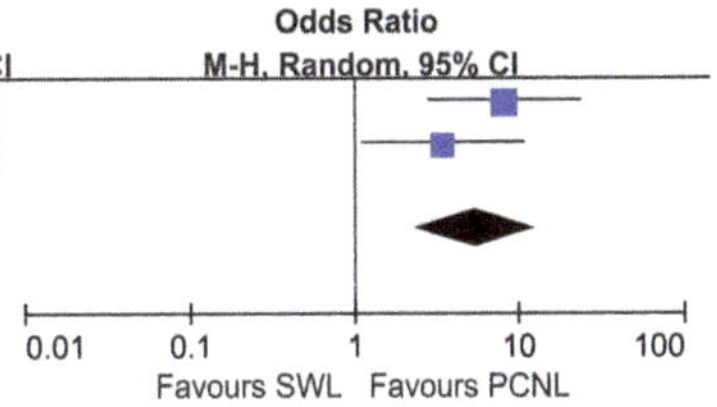

Complication rate

Study or Subgroup	PCNL Events	PCNL Total	SWL Events	SWL Total	Weight	Odds Ratio M-H, Random, 95% CI
Kumar 2015	22	106	4	106	80.1%	6.68 [2.21, 20.14]
Shokeir 2005	4	75	1	91	19.9%	5.07 [0.55, 46.37]
Total (95% CI)		**181**		**197**	**100.0%**	**6.32 [2.35, 16.98]**
Total events	26		5			

Heterogeneity: Tau² = 0.00; Chi² = 0.05, df = 1 (P = 0.83); I² = 0%
Test for overall effect: Z = 3.66 (P = 0.0003)

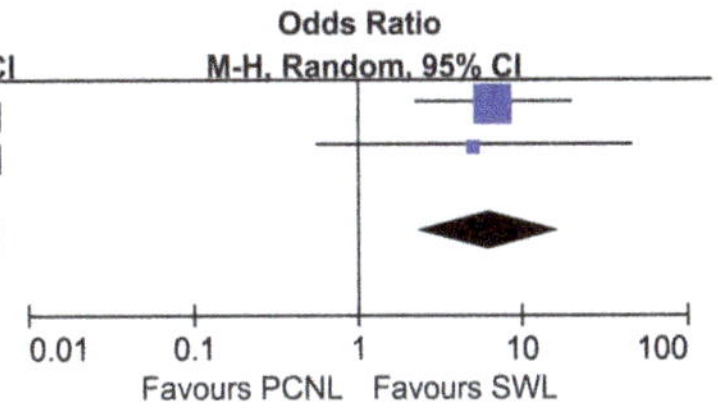

Minor complication rate

Study or Subgroup	PCNL Events	PCNL Total	SWL Events	SWL Total	Weight	Odds Ratio M-H, Random, 95% CI
Kumar 2015	18	106	3	106	85.5%	7.02 [2.00, 24.63]
Shokeir 2005	2	75	0	91	14.5%	6.22 [0.29, 131.67]
Total (95% CI)		**181**		**197**	**100.0%**	**6.90 [2.16, 22.03]**
Total events	20		3			

Heterogeneity: Tau² = 0.00; Chi² = 0.01, df = 1 (P = 0.94); I² = 0%
Test for overall effect: Z = 3.26 (P = 0.001)

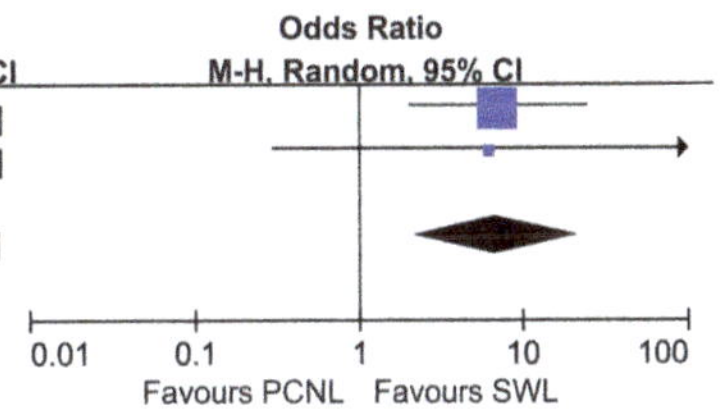

Major complication rate

Study or Subgroup	PCNL Events	PCNL Total	SWL Events	SWL Total	Weight	Odds Ratio M-H, Random, 95% CI
Kumar 2015	4	106	1	100	63.1%	4.12 [0.45, 37.47]
Shokeir 2005	0	75	1	91	36.9%	0.40 [0.02, 9.95]
Total (95% CI)		**181**		**197**	**100.0%**	**1.74 [0.19, 15.80]**
Total events	4		2			

Heterogeneity: Tau² = 0.74; Chi² = 1.37, df = 1 (P = 0.24); I² = 27%
Test for overall effect: Z = 0.49 (P = 0.62)

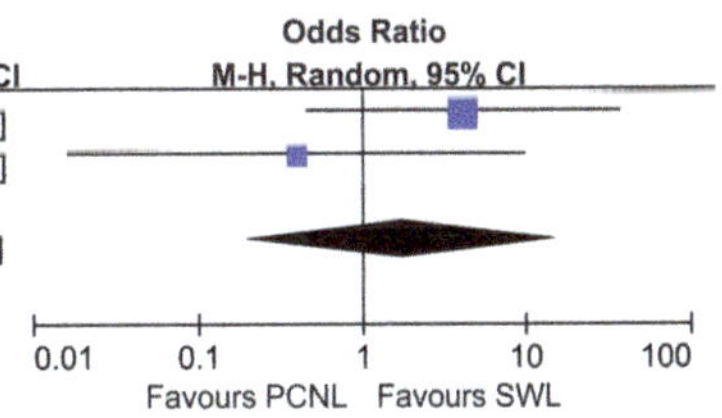

Retreatment rate

Study or Subgroup	PCNL Events	PCNL Total	SWL Events	SWL Total	Weight	Odds Ratio M-H, Random, 95% CI
ElSheemy 2016	3	43	23	52	23.3%	0.09 [0.03, 0.35]
Kumar 2015	3	106	44	106	26.6%	0.04 [0.01, 0.14]
Shokeir 2005	7	75	51	91	50.2%	0.08 [0.03, 0.19]
Total (95% CI)		**224**		**249**	**100.0%**	**0.07 [0.04, 0.13]**
Total events	13		118			

Heterogeneity: Tau² = 0.00; Chi² = 1.07, df = 2 (P = 0.58); I² = 0%
Test for overall effect: Z = 8.35 (P < 0.00001)

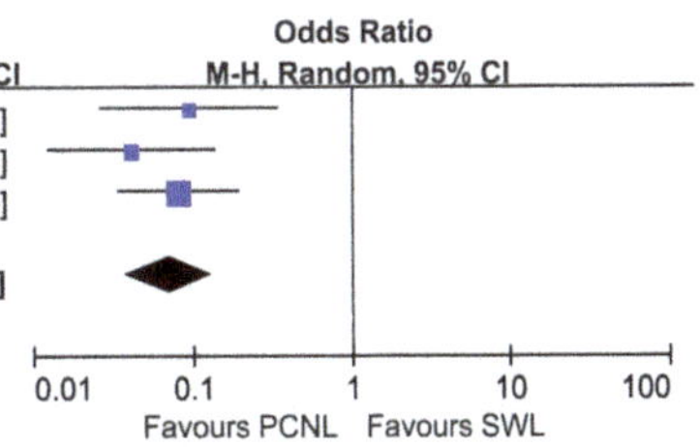

Auxiliary procedure rate

Study or Subgroup	PCNL Events	PCNL Total	SWL Events	SWL Total	Weight	Odds Ratio M-H, Random, 95% CI
Kumar 2015	6	106	15	106	61.1%	0.36 [0.14, 0.98]
Shokeir 2005	4	82	8	93	38.9%	0.54 [0.16, 1.88]
Total (95% CI)		**188**		**199**	**100.0%**	**0.43 [0.20, 0.92]**
Total events	10		23			

Heterogeneity: Tau² = 0.00; Chi² = 0.25, df = 1 (P = 0.62); I² = 0%
Test for overall effect: Z = 2.17 (P = 0.03)

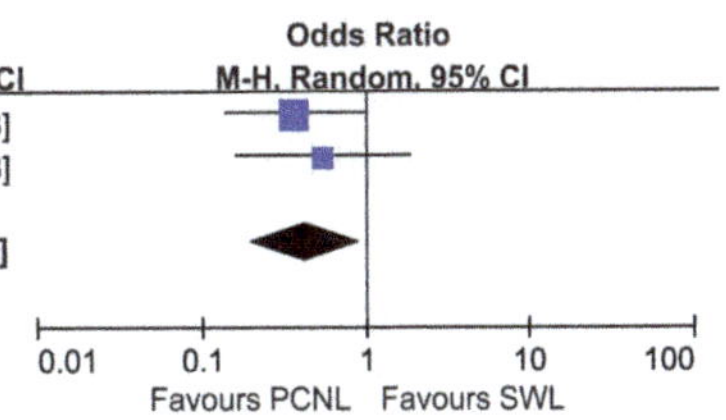

Fig. 7 Subgroup analyses results of PCNL vs SWL

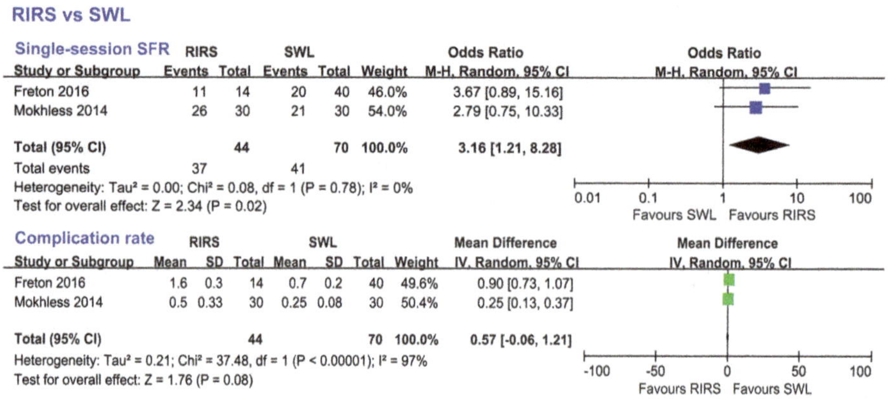

Fig. 8 Subgroup analyses results of RIRS vs SWL

PCNL (PCNL vs RIRS: 3.1 ± 1.2 vs 1.7 ± 0.6, days) [23]. PCNL requires the creation and dilation of an access tract through the renal parenchyma, and this is deemed to be more invasive than RIRS or SWL. However, the application of micro-PCNL or even super-mini PCNL can reduce complication events with a very high single session SFR.

SWL is considered the most minimally invasive procedure among these 3 treatment modalities, and it is still the first-line therapy for pediatric renal stones. In our analysis, RIRS is a more effective procedure than SWL according to the higher single-session SFR (OR 2.35, 95% CI 1.21 to 4.55, $p = 0.05$) and higher overall SFR in pediatric patients with upper urinary tract stone size ≤20 mm, although comparative studies of SWL vs RIRS included in this review had no positive result in SFR, including from an RCT [28]. Furthermore, the biological effects of SWL may induce acute injury of the renal parenchyma and adjacent tissues due to the acute effects of SWL, such as focal hemorrhage, rupture of small veins, extravasation and pooling of blood, necrosis in vasculature, disintegration in podocytes and mesangial cells, blood within Bowman's space and renal tubules, ischaemic changes, and infiltration by inflammatory cells [29]. Shock wave-induced transient tubular functional damage has been observed by Villanyi KK and colleagues [30]. Therefore, these authors recommended that consecutive treatments for pediatric renal stones should be spaced by at least 2 weeks. Although there is no clinical evidence about the long-term effect of SWL on pediatric kidneys [29], this effect should be kept in mind when SWL is chosen for pediatric renal stones due to the kidney still being in the growth and development stage.

In this review, higher overall complication rates and higher minor complication rates were only significantly found in the subgroup analyses of PCNL vs SWL. Although there was no significant difference in the various complication rates among the other subgroup analyses, blood transfusion was indicated exclusively in PCNL patients exclusively in our review. The highest transfusion rate, 13.64%, was reported by Saad KS, et al. [24]. Desoky EA and his colleagues [31] claimed that PCNL in the pediatric age group via the flank-free modified supine position was safe and effective in the management of renal pelvis stones of sizes 20–30 cm, and the SFR was similar to conventional PCNL in the prone position with only 1 (4.5%) blood transfusion.

Except for the results of subgroup analyses, there were no significant differences in all of the indexes of the complication rates comparing SWL with the other two treatments. This finding disagrees with the widespread recognition that SWL is the most minimally invasive procedure among these techniques. Moreover, steinstrasse formation was only observed in SWL (1.1–25%), except for 1 case of steinstrasse formation in PCNL [18] and another case in RIRS [22]. However, the fragment clearance after pediatric SWL is more efficient than in adults. D'Addessi A, et al. [28] indicated that, since the child's ureter is shorter than an adult's, this shorter length partially compensates for its narrower lumen, and the pediatric ureter is more elastic and distensible, promoting the passage of stone fragments. Finally, the small body volume of children reduces the loss of energy of the shockwaves in the process of release.

SWL had an undoubtedly shorter operative time than PCNL and RIRS, and it is usually performed as an outpatient treatment. All of the included studies preferred SWL over PCNL or RIRS, considering the operative time and hospital stay. However, with instrument miniaturization and other optimizations, RIRS has been increasingly performed, like SWL, as an outpatient procedure. The hospital stay of RIRS was also significantly shorter than PCNL, and this could reduce the medical cost, in spite of no significant difference being found in subgroup analyses. In addition to the relatively longer operative time and longer

PCNL vs RIRS

Overall SFR

Study or Subgroup	PCNL Events	PCNL Total	RIRS Events	RIRS Total	Weight	Odds Ratio M-H, Random, 95% CI
Bas 2016	36	45	31	36	61.8%	0.65 [0.20, 2.13]
Sen 2017	21	25	19	23	38.2%	1.11 [0.24, 5.05]
Total (95% CI)		**70**		**59**	**100.0%**	**0.79 [0.31, 2.03]**
Total events	57		50			

Heterogeneity: $Tau^2 = 0.00$; $Chi^2 = 0.30$, df = 1 (P = 0.58); $I^2 = 0\%$
Test for overall effect: Z = 0.49 (P = 0.63)

Single-session SFR

Study or Subgroup	PCNL Events	PCNL Total	RIRS Events	RIRS Total	Weight	Odds Ratio M-H, Random, 95% CI
Resorlu 2012	13	13	76	87	21.6%	4.06 [0.23, 73.03]
Sen 2017	21	25	19	23	78.4%	1.11 [0.24, 5.05]
Total (95% CI)		**38**		**110**	**100.0%**	**1.46 [0.38, 5.62]**
Total events	34		95			

Heterogeneity: $Tau^2 = 0.00$; $Chi^2 = 0.65$, df = 1 (P = 0.42); $I^2 = 0\%$
Test for overall effect: Z = 0.56 (P = 0.58)

Complication rate

Study or Subgroup	PCNL Events	PCNL Total	RIRS Events	RIRS Total	Weight	Odds Ratio M-H, Random, 95% CI
Bas 2016	6	45	6	36	63.5%	0.77 [0.23, 2.63]
Sen 2017	3	25	4	23	36.5%	0.65 [0.13, 3.27]
Total (95% CI)		**70**		**59**	**100.0%**	**0.72 [0.27, 1.92]**
Total events	9		10			

Heterogeneity: $Tau^2 = 0.00$; $Chi^2 = 0.03$, df = 1 (P = 0.87); $I^2 = 0\%$
Test for overall effect: Z = 0.65 (P = 0.51)

Minor complication rate

Study or Subgroup	PCNL Events	PCNL Total	RIRS Events	RIRS Total	Weight	Odds Ratio M-H, Random, 95% CI
Bas 2016	5	45	5	36	59.8%	0.78 [0.21, 2.92]
Sen 2017	3	25	4	23	40.2%	0.65 [0.13, 3.27]
Total (95% CI)		**70**		**59**	**100.0%**	**0.72 [0.26, 2.01]**
Total events	8		9			

Heterogeneity: $Tau^2 = 0.00$; $Chi^2 = 0.03$, df = 1 (P = 0.87); $I^2 = 0\%$
Test for overall effect: Z = 0.62 (P = 0.53)

Operative time

Study or Subgroup	PCNL Mean	PCNL SD	PCNL Total	RIRS Mean	RIRS SD	RIRS Total	Weight	Mean Difference IV, Random, 95% CI
Bas 2016	57.11	15.75	45	53.25	15.08	36	57.9%	3.86 [-2.88, 10.60]
Sen 2017	75.1	18.9	25	62.3	15.3	23	42.1%	12.80 [3.11, 22.49]
Total (95% CI)			**70**			**59**	**100.0%**	**7.62 [-1.03, 16.27]**

Heterogeneity: $Tau^2 = 21.81$; $Chi^2 = 2.20$, df = 1 (P = 0.14); $I^2 = 55\%$
Test for overall effect: Z = 1.73 (P = 0.08)

Fluoroscopy time

Study or Subgroup	PCNL Mean	PCNL SD	PCNL Total	RIRS Mean	RIRS SD	RIRS Total	Weight	Mean Difference IV, Random, 95% CI
Bas 2016	57.11	15.75	45	53.25	15.08	36	50.5%	3.86 [-2.88, 10.60]
Sen 2017	115	35.4	25	39.9	15.4	23	49.5%	75.10 [59.86, 90.34]
Total (95% CI)			**70**			**59**	**100.0%**	**39.14 [-30.67, 108.95]**

Heterogeneity: $Tau^2 = 2501.44$; $Chi^2 = 70.23$, df = 1 (P < 0.00001); $I^2 = 99\%$
Test for overall effect: Z = 1.10 (P = 0.27)

Hospital stay

Study or Subgroup	PCNL Mean	PCNL SD	PCNL Total	RIRS Mean	RIRS SD	RIRS Total	Weight	Mean Difference IV, Random, 95% CI
Bas 2016	2.29	0.92	45	1.55	0.77	36	49.0%	0.74 [0.37, 1.11]
Sen 2017	2.1	0.6	25	2.2	0.4	23	51.0%	-0.10 [-0.39, 0.19]
Total (95% CI)			**70**			**59**	**100.0%**	**0.31 [-0.51, 1.13]**

Heterogeneity: $Tau^2 = 0.32$; $Chi^2 = 12.46$, df = 1 (P = 0.0004); $I^2 = 92\%$
Test for overall effect: Z = 0.74 (P = 0.46)

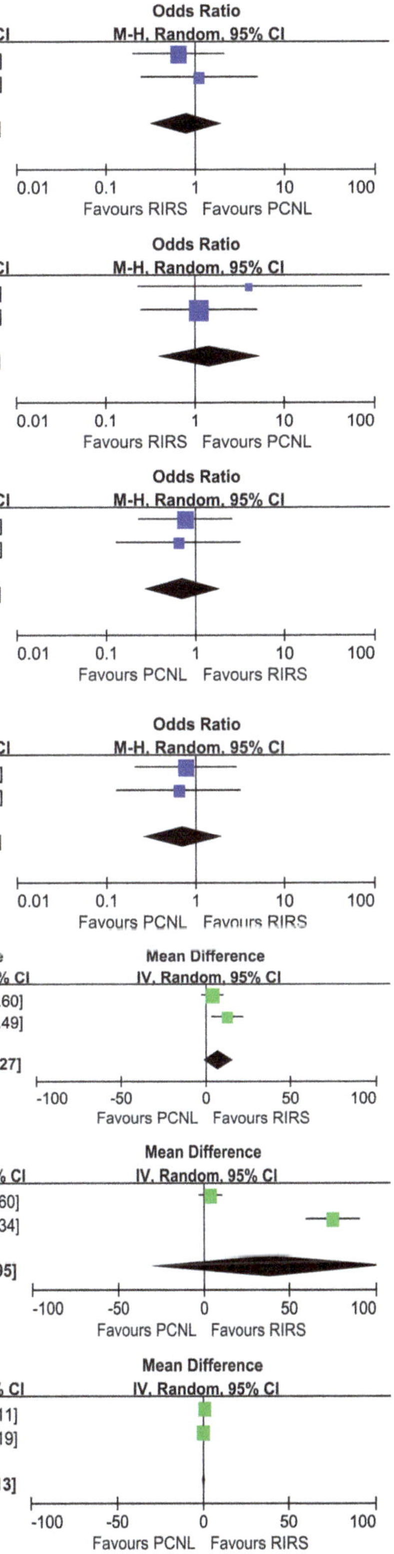

Fig. 9 Subgroup analyses results of PCNL vs RIRS

hospital stay, PCNL also presented a significantly longer fluoroscopy time than SWL or RIRS. Ristau BT and his colleagues [32] reported that radiation exposure was vital during treatment of pediatric stone disease, especially for defining the location of the stone when PCNL was performed. Therefore, these authors recommended that urologists should closely monitor the amount of radiation dose and limit the maximum effective dose to as low as reasonably achievable (ALARA) [33]. Specifically, ALARA principles mandated that the maximum effective dose should not exceed 50 mSv in any 1-year period, and an average dose less than 20 mSv per year over any 5-year period. In brief, the urologists should devote themselves to reducing the radiation hazard as much as possible.

Since SWL is mainly performed under ultrasonographic guidance, it becomes a more attractive option with lower radiation exposure than the other two treatments. However, SWL exhibited a significantly higher retreatment rate compared with the other two therapies, while the retreatment rate between PCNL and RIRS did not show any significant difference. Furthermore, SWL also caused a significantly higher auxiliary procedure rate than PCNL. Considering that the fragment clearance of children is more rapidly than that of adults after SWL, surgical approaches seem to be a last resort. Soygur T and his colleagues [34] suggested that expectant management was usually efficient even in patients who developed steinstrasse after SWL, except for patients with larger stones (> 20 mm), staghorn calculi or sepsis with an obstructed kidney. However, RIRS has a lower efficiency than SWL according to the EQ. In addition, every single EQ of RIRS from the included studies was less than 50% because the complete RIRS process includes one session for passive dilatation, one session for the lithotripsy and stent insertion, and one session for stent removal. Therefore, this technique requires more sessions under anaesthesia and more surgical risks.

When interpreting the results of our review, some limitations should be addressed. First, only 3 RCTs were available for final analysis, and more than half of the included studies were nonrandomized case control comparisons. Inevitably, patients and investigators cannot be double-blinded to the interventions. Allocation concealment was also not described in some RCTs. Furthermore, not all of the included articles were high-quality studies. A lack of more high-quality studies reduces the persuasiveness of our work. Second, no included study compared all three treatments head-to-head, and it was impossible to conduct a high-quality network meta-analysis since there were not enough relevant RCTs. Third, due to the nature of non-randomized studies, selection bias could be a major confounder, which might bias our conclusions. Finally, the heterogeneity among the studies was obvious for several parameters, which might be a result of the differences in pediatric inclusive criteria, physical environment, surgical skills, outcome definitions and standards, or imaging during follow-up. Even more concerning is the stone burdens were not similar among these included studies, and there was not enough data to execute a sufficient subgroup analysis.

In spite of these limitations, our study still has some merits and values. To the best of our knowledge, this is the first systematic review that has simultaneously analysed the efficacy and safety of SWL, PCNL, and RIRS simultaneously in the treatment of pediatric upper urinary tract stones. Furthermore, our work, updated with the most recent data, provides a newly reference for the selection of the ideal treatment modality in pediatric urolithiasis. However, it is noteworthy that making an optimal recommendation is unusually difficult, since the clinical option is based on the stone size, stone location, patient age, instrument caliber, previous interventions history, comorbidity, and other factors.

Conclusion

In summary, our review suggests that SWL performed as an outpatient procedure provides a shorter hospital stay and operative time, with a lower SFR, higher retreatment rate, higher auxiliary procedure rate, and relative lower EQ. PCNL presents a higher SFR than SWL and the highest EQ, but this is a technique accompanied by a longer fluoroscopy time and operative time than the other two modalities. RIRS offers a higher single-session SFR and lower retreatment rate than SWL but a lower EQ than SWL and PCNL, although a significantly shorter hospital stay than PCNL. Higher complication rates and higher minor complication rates were only significantly found in subgroup analyses of PCNL vs SWL. In other words, the complication rates are comparable among the three modalities, and most of these were minor complications.

The ultimate target of pediatric urinary stone management is to achieve extreme stone clearance with a safe and effective therapeutic regimen. To achieve this ideal target, urologists must choose the optimal individual modality, or combined other therapeutic regimens, according to the pediatric conditions and the goals of the parents.

Abbreviations

ALARA: As low as reasonably achievable; AUA: American Urological Association; CI: Confidence interval; EAU: Uropean Association of Urology; EQ: Effectiveness quotients; GFR: Glomerular filtration rate; LE: Level of evidence; NOS: Newcastle-Ottawa Scale; OR: Odds ratio; PCNL: Percutaneous nephrolithotomy; RCT: Randomized control trail; RIRS: Retrograde intrarenal surgery; SD: Standard deviation; SFR: Stone free rate; SWL: Extracorporeal shockwave lithotripsy; WMD: Weighted mean difference

Acknowledgements

We thank Dr. Hasan Serkan Dogan and Dr. Ephrem Odoy Olweny for providing very useful comments during the revision of this study.

Authors' contributions

QH and KWX carried out the literature search, quality assessment and data extraction, participated in the data analysis, drafted and revised the manuscript. YTC performed the statistical analysis and made the figures. BHL participated in the study design and supervised the project. HL and KJW conceived of the study and helped draft the manuscript. KJW is also the corresponding author for this manuscript. All authors read and approved the final manuscript.

References

1. Mahmud M, Zaidi Z. Percutaneous nephrolithotomy in children before school age: experience of a Pakistani Centre. BJU Int. 2004;94:1352–4.
2. Straub M, Gschwend J, Zorn C. Pediatric urolithiasis: the current surgical management. Pediatr Nephrol. 2010;25:1239–44.
3. Turk C, Petrik A, Sarica K, Seitz C, Skolarikos A, Straub M, et al. EAU guidelines on interventional treatment for urolithiasis. Eur Urol. 2016;69:475–82.
4. Assimos D, Krambeck A, Miller NL, Monga M, Murad MH, Nelson CP, et al. Surgical Management of Stones: American urological association/ Endourological society guideline, PART I. J Urol. 2016;196:1153–60.
5. Guven S, Istanbulluoglu O, Ozturk A, Ozturk B, Piskin M, Cicek T, et al. Percutaneous nephrolithotomy is highly efficient and safe in infants and children under 3 years of age. Urol Int. 2010;85:455–60.
6. Dogan HS, Kilicarslan H, Kordan Y, Celen S, Oktay B. Percutaneous nephrolithotomy in children: does age matter? World J Urol. 2011;29:725–9.
7. Dogan HS, Tekgul S. Minimally invasive surgical approaches to kidney stones in children. Curr Urol Rep. 2012;13:298–306.
8. Vanlangendonck R, Landman J. Ureteral access strategies: pro-access sheath. Urol Clin North Am. 2004;31:71–81.
9. Safwat AS, Bissada NK, Kumar U, Taha MI, Abdel-Hafez SES, Eltaher AM, et al. Experience with ureteroscopic holmium laser lithotripsy in children. Pediatr Surg Int. 2008;24:579–81.
10. Clavien PA, Barkun J, de Oliveira ML, Vauthey JN, Dindo D, Schulick RD, et al. The Clavien-Dindo classification of surgical complications: five-year experience. Ann Surg. 2009;250:187–96.
11. Clayman RV, McClennan BL, Garvin TJ, Denstedt JD, Andriole GL. Lithostar: an electromagnetic acoustic shock wave unit for extracorporeal lithotripsy. J Endourol. 1989;3:307–13.
12. B. Phillips, C. Ball, D. Sackett, D. Banenoch, S. Straus, B. Haynes MD. Oxford Centre for Evidencebased Medicine—Levels of Evidence 2009. [Internet]. Cent. Evidence-Based Med. [cited 2015 Jan 5]. Available from: http://www.cebm.net/index.aspx?o = 1025.
13. Oremus M, Wolfson C, Perrault A, Demers L, Momoli F, Moride Y. Interrater reliability of the modified Jadad quality scale for systematic reviews of Alzheimer's disease drug trials. Dement Geriatr Cogn Disord. 2001;12:232–6.
14. Wells GA, Shea B, O'Connell D, Peterson J, Welch V, Losos M, et al. The Newcastle-Ottawa scale (NOS) for assessing the quality of nonrandomized studies in meta-analyses. Ottawa Hosp Res Inst. 2013. Available: http://www.ohri.ca/programs/clinical_epidemiology/oxford.asp.
15. Zeng G, Jia J, Zhao Z, Wu W, Zhao Z, Zhong W. Treatment of renal stones in infants: comparing extracorporeal shock wave lithotripsy and mini-percutaneous nephrolithotomy. Urol Res. 2012;40:599–603.
16. Wadhwa P, Aron M, Bal CS, Dhanpatty B, Gupta NP. Critical prospective appraisal of renal morphology and function in children undergoing shockwave lithotripsy and percutaneous nephrolithotomy. J Endourol. 2007;21:961–6.
17. Kumar A, Kumar N, Vasudeva P, Kumar R, Jha SK, Singh H. A single center experience comparing Miniperc and shockwave lithotripsy for treatment of radiopaque 1-2 cm lower Caliceal renal calculi in children: a prospective randomized study. J Endourol. 2015;29:805–9.
18. Hatipoglu NK, Sancaktutar AA, Tepeler A, Bodakci MN, Penbegul N, Atar M, et al. Comparison of shockwave lithotripsy and microperc for treatment of kidney stones in children. J Endourol. 2013;27:1141–6.
19. Shokeir AA, Sheir KZ, El-Nahas AR, El-Assmy AM, Eassa W, El-Kappany HA. Treatment of renal stones in children: a comparison between percutaneous nephrolithotomy and shock wave lithotripsy. J Urol. 2006;176:706–10.
20. ElSheemy MS, Daw K, Habib E, Aboulela W, Fathy H, Shouman AM, et al. Lower calyceal and renal pelvic stones in preschool children: a comparative study of mini-percutaneous nephrolithotomy versus extracorporeal shockwave lithotripsy. Int J Urol. 2016;23:564–70.
21. Mokhless IA, Abdeldaeim HM, Saad A, Zahran AR. Retrograde intrarenal surgery monotherapy versus shock wave lithotripsy for stones 10 to 20 mm in preschool children: a prospective, randomized study. J Urol. 2014;191:1496–9.
22. Freton L, Peyronnet B, Arnaud A, Tondut L, Hascoet J, Pradere B, et al. Extracorporeal shockwave lithotripsy versus flexible Ureteroscopy for the Management of Upper Tract Urinary Stones in children. J Endourol. 2017;31:1–6.
23. Resorlu B, Unsal A, Tepeler A, Atis G, Tokatli Z, Oztuna D, et al. Comparison of retrograde intrarenal surgery and mini-percutaneous nephrolithotomy in children with moderate-size kidney stones: results of multi-institutional analysis. Urology. 2012;80:519–23.
24. Saad KSM, Youssif ME, Al Islam Nafis Hamdy S, Fahmy A, El Din Hanno AG, El-Nahas AR. Percutaneous Nephrolithotomy vs retrograde intrarenal surgery for large renal stones in pediatric patients: a randomized controlled trial. J Urol. 2015;194:1716–20.
25. Bas O, Dede O, Aydogmus Y, Utangac M, Yikilmaz TN, Damar E, et al. Comparison of retrograde intrarenal surgery and micro-percutaneous Nephrolithotomy in moderately sized pediatric kidney stones. J Endourol. 2016;30:765–70.
26. Sen H, Seckiner I, Bayrak O, Dogan K, Erturhan S. A comparison of micro-PERC and retrograde intrarenal surgery results in pediatric patients with renal stones. J Pediatr Urol. 2017;13:619.e1–5.
27. Pelit ES, Atis G, Kati B, Akin Y, Ciftci H, Culpan M, et al. Comparison of mini-percutaneous Nephrolithotomy and retrograde intrarenal surgery in preschool-aged children. Urology. 2017;101:21–5.
28. D'Addessi A, Bongiovanni L, Sasso F, Gulino G, Falabella R, Bassi P. Extracorporeal shockwave lithotripsy in pediatrics. J Endourol. 2008;22:1–12.
29. Akin Y, Yucel S. Long-term effects of pediatric extracorporeal shockwave lithotripsy on renal function. Res Rep Urol. 2014;6(1):21–5.
30. Villanyi KK, Szekely JG, Farkas LM, Javor E, Pusztai C. Short-term changes in renal function after extracorporeal shock wave lithotripsy in children. J Urol. 2001;166:222–4.
31. Desoky EAE, ElSayed ER, Eliwa A, Sleem M, Shabana W, Dawood T, et al. Flank-free modified supine percutaneous Nephrolithotomy in pediatric age group. Urology. 2015;85:1162–5.
32. Ristau BT, Dudley AG, Casella DP, Dwyer ME, Fox JA, Cannon GM, et al. Tracking of radiation exposure in pediatric stone patients: the time is now. J Pediatr Urol. 2015;11:339.e1–5.
33. Wrixon AD. New ICRP recommendations. J Radiol Prot. 2008;28(2):161–8.
34. Soygur T, Arikan N, Kilic O, Suer E. Extracorporeal shock wave lithotripsy in children: evaluation of the results considering the need for auxiliary procedures. J Pediatr Urol. 2006;2:459–63.

26

Relationship between plasma Atherogenic index and final pathology of Bosniak III-IV renal masses

Emre Karabay[1], Nejdet Karsiyakali[2*], Serdar Duvar[1], Cagatay Tosun[1], Ahmet Ruknettin Aslan[1] and Omer Ergin Yucebas[1]

Abstract

Background: There is an increased incidence of renal cell carcinoma (RCC) in patients with metabolic syndrome who usually have high levels of serum triglyceride (TG) and low high-density lipoprotein-cholesterol (HDL-C). Plasma atherogenic index (PAI) is the logarithmic ratio of serum TG level to HDL-C and related to cardiovascular diseases. In this study, we aimed to determine the accuracy of PAI in determining renal malignancy in localized renal masses preoperatively.

Methods: Totally 169 patients who were diagnosed with Bosniak III-IV lesions by imaging modalities and treated in our hospital with partial or radical nephrectomy were retrospectively analyzed using institutional renal cancer database between 2013 and 2018. Preoperative images were evaluated by two experienced radiologists. The patients were divided into two groups according to their postoperative pathological diagnosis as malignant or benign tumors. The PAI of each patient was calculated and the statistical significance of PAI in predicting malignancy for renal masses was analyzed using uni- and multivariable analyses.

Results: Of patients, 109 (64.5%) were males and 60 (35.5%) were females with a median age of 61 (33–84) years. Median tumor size was 6.5 (2–18) cm. Pathological diagnosis was malignant in 145 (85.8%) and benign in 24 (14.2%) patients. There was no statistically significant difference in serum TG levels between malignant and benign cases ($p > 0.05$). The HDL-C levels were significantly lower in malignant cases ($p = 0.001$). Median PAI value was 0.63 (0.34–1.58) and significantly higher in malignant cases ($p = 0.003$). The PAI cut-off value for malignancy was ≥0.34. The sensitivity was calculated as 88.2% and specificity as 45.8%, the positive predictive value as 90.8, negative predictive value as 39.3, and odds ratio as 6.37 (95% CI: 2.466–16.458). In multivariable analysis, gender, smoking status, and hypertension had no effect on malignancy, whereas PAI and HDL-C were independent risk factors ($p = 0.003$ and $p = 0.003$, respectively). The risk of malignancy was 5.019 times higher, when PAI was > 0.34 (95% CI: 1.744–14.445) in multivariable logistic regression analysis.

Conclusions: The PAI can be used as a predictive tool in suspicion of malignant renal masses. In case of a benign pathology, PAI levels may be encouraging for surgeons for nephron-sparing surgery.

Keywords: Atherogenic index of plasma (AIP), Benign, Carcinoma, Renal cell carcinoma

* Correspondence: nkarsiyakali@hotmail.com
[2]Department of Urology, Cukurca State Hospital, Cukurca Devlet Hastanesi, Uroloji Klinigi, Cukurca/, HAKKARI, Turkey
Full list of author information is available at the end of the article

Background

Renal cell carcinoma (RCC) is 2 to 4% of all newly diagnosed tumors in adults [1]. Renal masses are often found incidentally in ultrasonography (USG), computed tomography (CT), and magnetic resonance imaging (MRI) which are performed to evaluate other pathologies [2]. These are called localized renal masses and, although most of them are malignant in pathological examination, about 20 to 30% of specimens are still diagnosed with benign lesions [3]. Tumor biopsy is the only histological diagnostic method in the preoperative period, particularly in small renal masses. In addition, CT imaging is the standard tool to detec renal masses; however, it is not reliable in distinguishing different histological types of tumors [4]. Also, MRI and USG are helpful in evaluating complex renal masses, although they have some limitations [5, 6]. In a systematic review, overall median diagnostic sensitivity and specificity in predicting RCC were reported as 88% (IQR 81–94%) and as 75% (IQR 51–90%), respectively for CT and as 87.5% (IQR 75.25–100%) and as 89% (IQR 75–96%), respectively [7].

Well-defined risk factors for RCC include tobacco use, obesity, and hypertension (HT). Also, hyperglycemia, hypertrigliseridemia, low high-density lipoprotein HDL cholesterol (HDL-C) levels, and metabolic syndrome with obesity have been shown to be related with RCC [8]. Obesity is a known risk factor for renal cancer. Although lipid peroxidation and oxidative stress have been primarily blamed, the exact underlying biological mechanisms are still unclear [9, 10]. In addition, dyslipidemia has been shown to increase oxidative stress and chronic inflammation and to be associated with insulin resistance and metabolic syndrome [11]. Lipids which are the major cell membrane components promote cell growth and alterations in their concentrations may occur during carcinogenesis [12]. In general, RCC patients with hypertrigliseridemia have a lower progression-free and cancer-specific survival rates [13]. High triglyceride (TG)/HDL-C ratio indicates an atherogenic lipid profile, which is an independent risk factor for cardiovascular diseases [14, 15]. In recent studies, the Plasma Atherogenic Index (PAI) is used as a reliable indicator for cardiovascular diseases [16, 17] and has been shown to be associated with metabolic syndrome and high body weight [18, 19]. The PAI is the logarithmic ratio of the plasma TG to HDL-C levels [log (TG / HDL-C)] [20]. It is a simple calculation without an extra cost.

In the present study, we aimed to determine the accuracy of PAI in determining renal malignancy in localized renal masses preoperatively.

Methods

We retrospectively reviewed the medical records of patients with renal mass who underwent partial or radical nephrectomy in our hospital between the years 2013 and 2018. Approval was obtained from the institutional Ethics Committee. Patients were selected based on the existence of Bosniak III or IV lesions as evidenced by imaging modalities. Patients with incomplete data for lipid profiles before the operation, missing pre-operative diagnostic images, and those who were already on lipid-lowering agents, such as statin and fenofibrate, were excluded from the study. Metabolic syndrome was not considered an exclusion criterion. Although smoking may disrupt the lipid profile, smoking is a well-defined risk factor for RCC; therefore, it was not considered an exclusion criterion, either. A total of 169 patients who met the inclusion criteria and were randomly selected were included in the study. Two experienced radiologists evaluated preoperative images of the patients. Another experienced radiologist evaluated the images, when the diagnosis of malignancy was suspected. Two experienced uropathologists evaluated postoperative specimens of the patients. The patients were divided into two groups according to their pathological diagnosis as malignant or benign renal tumors. The PAI of each patient was calculated using the formula log [plasma TG level / plasma HDL-C level]. Multivariable logistic regression analysis was used to analyze the predictive factors for malignancy. The role of PAI in predicting malignancy of renal masses was evaluated.

A written informed consent was obtained from each patient. The study was conducted in accordance with the principles of the Declaration of Helsinki.

Statistical analysis

Statistical analysis was performed using the Number Cruncher Statistical System (NCSS) version 2007 software (NCSS LLC., Kaysville, UT, USA). Descriptive data were expressed in mean and standard deviation (SD), median (min-max), or number and frequency. Normal distribution of the quantitative data was analyzed using the Shapiro-Wilk test. The Student's t-test was used to compare two groups of quantitative variables showing normal distribution and Mann-Whitney U test was used to compare two groups of quantitative variables which did not show normal distribution. The analysis of variance (ANOVA) test was used in comparison of more than two groups of quantitative variables showing normal distribution. The Kruskal-Wallis test was used to compare more than two groups of quantitative variables which did not show normal distribution. The Pearson chi-square test was used to compare the qualitative data. Diagnostic scanning tests including sensitivity, specificity, positive predictive value (PPV), negative predictive value (NPV), and Receiver Operating Characteristics (ROC) analysis were carried out to determine the predictive value for the parameters. The correlation between age, gender, side, size, and localization of the tumor, smoking status, diabetes mellitus (DM), HT, body mass index (BMI), HDL-C, TG, and PAI and malignancy were evaluated in univariable analyses. The multivariable logistic regression analysis was used in four models to investigate the effect of HDL-C, PAI, and TG on malignancy. In all models, gender, BMI, smoking status, and HT were independent variables, while HDL-C in the first model, PAI in the second model, TG in the third model, and PAI in the fourth model was additionally included. In these analyses, the impact of PAI on malignancy was evaluated alone and combined with HDL-C and TG. The DeLong method of area under curve (AUC) of the ROC curve was conducted to analyze significant differences. A p value of < 0.05 was considered statistically significant.

Results

A total of 169 patients, 109 (64%) were males and 60 (36%) were females with a median age of 61 (33–84) years. Pathological diagnosis was a malignant renal lesion in 145 cases (85.8%) and a benign renal lesion in 24 cases (14.2%). The median tumor size was 6.5 (2–18) cm. The mean BMI was 29.00 ± 4.28 kg/m^2. The median value of PAI was 0.53 (0.15–1.58) (Table 1). Demographic and tumoral characteristics of the patients are summarized in Table 1.

There was no statistically significant relationship between malignancy and patient age, side, size, and localization of the tumor, and DM status of the patient. In male patients, malignancy rate was higher than females ($p = 0.039$). The BMI was significantly higher in malignant patients ($p = 0.023$). The number of smoker patients and those with HT was significantly higher in malignant group ($p = 0.009$ and $p = 0.026$, respectively). Plasma HDL-C levels were significantly lower in malignant cases ($p = 0.001$). There was no significant difference in plasma TG levels between malignant and benign cases ($p > 0.05$). The PAI of malignant cases was significantly higher than the PAI of benign cases ($p = 0.003$) (Table 2).

The ROC curve analysis showed that the cut-off value for malignancy was 0.34. The PAI cut-off value (0.34) had a sensitivity of 88.2% and a specificity of 45.8%. The PPV was 90.8 and NPV was 39.3. The AUC of the ROC curve was 69% and standard error was 5.8%. For the cut-off value of 0.34, the odds ratio was 6.37 (95% CI: 2.466–16.458).

Univariable analysis revealed that significant factors related to malignancy were gender, smoking status, HT, BMI, HDL-C level, and PAI. The effect of these variables was also evaluated by multivariable logistic regression analysis. According to the results of multivariable analyses, the effect of gender, smoking status, and HT on malignancy was not significant. A PAI of ≥0.34 increased the risk of malignancy by 5.019 folds (95% CI: 1.744–14.445) (Table 3 - Model 2). Similarly, low values of HDL-C (F < 55; M < 45) increased the risk of malignancy [5.019 folds (95% CI: 1.744–14.445) in Model 1 and 2.062 (95% CI: 0.738–5.767) in Model 4, respectively] (Table 3).

All models predicting malignancy revealed a statistically significant outcomes ($p < 0.001$, for all). Although the AUC of the ROC curve showed no statistically

Table 1 Demographics of Patients

Age (year)	median (min-max)	61 (33–84)
Gender (n, %)	Male	109 (64.5%)
	Female (n, %)	60 (35.5%)
Side (n, %)	Right (n, %)	84 (49.7%)
	Left (n, %)	85 (50.3%)
Body Mass Index (kg/m^2)	mean ± SD	29.00 ± 4.28
Tumour Size (cm)	median (min-max)	6.5 (2–18)
Tumour Localisation (n, %)	Lower Pole	26 (15.4%)
	Middle Pole	97 (57.4%)
	Upper Pole	46 (27.2%)
Tumour Type (n, %)	Clear Cell	114 (67.5%)
	Chromophobe Cell	16 (9.5%)
	Papillary	15 (8.9%)
	Angiomyolipoma	11 (6.5%)
	Oncocytoma	13 (7.7%)
Malignancy (n, %)	Malign	145 (85.8%)
	Benign	24 (14.2%)
Fuhrman Grade (n, %)	Grade 2	43 (33.3%)
	Grade 3	71 (55.0%)
	Grade 4	15 (11.6%)
Tumour Stage (n, %)	T1a	24 (16.7%)
	T1b	36 (25.0%)
	T2a	16 (11.1%)
	T2b	6 (4.2%)
	T3a	46 (31.9%)
	T3b	11 (7.6%)
	T4	5 (3.5%)
Smoking Status (n, %)	Exist	116 (68.6%)
	None	53 (31.4%)
Diabetes Mellitus (n, %)	Exist	67 (39.6%)
	None	102 (60.4%)
Hypertension (n, %)	Exist	105 (62.1%)
	None	64 (37.9%)
Triglyceride Value [mg/dl]	median (min-max)	145 (68–1019)
HDL-Cholesterol Value [mg/dl]	mean ± SD	41.12 ± 11.94
Plasma Atherogenic Index Value	median (min-max)	0.53 (0.15–1.58)

Table 2 Comparisons of Malignant and Benign Patients

		Malignancy		
		Malignant (n = 145, 85.8%)	Benign (n = 24, 14.2%)	p
Age (year)	median (min-max)	61 (33–84)	63 (39–76)	^{a}0.472
Gender (n, %)	Male	98 (89.9)	11 (10.1)	^{b}0.039*
	Female	47 (78.3)	13 (21.7)	
Side (n, %)	Right	73 (86.9)	11 (13.1)	^{b}0.682
	Left	72 (84.7)	13 (15.3)	
Size (cm)	median (min-max)	8 (2–18)	5 (3–11)	^{a}0.223
Localization (n, %)	Lower Pole	23 (88.5)	3 (11.5)	^{b}0.848
	Middle Pole	82 (84.5)	15 (15.5)	
	Upper Pole	40 (87.0)	6 (13.0)	
Smoking Status (n, %)	Exist	105 (90.5)	11 (9.5)	^{b}0.009**
	None	40 (75.5)	13 (24.5)	
Diabetes Mellitus (n, %)	Exist	57 (85.1%)	10 (14.9%)	^{b}0.827
	None	88 (86.3%)	14 (13.7%)	
Hypertension (n, %)	Exist	95 (90.5%)	10 (9.5%)	^{b}0.026*
	None	50 (78.1%)	14 (21.9%)	
Body Mass Index (kg/m^2)	mean ± SD	29.30 ± 4.36	27.16 ± 3.27	^{c}0.023*
Triglyceride Value [mg/dl]	median (min-max)	156 (68–1019)	164 (100–226)	^{a}0.383
HDL-Cholesterole Value [mg/dl]	mean ± SD	39.64 ± 11.53	50.04 ± 10.59	^{c}0.001**
Plasma Atherogenic Index Value	median (min-max)	0.63 (0.34–1.58)	0.62 (0.39–0.76	^{a}0.003**

^{a}*Mann Whitney U Test,* ^{b}*Pearson Chi-Square Test,* ^{c}*Student-t Test,* $^{*}p < 0.05$ $^{**}p < 0.01$

significant difference ($p > 0.05$, for all), the highest AUC of the ROC curve was observed in Model 2 which included PAI (Table 3 & Fig. 1). No significant difference was found in PAI between the Fuhrman grades ($p > 0.05$).

Discussion

In this retrospective study, we showed that PAI and low values HDL-C of the patients with pathologically proven malignant renal tumors were significantly higher, compared to PAI of patients with benign renal lesions. Based on the multivariable logistic regression analysis, the malignancy risk was 4.55 folds higher in the patients with a PAI of > 0.34.

Dobiasova et al. [20] were the first to publish about log (TG/HDL-C) formula which they named the PAI. They found that this ratio was directly proportional to fractional esterification of HDL-C, inversely proportional to the particle size of LDL-C, and there was a direct relation between the PAI and atherosclerosis risk. Later studies showed a correlation between PAI and acute coronary syndrome and other cardiovascular diseases [16, 17].

In an epidemiological study, Haggstrom et al. [21] reported that increased BMI, serum glucose, and TG levels were significant risk factors for renal cancer in male patients, while only increased BMI was found a significant risk factor in female patients. As the relationship between obesity and renal tumors is well-known and obesity has blamed for one of the underlying pathologies for impaired lipid metabolism, a number of studies have attempted to investigate the possible relationship between lipid levels and renal cancer. In the Metabolic Syndrome and Cancer project (Me-Can) examining the relationship between serum TG levels and cancer in patients with metabolic syndrome, a significant correlation was found between TG levels and renal cancer ($p = 0.001$ RR: 1.96 (1.51–2.46)) [22]. However, in another study conducted by the Vorarlberg Health Monitoring and Promotion Program (VHM&PP) Study Group, increased TG levels were not associated with an increased risk for cancer ($p = 0.105$ HR: 1.27 (0.95–1.69)) [23]. In the Apolipoprotein-related Mortality Risk (AMORIS) study, there was a significant correlation between TG and renal cancer risk ($p = 0.001$) and there was a negative correlation between total cholesterol and HDL-C and renal cancer risk ($p = 0.001$ and $p = 0.075$, respectively) [24]. In our study, although gender, HT, and smoking which are well-known risk factors for renal caner were found to be significant risk factors in the univariable analysis, we found no significant relationship between TG levels and renal cancer ($p > 0.05$). Although previous studies have shown a correlation between lipid levels and renal cancer, there is no study available in the literature comparing patients with suspected malignancy as

Table 3 Results of multivariable logistic regression analysis according to malignancy

Model		Odds Ratio (95%CI)	p	AuROC (95%CI)	p
1	Gender (M[a])	0.764 (0.246–2.367)	0.640	0.772 (0.672–0.873)	< 0.001*
	BMI	1.135 (1.002–1.287)	0.047*		
	Smoking Status	1.887 (0.63–5.65)	0.257		
	HT	2.296 (0.874–6.03)	0.092		
	HDL-Cholesterole (F[b] < 55; M[a] < 45)	5.019 (1.744–14.445)	0.003*		
2	Gender (M[a])	0.764 (0.246–2.367)	0.640	0.787 (0.687–0.887)	< 0.001*
	BMI	1.135 (1.002–1.287)	0.047*		
	Smoking Status	2.296 (0.874–6.03)	0.092		
	HT	1.887 (0.63–5.65)	0.257		
	Plasma Atherogenic Index (≥0.34)	5.019 (1.744–14.445)	0.003*		
3	Gender (M[a])	0.572 (0.2–1.633)	0.296	0.760 (0.663–0.857)	< 0.001*
	BMI	1.124 (0.996–1.269)	0.059		
	Smoking Status	2.157 (0.767–6.068)	0.145		
	HT	2.278 (0.902–5.753)	0.081		
	TG	1.003 (0.995–1.011)	0.456		
4	Gender (M[a])	0.516 (0.175–1.52)	0.230	0.773 (0.677–0.870)	< 0.001*
	BMI	1.13 (0.999–1.279)	0.052		
	Smoking Status	1.654 (0.538–5.084)	0.380		
	HT	2.181 (0.857–5.555)	0.102		
	HDL-Cholesterole (F[b] < 55; M[a] < 45)	2.062 (0.738–5.767)	0.168		
	TG	1.003 (0.995–1.011)	0.496		

[a] Male, [b] Female, *$p < 0.05$

assessed by imaging studies and those with a benign pathological diagnosis. In the AMORIS study, there was a significant correlation of the TG/HDL-C ratio with renal cancer, but not with cancer [24]. In this large-scale, comprehensive study, the cut-off value of the log (TG/HDL-C) to prevent cardiovascular diseases was calculated similar to previous studies (0.5) However, in our study, we used a cut-off value of 0.34, which suggested that PA with other variables was a predictor of renal cancer. Despite small sample size in our study, the reason for the discrepancy in our results and AMORIS findings may be due to different cut-off values used. Nonetheless, the use of different cut-off values for cardiovascular diseases and renal cancer is reasonable, since the pathophysiological mechanisms of both diseases are different.

Furthermore, it is well-established that systemic inflammatory response has a negative effect on survival of RCC patients [25]. Vivar et al. [26] reported that inflammation has a significant, negative impact on the prognosis and progression of clear-cell RCC. Systemic inflammation induces some alterations in lipid metabolism [27]. Changes in TG metabolism also affect HDL-C metabolism [28]. These alterations also modify PAI. Since renal malignancy may present with systemic inflammation and lipid metabolism changes, it is reasonable to use PAI to predict malignant renal masses in the preoperative period.

In addition, PAI has been shown to be related with metabolic syndrome and high body weight [18, 19]. Metabolic syndrome characterized by hyperglycemia, hypertension, hypertriglyceridemia, low HDL-C levels, and abdominal obesity has a strong correlation with RCC [8]. Progression-free and cancer-specific survival in RCC is worse, when TG levels are high [13]. In our study, there was no statistically significant difference between TG levels of malignant and benign cases ($p >$ 0.05). On the other hand, HDL-C levels of malignant cases were found to be significantly lower than benign cases ($p = 0.001$). Accordingly, PAI of malignant cases were significantly higher than benign cases ($p = 0.003$). Based on these findings, we believe that, in patients with suspected renal masses on their preoperative radiological images, PAI can be used as an additional predictive tool of malignancy and be helpful for planning the type of the operation (partial or radical nephrectomy).

Limitations

Nonetheless, there are some limitations to this study. First, it was a retrospective, observational study and the inherent retrospective and non-randomized nature

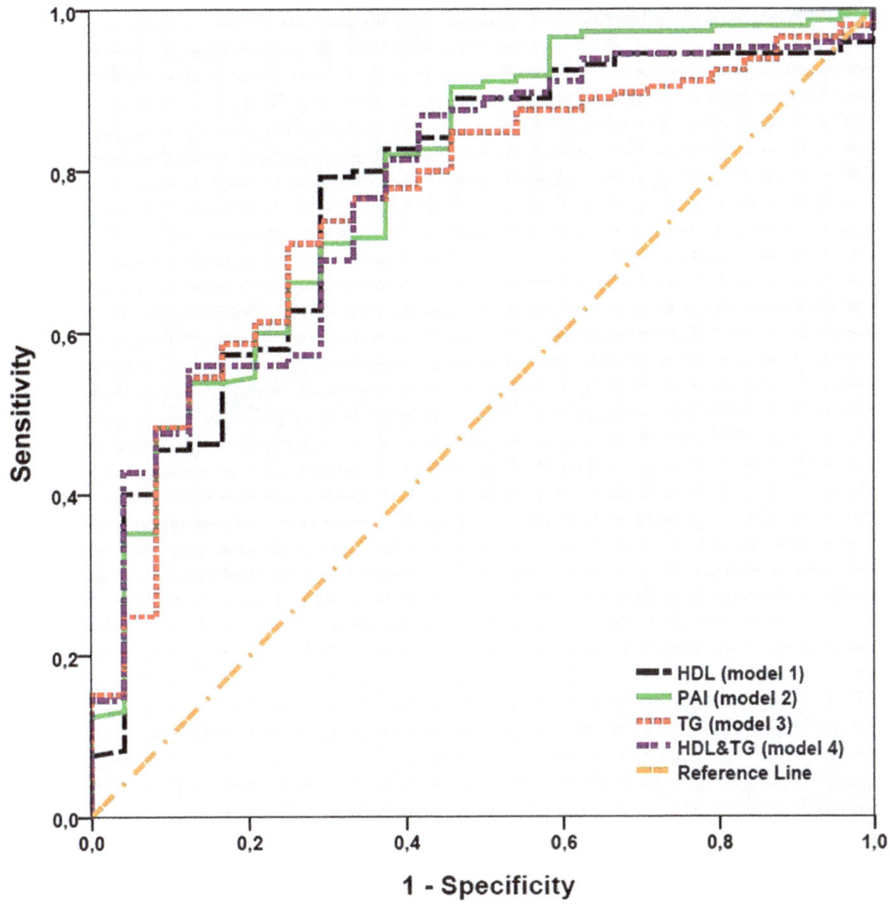

Fig. 1 ROC Curve for Models According to Malignancy

might have led to selection bias. Second, only patients of a single center were included and the sample size was small. Third, we evaluated only patients who underwent surgery for renal masses and we were unable to compare symptomatic and incidental cases. These conditions might have also led to selection bias and may be not representative of general population. Nevertheless, our study showed a direct correlation between PAI and malignant renal masses which should be investigated in further large-scale, prospective, multi-center studies.

Conclusions

In conclusion, the incidence of newly diagnosed localized renal masses has been increasing with the routine use of advanced imaging modalities. Our study results suggest that PAI can be used as a predictive tool preoperatively to distinguish benign cases from malignant ones and be encouraging for the surgeons to consider performing nephron-sparing surgery. However, further large-scale, prospective, and multi-center studies are needed to establish a definite conclusion.

Abbreviations

CT: Computed tomography; HDL-C: High-density lipoprotein cholesterol; MRI: Magnetic resonance imaging; MS: Metabolic syndrome; PAI: Plasma atherogenic index; RCC: Renal cell carcinoma; TG: Triglyceride; USG: Ultrasonography

Acknowledgements

Not applicable.

Authors' contributions

EK: Protocol/project development, Data management, Manuscript writing NK: Protocol/project development, Data management, Statistical analysis, Manuscript writing SD: Data Collection, Data analysis CT: Data Collection, Data analysis ARA: Critical revision of the manuscript for scientific and factual content, Manuscript editing OEY: Critical revision of the manuscript for scientific and factual content, Manuscript editing. All authors read and approved the final version of the manuscript.

Author details

[1]Department of Urology, Haydarpasa Numune Training and Research Hospital, University of Health Sciences, Tibbiye Street. No: 23 34668 Uskudar /, ISTANBUL, Turkey. [2]Department of Urology, Cukurca State Hospital, Cukurca Devlet Hastanesi, Uroloji Klinigi, Cukurca/, HAKKARI, Turkey.

References

1. Siegel R, Naishadham D, Jemal A. Cancer statistics, 2013. CA Cancer J Clin. 2013;63(1):11–30. https://doi.org/10.3322/caac.21166.

2. Dutcher JP. Update on the biology and management of renal cell carcinoma. J Investig Med. 2019;67(1):1-10. https://doi.org/10.1136/jim-2018-000918.
3. Frank I, Blute ML, Cheville JC, Lohse CM, Weaver AL, Zincke H. Solid renal tumors: an analysis of pathological features related to tumor size. J Urol. 2003;170(6 Pt 1):2217–20. https://doi.org/10.1097/01.ju.0000095475.12515.5e.
4. Pierorazio PM, Hyams ES, Tsai S, Feng Z, Trock BJ, Mullins JK, Johnson PT, Fishman EK, Allaf ME. Multiphasic enhancement patterns of small renal masses (</=4 cm) on preoperative computed tomography: utility for distinguishing subtypes of renal cell carcinoma, angiomyolipoma, and oncocytoma. Urology. 2013;81(6):1265–71. https://doi.org/10.1016/j.urology.2012.12.049.
5. Israel GM, Hindman N, Bosniak MA. Evaluation of cystic renal masses: comparison of CT and MR imaging by using the Bosniak classification system. Radiology. 2004;231(2):365–71. https://doi.org/10.1148/radiol.2312031025.
6. Gerst S, Hann LE, Li D, Gonen M, Tickoo S, Sohn MJ, Russo P. Evaluation of renal masses with contrast-enhanced ultrasound: initial experience. AJR Am J Roentgenol. 2011;197(4):897–906. https://doi.org/10.2214/AJR.10.6330.
7. Vogel C, Ziegelmuller B, Ljungberg B, Bensalah K, Bex A, Canfield S, Giles RH, Hora M, Kuczyk MA, Merseburger AS, Powles T, Albiges L, Stewart F, Volpe A, Graser A, Schlemmer M, Yuan C, Lam T, Staehler M. Imaging in suspected renal-cell carcinoma: systematic review. Clin Genitourin Cancer. 2019;17(2): e345-e355. https://doi.org/10.1016/j.clgc.2018.07.024.
8. Zhang GM, Zhu Y, Ye DW. Metabolic syndrome and renal cell carcinoma. World J Surg Oncol. 2014;12:236. https://doi.org/10.1186/1477-7819-12-236.
9. Don C. Atypical collapse of the right lung simulating combined right upper- and middle-lobe collapse. Can Assoc Radiol J. 1991;42(2):148.
10. Gago-Dominguez M, Castelao JE, Yuan JM, Ross RK, Yu MC. Lipid peroxidation: a novel and unifying concept of the etiology of renal cell carcinoma (United States). Cancer Causes Control. 2002;13(3):287–93.
11. Hsieh J, Hayashi AA, Webb J, Adeli K. Postprandial dyslipidemia in insulin resistance: mechanisms and role of intestinal insulin sensitivity. Atheroscler Suppl. 2008;9(2):7–13. https://doi.org/10.1016/j.atherosclerosissup.2008.05.011.
12. Vilchez JA, Martinez-Ruiz A, Sancho-Rodriguez N, Martinez-Hernandez P, Noguera-Velasco JA. The real role of prediagnostic high-density lipoprotein cholesterol and the cancer risk: a concise review. Eur J Clin Investig. 2014; 44(1):103–14. https://doi.org/10.1111/eci.12185.
13. Haddad AQ, Jiang L, Cadeddu JA, Lotan Y, Gahan JC, Hynan LS, Gupta N, Raj GV, Sagalowsky AI, Margulis V. Statin use and serum lipid levels are associated with survival outcomes after surgery for renal cell carcinoma. Urology. 2015;86(6):1146–52. https://doi.org/10.1016/j.urology.2015.09.015.
14. Krintus M, Koziński M, Kuligowska-Prusińska M, Laskowska E, Janiszewska E, Kubica J, Odrowąż-Sypniewska G. The performance of triglyceride to high-density lipoprotein cholesterol ratio in acute coronary syndromes using a diagnostic decision tree. Medical Research Journal. 2015;3(1):13–9.
15. da Luz PL, Favarato D, Faria-Neto JR Jr, Lemos P, Chagas AC. High ratio of triglycerides to HDL-cholesterol predicts extensive coronary disease. Clinics (Sao Paulo). 2008;63(4):427–32.
16. Zhan Y, Xu T, Tan X. Two parameters reflect lipid-driven inflammatory state in acute coronary syndrome: atherogenic index of plasma, neutrophil-lymphocyte ratio. BMC Cardiovasc Disord. 2016;16:96. https://doi.org/10.1186/s12872-016-0274-7.
17. Niroumand S, Khajedaluee M, Khadem-Rezaiyan M, Abrishami M, Juya M, Khodaee G, Dadgarmoghaddam M. Atherogenic index of plasma (AIP): a marker of cardiovascular disease. Med J Islam Repub Iran. 2015;29:240.
18. Shen S, Lu Y, Dang Y, Qi H, Shen Z, Wu L, Li F, Yang C, Qiang D, Yang Y, Shui K, Bao Y. Effect of aerobic exercise on the atherogenic index of plasma in middle-aged Chinese men with various body weights. Int J Cardiol. 2017; 230:1–5. https://doi.org/10.1016/j.ijcard.2016.12.132.
19. Pourfarzam M, Zadhoush F, Sadeghi M. The difference in correlation between insulin resistance index and chronic inflammation in type 2 diabetes with and without metabolic syndrome. Adv Biomed Res. 2016;5: 153. https://doi.org/10.4103/2277-9175.188489.
20. Dobiasova M, Frohlich J. The plasma parameter log (TG/HDL-C) as an atherogenic index: correlation with lipoprotein particle size and esterification rate in apoB-lipoprotein-depleted plasma (FER (HDL)). Clin Biochem. 2001;34(7):583–8.
21. Haggstrom C, Rapp K, Stocks T, Manjer J, Bjorge T, Ulmer H, Engeland A, Almqvist M, Concin H, Selmer R, Ljungberg B, Tretli S, Nagel G, Hallmans G, Jonsson H, Stattin P. Metabolic factors associated with risk of renal cell carcinoma. PLoS One. 2013;8(2):e57475. https://doi.org/10.1371/journal.pone.0057475.
22. Borena W, Stocks T, Jonsson H, Strohmaier S, Nagel G, Bjorge T, Manjer J, Hallmans G, Selmer R, Almquist M, Haggstrom C, Engeland A, Tretli S, Concin H, Strasak A, Stattin P, Ulmer H. Serum triglycerides and cancer risk in the metabolic syndrome and cancer (me-can) collaborative study. Cancer Causes Control. 2011;22(2):291–9. https://doi.org/10.1007/s10552-010-9697-0.
23. Ulmer H, Borena W, Rapp K, Klenk J, Strasak A, Diem G, Concin H, Nagel G. Serum triglyceride concentrations and cancer risk in a large cohort study in Austria. Br J Cancer. 2009;101(7):1202–6. https://doi.org/10.1038/sj.bjc.6605264.
24. Van Hemelrijck M, Garmo H, Hammar N, Jungner I, Walldius G, Lambe M, Holmberg L. The interplay between lipid profiles, glucose, BMI and risk of kidney cancer in the Swedish AMORIS study. Int J Cancer. 2012;130(9):2118–28. https://doi.org/10.1002/ijc.26212.
25. Wu Y, Fu X, Zhu X, He X, Zou C, Han Y, Xu M, Huang C, Lu X, Zhao Y. Prognostic role of systemic inflammatory response in renal cell carcinoma: a systematic review and meta-analysis. J Cancer Res Clin Oncol. 2011;137(5): 887–96. https://doi.org/10.1007/s00432-010-0951-3.
26. de Vivar Chevez AR, Finke J, Bukowski R. The role of inflammation in kidney cancer. Adv Exp Med Biol. 2014;816:197–234. https://doi.org/10.1007/978-3-0348-0837-8_9.
27. Khovidhunkit W, Kim MS, Memon RA, Shigenaga JK, Moser AH, Feingold KR, Grunfeld C. Effects of infection and inflammation on lipid and lipoprotein metabolism: mechanisms and consequences to the host. J Lipid Res. 2004; 45(7):1169–96. https://doi.org/10.1194/jlr.R300019-JLR200.
28. de Carvalho JF, Borba EF, Viana VS, Bueno C, Leon EP, Bonfa E. Anti-lipoprotein lipase antibodies: a new player in the complex atherosclerotic process in systemic lupus erythematosus? Arthritis Rheum. 2004;50(11): 3610–5. https://doi.org/10.1002/art.20630.

27

The role of RENAL, PADUA, C-index, CSA nephrometry systems in predicting ipsilateral renal function after partial nephrectomy

Yu-De Wang[1], Chi-Ping Huang[1,2], Chao-Hsiang Chang[1,2], Hsi-Chin Wu[2,3], Che-Rei Yang[1], Yu-Ping Wang[4] and Po-Fan Hsieh[1,2*]

Abstract

Background: Functional outcome is an important issue in nephron-sparing surgery. Various nephrometries have been developed to predict renal function preservation. The aim of this study was to examine the applicability of R.E.N.A.L., PADUA, C-index, and mathematical tumor contact surface area (CSA) in predicting ipsilateral renal function after partial nephrectomy using radio-isotope scans.

Methods: We performed this retrospective study in patients who underwent partial nephrectomy between May 2013 and April 2017, and used abdominopelvic computerized tomography or magnetic resonance imaging to obtain R.E.N.A.L., C-index, and CSA. Renal function was measured by 99mTc mercaptoacetyltriglycine (MAG3). We evaluated correlations between nephrometries and perioperative parameters, and comparatively analyzed different nephrometries to determine the predictive ability in the percent change of effective renal plasma flow of the affected kidney.

Results: Three, two, and 35 patients received partial nephrectomy in open, laparoscopic, and robotic approaches, respectively. The median (IQR) tumor size was 3.13 (2.4) cm. The median (IQR) R.E.N.A.L., PADUA, C index, and CSA scores were 7 (3), 8 (2), 2.01 (1.87), and 14.14 (19.25) cm^2, respectively. Spearman correlation analysis showed that four nephrometries were correlated with each other. The strongest correlations were between CSA and C-index (coefficient: − 0.885, $p < 0.001$), followed by R.E.N.A.L. and PADUA (coefficient: 0.778, $p < 0.001$). Ischemia time was significantly correlated with R.EN.A.L. (coefficient: 0.35, $p = 0.025$), PADUA (coefficient: 0.42, $p = 0.007$), C-index (coefficient: − 0.45, $p = 0.004$), and CSA (coefficient: 0.41, $p = 0.009$). In multivariate analysis, PADUA significantly affected ischemia time ($p = 0.04$). The percent change in effective renal plasma flow (PCE) of the operated kidney was correlated with PADUA (coefficient: 0.48 $p = 0.002$), C-index (coefficient: − 0.74, $p < 0.001$), and CSA (coefficient: 0.75, $p < 0.001$). Only CSA and C-index independently affected PCE (both $p < 0.05$) in multivariate analysis. In ROC curve analysis, both C-index and CSA could predict 20% change in effective renal plasma flow (AUC: 0.91 vs 0.86, $p = 0.2$) of the affected kidney.

Conclusions: We suggest using PADUA to evaluate surgical complexity and ischemia time. Regarding the accuracy of the prediction of post-operative ipsilateral renal function, both CSA and C-index outperformed R.E.N.A.L. and PADUA nephrometries.

Keywords: Contact surface area, Partial nephrectomy, Renal function, Nephrometry, Renal scintigraphy

* Correspondence: d17341@mail.cmuh.org.tw
[1]Department of Urology, China Medical University Hospital, No. 2, Yu-De Rd., Taichung City 404, Taiwan, Republic of China
[2]School of Medicine, China Medical University, No. 91, Xueshi Rd., North Dist, Taichung City 404, Taiwan, Republic of China
Full list of author information is available at the end of the article

Background

Partial nephrectomy (PN) is the gold standard treatment for T1 renal tumors and even some T2 renal tumors in present clinical practice [1, 2]. Compared to radical nephrectomy, PN can decrease the incidence of renal dysfunction which may lower the incidence of non-cancer mortality [3, 4]. In order to improve rates of achieving of trifecta or pentafecta in PN, comprehensive evaluation of the tumor's complexity is necessary before surgery. Therefore, using an adequate tool to evaluate the feasibility of PN and even predict the post-operative outcome is a critical issue in the treatment of localized renal tumors.

Various nephrometry systems have proposed to standardize the description and academic recording of renal tumors. The R.E.N.A.L. nephrometry system was the first to be proposed, followed by the PADUA classification system. These two systems use similar semi-quantitative anatomical factors and methodologies [5, 6]. In the contrast, C-index and mathematical tumor contact surface area (CSA) yield continuous variables which describe the geometric relationship between the tumor and kidney [7, 8]. These four nephrometry systems have been validated externally and they have all been associated with peri-operative outcomes [8–10].

Previous studies have tried to clarify the correlations between nephrometry systems and global functional outcomes assessed by estimated glomerular filtration rate (eGFR) [9, 11]. However inconsistencies and inaccuracies have been reported when using eGFR in patients undergoing PN because of compensatory hypertrophy of the contralateral kidney [12]. Split renal function assessed by radio-isotope scans has been shown to be more precise than eGFR to estimate renal function [13, 14]. In addition 99mTc mercaptoacetyltriglycine (MAG3) is preferred over 99mTc diethylene triamine penta-acetic acid (DTPA) in patients with impaired renal function.[15]. R.E.N.A.L. score and its individual constituents "R,E,N" have been reported to be relevant to ipsilateral post-operative renal function (IPRF) [16]. However, little is known about head-to-head comparisons of the predictive ability of IPRF using different nephrometries. In this study, we aimed to evaluate correlations between R.E.N.A.L, PADUA, C-index, and CSA and perioperative and renal functional outcomes assessed by radio-isotope scans.

Methods

Patients and data collection

After Institutional Review Board approval, we evaluated consecutive patients who underwent PN via open (OPN), laparoscopic (LPN), or robotic assisted (RPN) approaches for localized renal tumors between May 2013 and April 2017 at a tertiary referral center. We excluded patients with multiple renal tumors within one kidney, solitary kidneys, or end-stage kidney disease. The choice of surgical approach and resection and repair techniques were based on the surgeons' expertise and the patients' preference. All PN procedures were performed with the conventional on-clamp technique with clamping of both the renal artery and renal vein. All of the patients had pre-operative imaging with either computed tomography or magnetic resonance imaging. Cold ischemia was used only in OPN, and warm ischemia was used in both LPN and RPN. The patients' demographics, clinical data, and imaging studies were obtained electronically and analyzed retrospectively.

Preoperative demographics data (sex, age, American Society of Anesthesiologists score, Charlson Comorbidity Index), perioperative outcomes (operative time, ischemia time, estimated blood loss, perioperative complications, length of hospitalization), and pathology features were recorded and evaluated. Nephrometry score including R.E.N.A.L., PADUA, C-index, CSA were obtained according to the original studies [5–8]. Global renal function was assessed according to eGFR. Split renal function represented by effective renal plasma flow (ERPF) was measured by 99mTc-MAG3 pre-operatively and 1 year after surgery. IPRF was reported as the absolute change of ERPF (ACE), and percent change of ERPF (PCE) of the operated kidney.

Statistical analysis

Continuous variables are shown as median (IQR). Categorical variables, including those with a > 20% change of ERPF (PCE20) are shown as percentage. Spearman correlation analysis was used to evaluate the relationships among R.E.N.A.L. score, PADUA, C-index, and CSA and perioperative outcomes. Univariate and multivariate analyses of various clinical variables including nephrometries and PCE of the operated kidney were performed using linear regression models. The predive ability of nephrometries for PCE of the operated kidney was evaluated and compared using ROC curve analysis. All analyses was performed using SPSS v.22 (SPSS, Chicago,IL,USA), and a *P* value < 0.05 was considered to be statistically significant.

Results

Three, two, and 35 patients received PN via open, laparoscopic, and robotic approaches, respectively. The median (IQR) tumor size was 3.13 (2.4) cm. The median (IQR) R.E.N.A.L., PADUA, C-index, and CSA were 7 (3), 8 (2), 2.01 (1.87), and 14.14 (19.25) cm^2, respectively. The median (IQR) cold ischemia times and warm ischemia times were 28 (3) minutes and 20.5 (6.38) minutes, respectively (Table 1). The overall complication rate was 22.5%. Of the complications, four patients had urinary

Table 1 Demographic information of the study population

Variables	$N = 40$
Age, years	58 (11.25)
Male gender	23 (57.5)
ASA	2 (0)
CCI	0 (1.75)
Tumor size, cm	3.13 (2.4)
Depth of invasion, cm	1.6 (1.02)
RENAL score	7 (3)
PADUA	8 (2)
C-index	2.01 (1.87)
CSA, cm^2	14.14 (19.25)
Minimal invasive surgery	37 (92.5)
Time from pre-operative ERPF to surgery, days	15 (8)
Time from surgery to post-operative ERPF, months	15 (1.5)

Data are expressed as median (IQR), or n (%)
ASA American Society of Anesthesiologists score, *CCI* Charlson Comorbidity Index, *CSA* Mathematical Contact Surface Area, *ERPF* effective renal plasma flow

Table 2 Perioperative features and change in renal function

Operative time, minutes	207.5 (101.75)
Ischemia time, minutes	21.02 (8.38)
Cold ischemia time, minutes	28 (3)
Warm ischemia time, minutes	20.5 (6.38)
EBL, mL	100 (237.5)
Complication	
Major, Clavien-Dindo grade 3 or more	0 (0)
Minor, Clavien-Dindo grade 2 or less	9 (22.5)
Length of stay, days	6 (1.75)
Pathological features	
RCC	23 (57.5)
T1a	16 (69.57)
T1b	5 (21.74)
T2	2 (8.7)
Oncocytoma	2 (5)
Angiomyolipoma	14 (35)
Carcinoid	1 (2.5)
Pre-operative	
Global eGFR, ml/min/1.73m^2	94 (27)
ERPF of affected kidney, ml/min/1.73m^2	187.08 (76.11)
Post-operative	
Global eGFR, ml/min/1.73m^2	82 (31)
ERPF of affected kidney, ml/min/1.73m^2	149.41 (169.45)
Functional change	
Percent change of eGFR	23.2 (12.51)
Absolute change of ERPF	47.65 (69.39)
Percent change of ERPF	22.16 (34.45)

Data are expressed as median (IQR), or n (%)
EBL estimated blood loss, *RCC* renal cell carcinoma, *eGFR* estimated glomerular filtration rate, *ERPF* effective renal plasma flow

infections, two had pneumonia which was cured by antibiotics, two had anemia and received blood transfusions and 1 had a stress ulcer which was treated with a proton pump inhibitor. None of the patients had Clavien-Dindo grade 3 or higher complications. Pathological features demonstrated that renal cell carcinoma accounted for 57.5% of all tumors. Among them, 69.6% were pT1a, 21.7% were pT1b, and 8.7% were pT2 (Table 2).

The median (IQR) time from preoperative ERPF to surgery was 15 (8) days, and the median (IQR) time from surgery to postoperative ERPF was 15 (1.5) months. The median (IQR) ACE was 47.65 (69.39) ml/min/1.73 m^2, and the median (IQR) PCE was 22.16 (34.45) % (Table 2). Spearman correlation analysis showed that four nephrometries were moderately to strongly correlated with each other. The strongest correlations were between CSA and C-index (coefficient: − 0.885, $p < 0.001$), followed by R.E.N.A.L. and PADUA (coefficient: 0.778, $p < 0.001$). Ischemia time was significantly correlated with R.EN.A.L. (coefficient: 0.35, $p = 0.025$), PADUA (coefficient:0.42, $p = 0.007$), C-index (coefficient: − 0.45, $p = 0.004$), and CSA (coefficient: 0.41, $p = 0.009$). Operative time was correlated with C-index (coefficient: − 0.34, $p = 0.037$) and CSA (coefficient: 0.37, $p = 0.018$), and PCE of the operated kidney was correlated with PADUA (coefficient: 0.48 $p = 0.002$), C-index (coefficient: − 0.74, $p < 0.001$), and CSA (coefficient: 0.75, $p < 0.001$). However weaker correlation coefficients for PCE/ ACE were noted in PADUA compared with C-index and CSA (Table 3).

In univariate analysis, operative time, R.E.N.A.L., PADUA, and C-index significantly affected ischemia time. However, only PADUA ($p = 0.04$) significantly affected ischemia time in multivariate analysis (Table 4). Ischemia time, PADUA, C-index, and CSA affected PCE of the operated kidney in univariate analysis, while only C-index ($p = 0.03$) and CSA ($p = 0.005$) influenced PCE of the operated kidney independently (Table 5). The predictive value for PCE20 of C-index and CSA were evaluated via ROC curve analysis, in which both C-index and CSA were equally able to predict the PCE20 (AUC: 0.91 vs 0.86, $p = 0.2$). The cut off values of PCE20 derived from Youden's index were 2.11 for C-index and 10.37 cm^2 for CSA.

Discussion

In recent decades, a few studies have focused on factors impacting functional changes after PN, and identified both unmodifiable and modifiable factors [17]. The two most important modifiable factors, ischemia time and renal volume preservation, indicate the quality and

Table 3 Correlation between nephrometries and peri-operative features

Variables	RENAL		PADUA		C-index		CSA	
	coefficient	*P*-value	coefficient	*P*-value	coefficient	*P*-value	coefficient	*P*-value
RENAL			0.778	< 0.001	−0.372	0.02	0.44	0.005
PADUA	0.778	< 0.001			− 0.622	< 0.001	0.647	< 0.001
C-index	− 0.372	0.02	− 0.622	< 0.001			−0.885	< 0.001
CSA (cm^2)	0.44	0.005	0.647	< 0.001	−0.885	< 0.001		
EBL (ml)	0.179	0.269	0.082	0.616	−0.115	0.485	0.161	0.321
Operative time (minutes)	0.278	0.082	0.218	0.176	−0.336	0.037	0.373	0.018
Length of stay (days)	0.178	0.272	0.256	0.11	−0.187	0.254	0.107	0.511
Complication (Clavien-Dindo classification)	−0.137	0.399	0.075	0.647	−0.147	0.373	0.163	0.314
Ischemia time (minutes)	0.354	0.025	0.421	0.007	−0.453	0.004	0.409	0.009
Absolute change of ERPF ($ml/min/1.73m^2$)	0.195	0.235	0.369	0.021	−0.687	< 0.001	0.680	< 0.001
Percent change of ERPF (%)	0.263	0.106	0.476	0.002	−0.740	< 0.001	0.747	< 0.001

CSA Mathematical Contact Surface Area, *EBL* estimated blood loss, *ERPF* effective renal plasma flow

quantity of the affected kidney, respectively [18]. The correlation between post-operative global renal function and different nephrometry systems varies from study to study [9, 11]. Furthermore, few head-to-head comparisons of the predictive ability of IPRF between different nephrometries have been reported. To the best of our knowledge, this is the first study to compare correlations between different nephrometries and IPRF. In this study, the four nephrometries were correlated with peri-operative outcomes and IPRF. In addition, we found that PADUA could significantly predict the ischemia time, while C-index and CSA independently affected IPRF.

The indication for PN has progressed from small renal masses to renal tumors < 7 cm in size [1, 2]. Contralateral kidney compensation becomes significant with greater parenchymal loss in patients with larger renal tumors [12]. Traditional models used to calculate eGFR according to serum creatinine have limitations such as estimation errors and inconsistencies, and therefore eGFR is suboptimal to assess functional outcomes [13]. Thus, assessing ipsilateral renal function using radio-isotope scans has become the standard evaluation method [1, 2]. Takagi et al. studied patients with small renal masses with a median size of 3.5 cm, which is similar to our study. In their study, the percent eGFR changes in operated and contralateral kidneys were − 24.4 and + 2.29%, respectively [12]. Other series have also reported that about 72–80% renal function preservation in the operated kidney [14]. The volume of renal preservation has been shown to be more important than ischemia time for long-term renal function in recent studies [17, 19].

Perioperative outcomes and different nephrometries have been highly correlated [9]. Borgmann et al. demonstrated that surgical complexity and trifecta of PN were better assessed by R.E.N.A.L score than C-index [20]. In

Table 4 Regression analysis in ischemia time

Variables	Univariate			Multivariate analysis		
	B	(95% CI)	*P*-value	B	(95% CI)	*P*-value
Age	− 0.07	(−3,0.15)	0.52			
Sex	−1.45	(−6.2,3.3)	0.54			
ASA	−0.95	(−5.92,4.02)	0.7			
CCI	−0.3	(−2.11,1.5)	0.74			
Operative method	−2.14	(− 6.35,2.06)	0.31	0.5	(−4.14,5.15)	0.83
Operative time	0.04	(0.01,0.07)	0.03	0.02	(−0.01,0.06)	0.23
R.E.N.A.L.	1.69	(0.46,2.92)	0.009	−0.32	(−0.34,1.71)	0.75
PADUA	2.63	(1.27,34)	< 0.001	2.85	(0.09,5.62)	0.04
C-index	−1.6	(−3, −0.21)	0.03	−0.16	(− 3.12,0.8)	0.24
CSA	0.17	(−0.04,0.39)	0.11	−0.18	(0.47,0.11)	0.22

ASA American Society of Anesthesiologists score
CCI Charlson Comorbidity Index
CSA Mathematical Contact Surface Area

Table 5 Regression analysis in ERPF

Variables	Univariate analysis			Multivariate analysis		
	B	(95% CI)	*P*-value	B	(95% CI)	*P*-value
Age	−0.04	(− 0.77,0.69)	0.91			
Sex	−1.09	(− 16.76,14.59)	0.89			
ASA	3.55	(−12.4,19.49)	0.66			
CCI	−0.29	(−6.53,5.95)	0.93			
Operative method	−2.16	(−18.13,13.81)	0.79			
Ischemia time (minutes)	1.23	(0.22,2.17)	0.01	0.57	(−0.34,1.48)	0.21
Operative time (minutes)	0.02	(−0.1,1.35)	0.76			
Complication (Clavien-Dindo classification)	10.93	(−7.82,29.67)	0.25	−0.47	(−15.12,14.17)	0.95
EBL	0.02	(−0.02,0.05)	0.34	< 0.001	(−0.020.02)	1
R.E.N.A.L.	3.43	(−0.9,7.76)	0.12	0.78	(−4.46,6.18)	0.77
PADUA	6.21	(1.45,10.96)	0.01	−2.9	(−10.39,4.59)	0.44
C-index	−9.71	(−13.17, −6.25)	< 0.001	−5.14	(−9.8, −0.48)	0.03
CSA	1.57	(1.06,2.08)	< 0.001	1.1	(0.36,1.86)	0.005
ERPF of affected kidney (pre-operative)	0.03	(−0.12, 0.18)	0.71			

ASA American Society of Anesthesiologists score
CCI Charlson Comorbidity Index
EBL estimated blood loss
CSA Mathematical Contact Surface Area
ERPF effective renal plasma flow

the current study, PADUA nephrometry significantly affected ischemia time, while C-index and CSA did not. This may be because ischemia time reflects the surgical complexity, which involves the tumor location and sinus or collecting system invasion. In addition, it is better described by the comprehensive multiple anatomical factors included in PADUA. Recently Ficarra et al. proposed an updated version of PADUA, the Simplified PADUA REnal (SPARE) nephrometry, which exerts similar predictive ability of complication. Compared with CSA, SPARE nephrometry is not an independent predictor of renal function impairment [21]. It is possible that multiple factors with equal weights in the PADUA system may weaken the power in predicting IPRF.

Kwon et al. and Yoo et al. reported that R.E.N.A.L. was an independent predictor of IPRF as measured by 99mTc DTPA [22, 23]. In contrast to their study, R.E.N.A.L. score in our cohort was not a significant predictor of IPRF. The difference may be because the previous study treated the R.E.N.A.L. score as a binary variable and analyzed it with different ischemic types in linear multivariate analysis [22]. More importantly, the quality of 99mTc MAG3 images as used in our study has been reported to be superior to scans obtained using 99mTc DTPA in patients with diseased kidneys [15, 18]. A recent study further revealed that only the constituents of "R" and "E" in R.E.N.A.L nephrometry instead of total score were associate with ipsilateral renal function [16]. These two constituents are included in CSA and C-index.

Simmon et al. reported that C-index affected the nadir and late eGFR [24]. Samplaski et al. further reported that a C-index cut-off value < 2.5 increased the probability of a 30% decline in global renal function by 2.2-fold [25]. Another study reported that C-index outperformed R.E.N.A.L. score in predicting global renal function loss [10, 26]. To the best of our knowledge, this study is the first cohort study to evaluate the predictive ability of IPRF using C-index. Several potential reasons may explain the difference in cut-off value (2.5 vs 2.1) to predict renal functional loss. First, different methodologies were applied to yield cut-off values in the previous study [25]. Second, greater global function loss was reported in the previous study compared to in our cohort [25]. Third, split renal function is more sensitive than eGFR, so the cut-off value for the same percentage of functional reduction may be smaller.

Both CSA and C-index described the degree of tumor invasion and had the common factor of tumor size. Moreover, depth(d) in CSA and distance(c) in C-index are very closely related. Our study further proved this concept because these two nephrometries were highly correlated (coefficient: − 0.885, $p < 0.001$). The impact of CSA and C- index on IPRF is supported by evidence showing that tumor size and depth are the most important prognostic factors of ipsilateral renal function [27]. The interplay between volume, CSA, and C-index is described in Fig. 1. The distance between tumor and kidney center (c) consists of tumor radius (r) and nearest distance between tumor margin and kidney center (k).

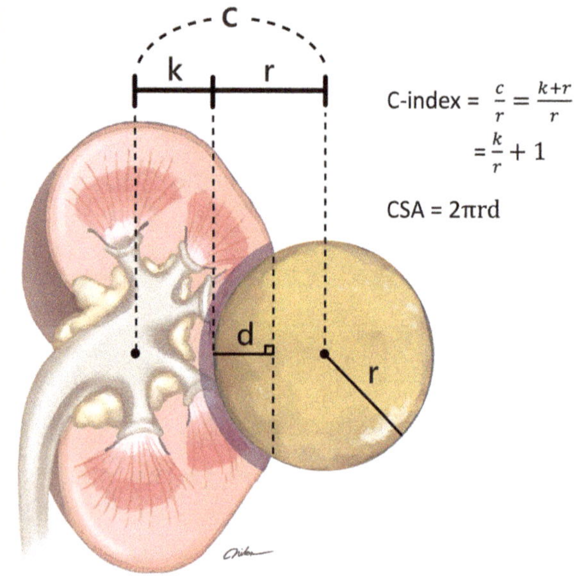

Fig. 1 Geometric interplay between renal volume, C-index, and CSA; r: tumor radius, d: depth of invasion, k: nearest distance between tumor margin and kidney center; This figure is created by YPW

Depth (d) implies the volume of resected renal parenchyma, and CSA was shown to be correlated with resected and ischemic renal volume in our previous study [28]. In addition, "k" implies the thickness of residual renal parenchyma, and C-index has been shown to be correlated with percent functional volume preservation [24]. Lee et al. found that CSA and C-index independently affected the percent reduction in renal cortical volume. [29] Therefore, both CSA and C-index were effective in predicting IPRF based on mathematical volume theory.

The strength of this study is that it is the first cohort study to compare ipsilateral functional outcomes among four nephrometries. In contrast to previous studies we provided more precise data derived from 99mTc MAG3 studies. Moreover, we directly compared the ability and provided cut-off values to predict functional changes for both CSA and C-index. There are also several limitations in this study. First, it was a retrospective design with a relatively small number of cases, and therefore selection bias was possible which may have resulted in confined tumor complexity and may be not representative the experience of other centers. However, the tumor complexity in our cohort was similar to previous studies [11, 20]. Although the follow-up time was only 1 year, Porpiglia et al. showed that ERPF remained stable 3 months after surgery [30]. Second, some of the renal tumors in our study were angiomyolipoma or other benign histology. However, the degree of global renal functional change in patients with angiomyolipoma after PN has shown to be similar to RCC [31]. Third, the PN technique such as enucleation and wedge resection was not unified. Therefore, further studies are needed to evaluate relationships among different nephrometries and pathologic or radiographic renal volume.

Conclusions

Based on the results of this study and the different characteristics of each nephrometry systems, we suggest using PADUA nephrometry to evaluate surgical complexity and ischemia time. Regarding the precise prediction of IPRF, we recommend using both CSA and C-index, as this may have greater predictive ability than R.E.N.A.L. and PADUA nephrometries.

Abbreviations

ACE: Absolute change of ERPF; CSA: Mathematical tumor contact surface area; DTPA: Diethylene triamine penta-acetic acid; eGFR: estimated glomerular filtration rates; ERPF: Effective renal plasma flow; IPRF: Ipsilateral post-operative renal function; LPN: Laparoscopic partial nephrectomy; MAG3: Tc-99 m mercaptoacetyltriglycine; OPN: Open partial nephrectomy; PCE: Percent change of ERPF; PN: Partial nephrectomy; RPN: Robotic-assisted laparoscopic partial nephrectom

Acknowledgments

The authors would like to thank China Medical University Hospital for providing the opportunity to conduct this study.

Authors' contributions

YDW designed the study, collected the data, analyzed and interpreted the results, and drafted the manuscript. CPH developed the protocol and collected the data. CHC, HCW and CRY collected the data. YDW, YPW, and PHF analyzed the data. YPW drew the figure. PFH conceived the study, interpreted the data, and reviewed the manuscript. All authors read and approved the final manuscript.

Author details

[1]Department of Urology, China Medical University Hospital, No. 2, Yu-De Rd., Taichung City 404, Taiwan, Republic of China. [2]School of Medicine, China Medical University, No. 91, Xueshi Rd., North Dist, Taichung City 404, Taiwan, Republic of China. [3]Department of Urology, China Medical University Beigang Hospital, No. 123, Xinde Rd., Beigang Township, Yunlin County 651, Taiwan, Republic of China. [4]Department of Radiology, Taichung Veterans General Hospital, No. 1650, Sec. 4, Taiwan Blvd., Xitun Dist., Taichung City 407, Taiwan, Republic of China.

References

1. Ljungberg B, Albiges L, Bensalah K, Bex A, Giles RH, Hora M, Kuczyk MA, Lam T, Marconi L, Merseburger AS, et al. EAU Guidelines on Renal Cell Carcinoma 2018. In: European Association of Urology guidelines 2018 edition. Volume presented at the EAU annual congress Copenhagen 2018, edn. Arnhem. The Netherlands: European Association of Urology Guidelines Office; 2018.
2. NCCN Guidlines Version 2.2019 Kidney Cancer [https://www.nccn.org/professionals/physician_gls/pdf/kidney.pdf].
3. Capitanio U, Terrone C, Antonelli A, Minervini A, Volpe A, Furlan M, Matloob R, Regis F, Fiori C, Porpiglia F, et al. Nephron-sparing techniques independently decrease the risk of cardiovascular events relative to radical nephrectomy in patients with a T1a-T1b renal mass and normal preoperative renal function. Eur Urol. 2015;67(4):683–9.
4. Tan HJ, Norton EC, Ye Z, Hafez KS, Gore JL, Miller DC. Long-term survival following partial vs radical nephrectomy among older patients with early-stage kidney cancer. JAMA. 2012;307(15):1629–35.
5. Kutikov A, Uzzo RG. The R.E.N.A.L. nephrometry score: a comprehensive standardized system for quantitating renal tumor size, location and depth. J Urol. 2009;182(3):844–53.

6. Ficarra V, Novara G, Secco S, Macchi V, Porzionato A, De Caro R, Artibani W. Preoperative aspects and dimensions used for an anatomical (PADUA) classification of renal tumours in patients who are candidates for nephron-sparing surgery. Eur Urol. 2009;56(5):786–93.
7. Simmons MN, Ching CB, Samplaski MK, Park CH, Gill IS. Kidney tumor location measurement using the C index method. J Urol. 2010;183(5): 1708–13.
8. Hsieh PF, Wang YD, Huang CP, Wu HC, Yang CR, Chen GH, Chang CH. A mathematical method to calculate tumor contact surface area: an effective parameter to predict renal function after partial nephrectomy. J Urol. 2016; 196(1):33–40.
9. Bylund JR, Gayheart D, Fleming T, Venkatesh R, Preston DM, Strup SE, Crispen PL. Association of tumor size, location, R.E.N.A.L., PADUA and centrality index score with perioperative outcomes and postoperative renal function. J Urol. 2012;188(5):1684–9.
10. Spaliviero M, Poon BY, Aras O, Di Paolo PL, Guglielmetti GB, Coleman CZ, Karlo CA, Bernstein ML, Sjoberg DD, Russo P, et al. Interobserver variability of R.E.N.A.L., PADUA, and centrality index nephrometry score systems. World J Urol. 2015;33(6):853–8.
11. Gupta R, Tori M, Babitz SK, Tobert CM, Anema JG, Noyes SL, Lane BR. Comparison of RENAL, PADUA, CSA, and PAVP Nephrometry scores in predicting functional outcomes after partial nephrectomy. Urology. 2019; 124:160–7.
12. Takagi T, Mir MC, Sharma N, Remer EM, Li J, Demirjian S, Kaouk JH, Campbell SC. Compensatory hypertrophy after partial and radical nephrectomy in adults. J Urol. 2014;192(6):1612–9.
13. Sankin A, Sfakianos JP, Schiff J, Sjoberg D, Coleman JA. Assessing renal function after partial nephrectomy using renal nuclear scintigraphy and estimated glomerular filtration rate. Urology. 2012;80(2):343–6.
14. Zargar H, Akca O, Autorino R, Brandao LF, Laydner H, Krishnan J, Samarasekera D, Stein RJ, Kaouk JH. Ipsilateral renal function preservation after robot-assisted partial nephrectomy (RAPN): an objective analysis using mercapto-acetyltriglycine (MAG3) renal scan data and volumetric assessment. BJU Int. 2015;115(5):787–95.
15. Taylor AT. Radionuclides in nephrourology, part 1: radiopharmaceuticals, quality control, and quantitative indices. J Nucl Med. 2014;55(4):608–15.
16. Watts KL, Ghosh P, Stein S, Ghavamian R. Value of Nephrometry score constituents on perioperative outcomes and Split renal function in patients undergoing minimally invasive partial nephrectomy. Urology. 2017;99:112–7.
17. Mir MC, Ercole C, Takagi T, Zhang Z, Velet L, Remer EM, Demirjian S, Campbell SC. Decline in renal function after partial nephrectomy: etiology and prevention. J Urol. 2015;193(6):1889–98.
18. Volpe A, Blute ML, Ficarra V, Gill IS, Kutikov A, Porpiglia F, Rogers C, Touijer KA, Van Poppel H, Thompson RH. Renal ischemia and function after partial nephrectomy: a collaborative review of the literature. Eur Urol. 2015;68(1):61–74.
19. Ginzburg S, Uzzo R, Walton J, Miller C, Kurz D, Li T, Handorf E, Gor R, Corcoran A, Viterbo R, et al. Residual parenchymal volume, not warm ischemia time, predicts ultimate renal functional outcomes in patients undergoing partial nephrectomy. Urology. 2015;86(2):300–5.
20. Borgmann H, Reiss AK, Kurosch M, Filmann N, Frees S, Mager R, Tsaur I, Haferkamp A. R.E.N.A.L. score outperforms PADUA score, C-index and DAP score for outcome prediction of nephron sparing surgery in a selected cohort. J Urol. 2016;196(3):664–71.
21. Ficarra V, Porpiglia F, Crestani A, Minervini A, Antonelli A, Longo N, Novara G, Giannarini G, Fiori C, Simeone C, et al. The simplified PADUA REnal (SPARE) nephrometry system: a novel classification of parenchymal renal tumours suitable for partial nephrectomy. BJU Int. 2019; https://doi.org/10.1111/bju.14772.
22. Kwon T, Jeong IG, Ryu J, Lee C, Lee C, You D, Kim CS. Renal function is associated with Nephrometry score after partial nephrectomy: a study using diethylene Triamine Penta-acetic acid (DTPA) renal scanning. Ann Surg Oncol. 2015;22(Suppl 3):S1594–600.
23. Yoo S, Lee C, You D, Jeong IG, Kim CS. Comparison of renal functional outcomes in exactly matched pairs between robot-assisted partial nephrectomy using warm ischemia and open partial nephrectomy using cold ischemia using diethylene triamine penta-acetic acid renal scintigraphy. Int Urol Nephrol. 2016;48(5):687–93.
24. Simmons MN, Hillyer SP, Lee BH, Fergany AF, Kaouk J, Campbell SC. Nephrometry score is associated with volume loss and functional recovery after partial nephrectomy. J Urol. 2012;188(1):39–44.
25. Samplaski MK, Hernandez A, Gill IS, Simmons MN. C-index is associated with functional outcomes after laparoscopic partial nephrectomy. J Urol. 2010; 184(6):2259–63.
26. Sugiura M, Suyama T, Kanesaka M, Fujimoto A, Hou K, Araki K, Masuda H, Kojima S, Naya Y. Usefulness of R.E.N.a.L Nephrometry scoring system and centrality index score for predicting outcome of laparoscopic partial nephrectomy. J Laparoendosc Adv Surg Tech A. 2016;26(10):784–8.
27. Chan AA, Wood CG, Caicedo J, Munsell MF, Matin SF. Predictors of unilateral renal function after open and laparoscopic partial nephrectomy. Urology. 2010;75(2):295–302.
28. Wang YD, Chang CH, Huang CP, Wu HC, Yang CR, Hsieh PF. New-generation nephrometry systems: head-to-head comparison of tumor contact surface area and resected and ischemic volume. Urol Sci. 2017; 28(2):84–8.
29. Lee CH, Ku JY, Park YJ, Seo WI, Ha HK. The superiority of contact surface area as a predictor of renal cortical volume change after partial nephrectomy compared to RENAL, PADUA and C-index: an approach using computed tomography-based renal volumetry. Scand J Urol. 2019;53(2–3):129–33.
30. Porpiglia F, Fiori C, Bertolo R, Morra I, Russo R, Piccoli G, Angusti T, Podio V. Long-term functional evaluation of the treated kidney in a prospective series of patients who underwent laparoscopic partial nephrectomy for small renal tumors. Eur Urol. 2012;62(1):130–5.
31. Lin CY, Yang CK, Ou YC, Chiu KY, Cheng CL, Ho HC, Wang SS, Chen CS, Li JR. Long-term outcome of robotic partial nephrectomy for renal angiomyolipoma. Asian J Surg. 2018;41(2):187–91.

Long-term response of metastatic hereditary leiomyomatosis and renal cell carcinoma syndrome associated renal cell carcinoma to bevacizumab plus erlotinib after temsirolimus and axitinib treatment failures

Inkeun Park[1*], Young Sup Shim[2], Heounjeong Go[3], Bum Sik Hong[4] and Jae Lyun Lee[5]

Abstract

Background: Hereditary leiomyomatosis and renal cell carcinoma (HLRCC) is a rare hereditary kidney cancer syndrome in which affected individuals are at risk of skin and uterine leiomyomatosis and kidney cancer. HLRCC-associated kidney cancer is a lethal disease with a highly aggressive behavior, and there is no standard treatment option for metastatic disease.

Case presentation: Here, we report a 29-year-old patient with a locally advanced HLRCC-assiciated RCC. He was administrated temsirolimus initially, then underwent surgical removal of kidney, retroperitoneal lymph nodes, inferior vena cava and tumor thrombi. Unfortunately, multiple liver metastases were confirmed 1 month after surgery, so axitinib was given but failed immediately. We tried bevacizumab plus erlotinib, which achieved long-term good response lasting more than 18 months. He is alive with disease and maintains bevacizumab plus erlotinib treatment.

Conclusion: The promising results obtained in this patient suggest that combined bevacizumab plus erlotinib may offer a valid treatment option for advanced HLRCC-associated kidney cancer, even after failures of mTOR inhibitor and/or VEGFR TKI based therapies.

Keywords: Hereditary leiomyomatosis and renal cell carcinoma, Metastasis, Bevacizumab, Erlotinib

Background

Hereditary leiomyomatosis and renal cell carcinoma (HLRCC) syndrome is a rare autosomal-dominant hereditary syndrome caused by germline mutation in the fumarate hydratase (*FH*) gene [1]. The phenotypic manifestations of this syndrome include cutaneous leiomyomatosis, uterine leiomyomatosis, and renal cell carcinoma. Renal cell carcinoma in HLRCC has a penetrance rate of 10–20%, and used to be categorized as a form of type 2 papillary RCC, but now is classified separately as HLRCC-associated RCC [2]. This type of RCC is a lethal disease with tendencies toward early metastasis and rapid progression, and thus, immediate surgical excision is recommended after its detection even when tumors are small [3]. Currently, the only curative option for HLRCC-associated RCC is early detection by routine screening in affected individual and immediate surgery. No standard systemic treatment option is available for metastatic disease, though most medical oncologists prescribe vascular endothelial growth factor receptor tyrosine kinase inhibitors (VEGFR TKIs) or mammalian

* Correspondence: Ingni79@gilhospital.com
[1]Division of Medical Oncology, Department of Internal Medicine, Gachon University Gil Medical Center, 1198 Guwol-dong, Namdong-gu, Incheon 21565, Republic of Korea
Full list of author information is available at the end of the article

target of rapamycin (mTOR) inhibitors. Here we report a case of metastatic HLRCC-associated RCC, which exhibited long-term response to bevacizumab plus erlotinib after failure of temsirolimus and of axitinib.

Case presentation

A 29 year-old male presented a right flank mass and lower extremity edema in August 2015. He had no past medical history of illness, but a family history of uterine myoma in his sister, aunt, cousin, and grandmother and of skin leiomyomatosis in his grandmother, father, and uncle. His sister was later diagnosed with RCC in May 2016 (Fig. 1). Magnetic resonance imaging (MRI) of the abdomen revealed an 8 cm-sized mass in the right kidney that invaded the renal vein into infra-diaphragmatic IVC, obstructing and causing thrombosis of the infrarenal inferior vena cava and both iliac veins, with conglomerated lymph nodes (LNs) at retrocaval and aortocaval stations (Fig. 2a). Kidney mass biopsy revealed type 2 papillary renal cell carcinoma.

Because the massive thrombus and lymph nodes were deemed unresectable, he was administered temsirolimus from September 2015, but best response was stable disease. However, the primary mass and lymph node had enlarged in March 2016, indicating progressive disease (Fig. 2b).

Because there is no standard treatment after temsirolimus in non-clear cell RCC and he maintained a good performance status, he underwent retroperitoneal lymph node dissection, IVC tumor thrombectomy, and radical nephrectomy in March 2016. Pathologic diagnosis was papillary type 2 RCC (Fig. 3). However, 1 month after surgery, follow-up CT demonstrated multiple liver metastases (Fig. 2c). Axitinib was started in May 2016, but the disease progressed, in liver, retroperitoneal LNs, and spine (Fig. 2d).

Considering his age at onset and family history of skin disease and uterine myoma, and tumor histology, HLRCC was suspected, and thus he and his family underwent germline *FH* mutation testing, which demonstrated the presence of mutation in *FH* exon 5 (c.688A > G, p.Lys230Glu). Although this specific mutation has not been reported in HLRCC, mutation in *FH* c. 689 A > G (p.Lys203Arg) had been reported to be pathogenic (rs752232718), and thus, we considered his kidney cancer was HLRCC-associated RCC. Immunohistochemical staining with anti-FH antibody (mousemonoclonal, clone J-13, 1:10000, SC-100743, SANTACRUZ, CA, USA) demonstrated no expression of FH in tumor cells (Fig. 3d). Based on a preliminary report, in which it was suggested bevacizumab and erlotinib in combination may be effective in HLRCC-associated RCC [4], we administrated bevacizumab (10 mg/kg every 2 weeks) and erlotinib (150 mg daily) from June 2016. After treatment, metastatic lesions in liver, LNs, and bone decreased rapidly, achieving partial response (Fig. 2e). As of Dec 2017, 18 months after start of bevacizumab plus erlotinib, this good response is maintained and the patient remains symptom free.

Discussion and conclusions

In this case, we report long lasting response to bevacizumab plus erlotinib after temsirolimus and axitinib had both failed. Currently, temsirolimus is the only treatment option in non-clear cell RCC (nccRCC) that prolonged overall survival (OS) in a randomized controlled phase 3 trial [5]. However, this trial was not

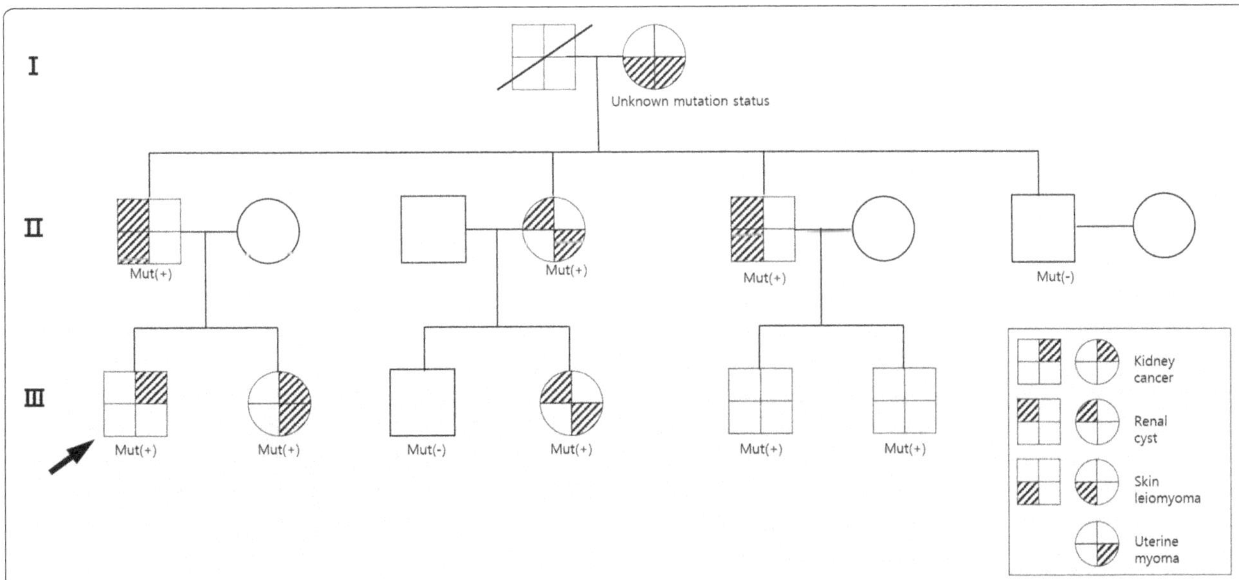

Fig. 1 Patient pedigree showing individuals with uterine myoma, skin leiomyoma, renal cysts, and renal cell carcinoma

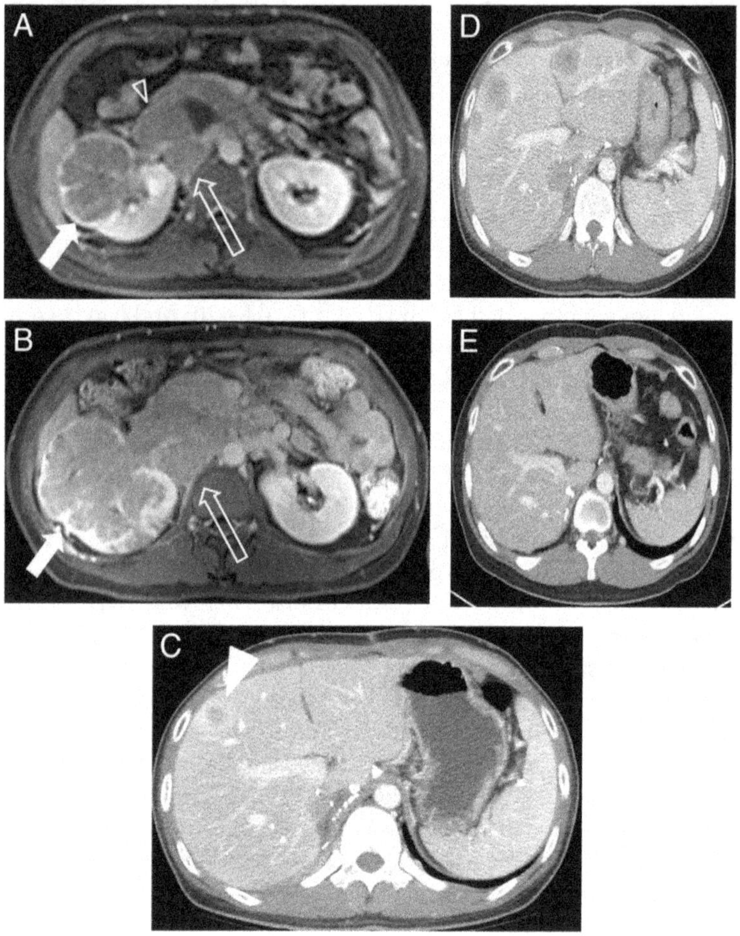

Fig. 2 Serial CT and MRI images. **a** Axial fat saturated T1-weighted MRI image with contrast enhancement showing a lobulated contoured poorly enhancing tumor (arrow) in the right kidney. Tumor invasion was observed at IVC (arrow head) and metastatic lymph nodes (open arrow) were noted. **b** Despite temsirolimus treatment, primary tumor and metastatic lymph node size increased. **c** After radical nephrectomy, hepatic metastasis (arrowhead) was noted on a follow up CT scan, which (**d**) became aggravated despite axitinib therapy. **e** However, at 2 months after bevacizumab plus erlotinib therapy, the multiple hepatic metastases had nearly disappeared

specifically designed for nccRCC, and included mostly clear cell RCC patients with poor prognostic risk group (n = 502, 80%), while the remaining 20% was composed of non-clear cell or indeterminated histology RCC (n = 124, 20%). Although statistically significant, the efficacy of temsirolimus was not impressive in this trial, as median OS was 10.9 months in the temsirolimus group compared to 7.3 months in the interferon group. Other than temsirolimus, VEGFR TKI can be an option. The randomized phase 2 trials, A Randomized Phase II study of Afinitor vs. Sutent in Patients With Metastatic Non-Clear Cell Renal Cell Carcinoma (ASPEN) and Everolimus Versus Sunitinib Prospective Evaluation in Metastatic Non-Clear Cell Renal Cell Carcinoma (ESPN), showed sunitinib appears to be more effective and numerically better than everolimus in nccRCC [6, 7]. Although sunitinib is the most widely studied VEGFR TKI in patient with nccRCC, the best VEGFR TKI for nccRCC have not been determined, as phase II trials on pazopanib and axitinib for nccRCC showed similar or better outcome compared to sunitinib [8, 9].

Trials on temsirolimus and VEGFR TKIs were conducted on a mixture of nccRCC variants, which included sarcomatoid, papillary type 1, papillary type 2, chromophobe, unclassified, and MiT family translocation RCC. Furthermore, multi-omics has recently revealed these variants are completely different disease entities with unique molecular pathobiologies [10, 11]. Therefore, ideally, a genomics-based clinical trial is required to determine the best treatment option for each of nccRCC variants. As HLRCC-associated RCC is a very rare, it is unlikely that any large-scale clinical trial dedicated to this cancer will ever be performed.

HLRCC is caused by a germline mutation in *FH* which encodes fumarate hydratase that converts fumarate into

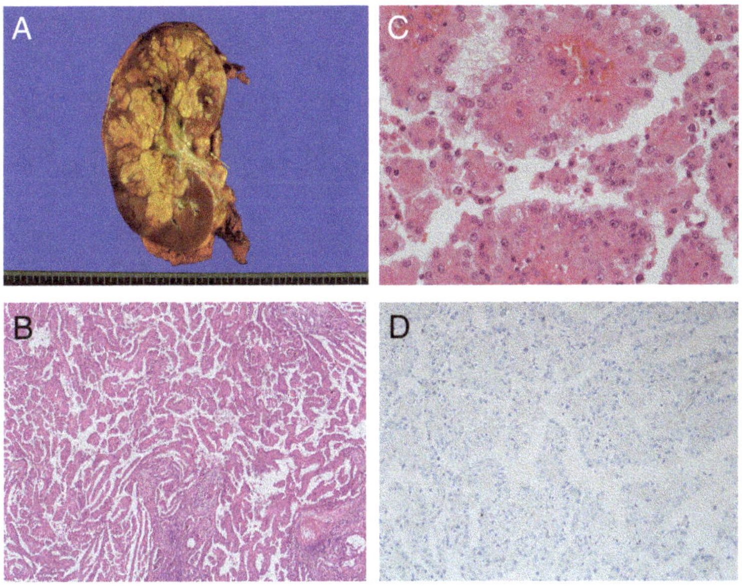

Fig. 3 Gross and histologic characteristics of the primary tumor. **a** Nephrectomy specimen, the 11.8x7x7 cm sized well-demarcated, multilobulated mass in the right kidney had a whitish yellow, soft, friable papillary cut surface with renal vein thrombi (arrow). **b** Renal tumors exhibited infiltrative, tubulopapillary architectural growth intermixed with tumoral renal parenchyma (× 40). **c** Tumors were composed of large cells with abundant eosinophilic cytoplasm, large nuclei, and prominent inclusion-like eosinophilic nucleoli with perinuclear halos (× 400). **d** No expression of fumarate hydrate in tumor cells on immnohistochemical staining (× 200)

malate in the Krebs cycle. Consequently, HLRCC-associated RCC exhibits an impaired Krebs cycle and characteristic dependency on aerobic glycolysis. As fumarate accumulates, increased levels of fumarate inhibit hypoxia-inducible factor (HIF) prolyl hydroxylase which facilitates degradation of HIF-1α and HIF-2α. As a result, stabilization of HIF-1α leads to increased level of VEGF and GLUT1, which are necessary for aerobic glycolysis [12]. A mechanism-based clinical trial of bevacizumab plus erlotinib in papillary renal cell carcinoma is currently underway (NCT01130519). Interim results are promising, especially in patients with HLRCC-associated RCC [4]; response rate and median progression-free survival were 29% and 7.4 months, respectively, in non-hereditary papillary RCC, whereas 60% and 24.2 months, respectively, in HLRCC-associated RCC.

In conclusion, we suggest bevacizumab plus erlotinib be considered a treatment option in patients with metastatic HLRCC-associated RCC, even after failures of mTOR inhibitor and/or VEGFR TKI based therapies.

Abbreviations

FH: Fumarate hydratase; GLUT: Glucose transporter; HIF: Hypoxia-inducble factor; HLRCC: Hereditrary leiomyomatosis and renal cell carcinoma; mTOR: mammalian target of rapamycin; RCC: Renal cell carcinoma; VEGFR TKI: Vascular endothelial growth factor receptor tyrosine kinase inhibitor

Acknowledgements

None.

Authors' contributions

IKP and JLL wrote the manuscript and made the revisions. YSS, HJG, and BSH participated in data collection and interpretation. All authors read and approved the final manuscript.

Author details

[1]Division of Medical Oncology, Department of Internal Medicine, Gachon University Gil Medical Center, 1198 Guwol-dong, Namdong-gu, Incheon 21565, Republic of Korea. [2]Department of Radiology, Gachon University Gil Medical Center, Incheon, Republic of Korea. [3]Department of Pathology, Ulsan University Asan Medical Center, Seoul, Republic of Korea. [4]Department of Urology, Ulsan University Asan Medical Center, Seoul, Republic of Korea. [5]Department of Oncology, Ulsan University Asan Medical Center, Seoul, Republic of Korea.

References

1. Schmidt LS, Linehan WM. Hereditary leiomyomatosis and renal cell carcinoma. Int J Nephrol Renovasc Dis. 2014;7:253–60.
2. Moch H, Cubilla AL, Humphrey PA, Reuter VE, Ulbright TM. The 2016 WHO classification of Tumours of the urinary system and male genital organs-part a: renal, penile, and testicular Tumours. Eur Urol. 2016;70(1):93–105.
3. Schmidt LS, Linehan WM. Genetic predisposition to kidney cancer. Semin Oncol. 2016;43(5):566–74.
4. Srinivasan R, Su D, Stamatakis L, Siddiqui MM, Singer E, Shuch B, Nix J, Friend J, Hawks G, Shih J, et al. 5 mechanism based targeted therapy for hereditary leiomyomatosis and renal cell cancer (HLRCC) and sporadic papillary renal cell carcinoma: interim results from a phase 2 study of bevacizumab and erlotinib. Eur J Cancer. 2014;50:8.
5. Hudes G, Carducci M, Tomczak P, Dutcher J, Figlin R, Kapoor A, Staroslawska E, Sosman J, McDermott D, Bodrogi I, et al. Temsirolimus, interferon alfa, or both for advanced renal-cell carcinoma. N Engl J Med. 2007;356(22):2271–81.
6. Tannir NM, Jonasch E, Albiges L, Altinmakas E, Ng CS, Matin SF, Wang X, Qiao W, Dubauskas Lim Z, Tamboli P, et al. Everolimus versus Sunitinib prospective evaluation in metastatic non-clear cell renal cell carcinoma (ESPN): a randomized multicenter phase 2 trial. Eur Urol. 2016;69(5):866–74.

7. Armstrong AJ, Halabi S, Eisen T, Broderick S, Stadler WM, Jones RJ, Garcia JA, Vaishampayan UN, Picus J, Hawkins RE, et al. Everolimus versus sunitinib for patients with metastatic non-clear cell renal cell carcinoma (ASPEN): a multicentre, open-label, randomised phase 2 trial. Lancet Oncol. 2016;17(3):378–88.
8. Jung KS, Lee SJ, Park SH, Lee JL, Lee SH, Lim JY, Kang JH, Lee S, Rha SY, Lee KH, et al. Pazopanib for the treatment of non-clear cell renal cell carcinoma: a single-arm, open-label, multicenter, phase II study. Cancer Res Treat. 2018; 50:488–94.
9. Park I, Lee SH, Lee JL. A multicenter phase II trial of Axitinib in patients with recurrent or metastatic non-clear-cell renal cell carcinoma who had failed prior treatment with Temsirolimus. Clin Genitourin Cancer. 2018;16(5):e997–e1002.
10. Cancer Genome Atlas Research N, Linehan WM, Spellman PT, Ricketts CJ, Creighton CJ, Fei SS, Davis C, Wheeler DA, Murray BA, Schmidt L, et al. Comprehensive molecular characterization of papillary renal-cell carcinoma. N Engl J Med. 2016;374(2):135–45.
11. Durinck S, Stawiski EW, Pavia-Jimenez A, Modrusan Z, Kapur P, Jaiswal BS, Zhang N, Toffessi-Tcheuyap V, Nguyen TT, Pahuja KB, et al. Spectrum of diverse genomic alterations define non-clear cell renal carcinoma subtypes. Nat Genet. 2015;47(1):13–21.
12. Linehan WM, Rouault TA. Molecular pathways: fumarate hydratase-deficient kidney cancer--targeting the Warburg effect in cancer. Clin Cancer Res. 2013;19(13):3345–52.

29

Comparison of survival benefits of nephron-sparing intervention or active surveillance for patients with localized renal masses

Run-Qi Guo and Xiao-Guang Li*

Abstract

Background: Strong evidence comparing effectiveness between nephron-sparing intervention (NSI) and active surveillance (AS) is lacking. Thus, we aim to compare the outcomes of survival, including cancer-specific survival (CSS), overall survival (OS), and cardiovascular-specific survival (CVSS), in patients with renal masses who underwent NSI or AS.

Methods: A systematic literature search of PubMed, Web of Science, and EMBASE was performed for citations published prior to September 2018 that described NSI, partial nephrectomy and thermal ablation included, and AS for patients with renal masses and a standard meta-analysis on survival outcomes was then conducted.

Results: The meta-analysis included seven studies containing 5809 patients. The results comparing NSI with AS were as follows: CSS (hazard ratio (HR) = 0.64, 95% confidence interval (CI): 0.46–0.89, $P < 0.001$), OS (HR = 0.46, 95%CI: 0.39–0.53, $P < 0.001$), and CVSS (HR = 0.37, 95%CI: 0.24–0.57, $P < 0.001$).

Conclusions: This systematic review and meta-analysis indicates that NSI is associated with better OS, CSS and CVSS when compared with AS for patients with renal masses. Further better prospective cohort studies are needed to make definitive statements about these different treatment methods.

Keywords: Ablation, Active surveillance, Renal mass, Partial nephrectomy, Survival

Background

Renal masses range from benign tumors to cancers that can be indolent or aggressive, of which 80–90% are renal cell carcinoma (RCC) [1, 2]. RCC represents 2–3% of all cancers, with the highest incidence occurring in Western countries [3, 4]. Surgical resection, including radical nephrectomy and partial nephrectomy (PN), remains an effective treatment for clinically localized RCC. Given a low RCC-specific mortality for the elderly and those with small renal masses and other competing-cause mortality [5], active surveillance (AS) and thermal ablation (TA) such as cryoablation or radiofrequency ablation are alternative options for selected patients. Cardiovascular comorbidity and survival is especially relevant for RCC patients [6–8]. Thus, these approaches are being progressively supported by professional organizations, especially for patients with extensive comorbidities or decreased life expectancy. Each of the management options has its own relative risks and advantages in different patients, and no strict criteria for patient selection have been advocated by current guidelines. Furthermore, strong evidence comparing effectiveness between nephron-sparing intervention (NSI) (PN and TA included) and AS is lacking.

Given the need to clarify existing management algorithms for renal masses, the objective of present study was to compare the outcomes of survival, including cancer-specific survival (CSS), overall survival (OS), and

* Correspondence: xglee88@126.com
Minimally Invasive Tumor Therapies Center, Beijing Hospital, National Center of Gerontology, No.1 Dongdan Dahua Street, Beijing 100370, People's Republic of China

cardiovascular-specific survival (CVSS), in patients with renal masses undergoing NSI or AS.

Methods

Search strategy

A bibliographic search was from January 2000 to September 2018 on PubMed, EMBASE and Web of Science. Institutional Review Board approval was not required as this study was evidenced-based review. All the records are written in English. The main key words used for the search were "ablation" or "cryoablation" or "radiofrequency ablation" or "microwave ablation" or "partial nephrectomy", "active surveillance" or "watchful waiting" or "expectant management", "prognosis" or "survival" or "oncological outcome", and "kidney cancer" or "renal tumor". Besides, we reviewed the reference lists from the related articles manually. Only full-text articles published in peer-reviewed journals were identified.

Eligibility criteria

The identified studies were screened in accordance with the following criteria: (1) studies comparing the effectiveness or survival between NSI (enucleation, PN, and TA, like radiofrequency ablation, cryoablation, microwave ablation, etc.) and AS; (2) studies that clearly described outcome assessment by representing it in OS or CSS or CVSS; (3) survival outcome further demonstrated hazard ratio (HR) and corresponding 95% confidence interval (CI) or adequate data to achieve an estimated HR and 95% CI by using the methods reported by Tierney et al [9]; (4) prospective cohort or retrospective study; and (5) median follow-up of at least 12 months.

The exclusion criteria were as follow: (1) The literature was review, letter, case reports and meta-analysis; (2) The data were not available; (3) The literature deal with recurrent RCC, metastatic carcinoma, or urothelial carcinoma; and (4) Duplicate publication.

Two researchers identified all the publications that fit the criteria for the assessment of the titles and abstracts and full review. Divergences were settled through discussion.

Data extraction

The two reviewers extracted data from full length articles independently. The extracted data included the followings: name of the author, publication year, study region, study period, study design, sample size, intervention, median age, median follow-up duration, number of patients received intervention or active surveillance, median tumor size, outcomes including CSS or OS or CVSS. Any differences were settled by consensus.

Quality assessment

The quality of each study was determined using the modified Newcastle-Ottawa Scale [10]. This scale evaluates the risk in three aspects: selection of patients, comparability of NSI and AS groups and evaluation of the treatment outcome. Studies with scores less than 4 were considered to have a high risk of bias, scores of 4–6 to have a moderate risk of bias, and scores over 6 to have a low risk of bias. Each study was evaluated by two researchers independently. Disagreement was reassessed by both the researchers until consensus was reached.

Data analysis and synthesis

Log HR and the variance were utilized as the summary outcome measure from all studies in the meta-analysis. For each study, HR with the 95%CI of the survival rate was derived to compare the effectiveness between NSI and AS for patients with renal masses. Each meta-analysis was repeated after excluding Surveillance, Epidemiology, and End Results (SEER) data. Fixed-effects model, namely Mantel-Haenszel method, was applied to pool the results when there was no evident heterogeneity ($I^2 > 50\%$ and P value < 0.1 suggested obvious heterogeneity) [11], otherwise, the random-effects model (DerSimonian and Laird method) was utilized, which provided more conservative estimates when there was significant heterogeneity [12]. Meta-regression analysis and subgroup analysis were conducted for potential sources of inter-study heterogeneity.

The funnel plot was constructed for each meta-analysis to detect the publication bias, and the Egger's test was utilized to assess publication bias statistically [13]. All analyses were performed using Review manager version 5.3 (Cochrane Collaboration, Oxford, UK) and STATA version 14.0 (State Corporation, College Station, TX, USA). A P value was regarded as statistical significance when less than 0.05.

Results

Literature search and characteristics of studies

A total of 311 potentially relevant studies were identified. 142 duplicated publications were excluded through literature manager software (Endnote). According to the titles and abstracts, 141 were precluded: 52 were irrelevant studies, eight were case/series/case reports, 74 were letters/reviews/comments, seven were not in English or Chinese. After reviewed in depth, 15 publications were excluded due to inadequate outcome and five was excluded due to potentially overlapping populations. Additionally, one study was excluded because only this study focused on chronic kidney disease upstaging free survival. Finally, seven studies were included in the present meta-analysis [14–20] (Fig. 1). Table 1 summarized the study design characteristics [14–20].

The seven studies contained 5809 patients with renal mass, including 3112 patients who received NSI and 2697 patients in AS group. Of the seven studies, all seven

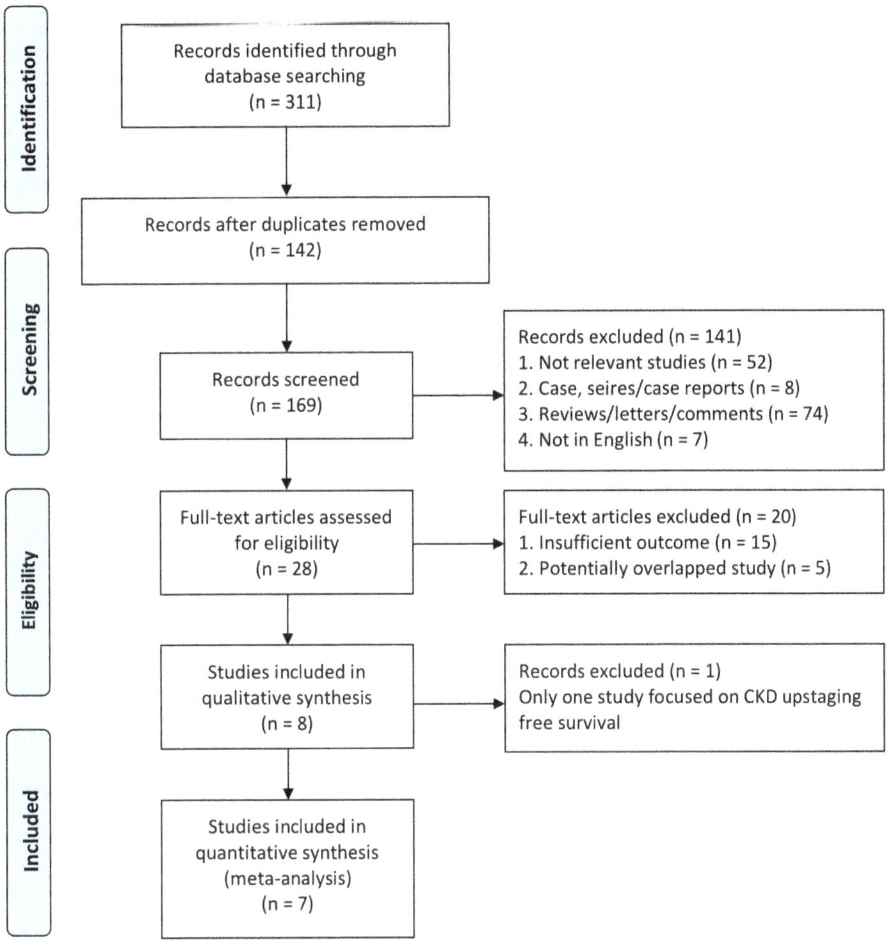

Fig. 1 Flowchart of study selection

studies were conducted to compare the CSS between NSI group and AS group [14–20], six studies containing 3949 patients compared the OS [14–16, 18–20], and two studies containing 2994 patients compared CVSS [18, 20].

Study qualities were assessed based on the modified Newcastle-Ottawa scale. All the seven studies reached stars ranging from seven to nine and were identified as moderate to high quality (Table 1). The baseline characteristics of included studies (number of patients received NSI or AS, gender, median age, tumor size and follow-up duration) were shown in Table 2.

Meta-analysis results

Cancer-specific survival

Seven studies addressed to CSS, of which two were studies of the SEER dataset [17, 18]. The combined HR of these studies revealed that NSI was associated with a statistically significant CSS benefit compared with AS for patients with renal masses (HR = 0.64, 95%CI: 0.46–0.89, $P < 0.001$) with apparent inter-study heterogeneity ($I^2 = 54\%$, $Chi^2 = 13.10$, $P = 0.04$) (Fig. 2a). To explore the source of the heterogeneity, meta-regression analysis and subgroup analysis were conducted by quality of the study, publication year, patient sample, type of intervention, and tumor size. The results showed that patient sample ($P = 0.030$) and tumor size ($P = 0.046$) might have significant association with the heterogeneity, while other factors did not (Table 3). Both population-based SEER and non-SEER studies demonstrated a CSS advantage of NSI over AS (HR = 0.39, 95%CI: 0.26–0.60, $P < 0.001$; HR = 0.78, 95%CI: 0.63–0.96, $P = 0.02$, respectively). Furthermore, subgroup analysis showed that both PN and TA were associated with better CSS when compared with AS (HR = 0.67, 95%CI: 0.49–0.90, $P = 0.008$; HR = 0.68, 95%CI: 0.52–0.89, $P = 0.005$, respectively). When confined to studies with T1a renal tumor, patients undergoing NSI showed a better CSS than those in AS (HR = 0.68, 95%CI: 0.56–0.82, $P < 0.001$).

Overall survival

Six studies including one SEER study [18] reported data for OS, and there was significant heterogeneity ($I^2 = 79\%$,

Table 1 Study design characteristics of included studies in meta-analysis

Study	Year	Region/ Country	Study period	Study design	Database	No. of patients	Intervention	Control	Inclusion criteria	Exclusion criteria	Outcome	Quality score
Alam R et al [14]	2018	USA	2009-NA	Prospective cohort	Delayed Intervention and Surveillance for Small Renal Masses Registry	597	PN, TA (CA, RFA)	AS	Age > 18, cT1a renal mass	History of RCC, familial RCC syndrome, or suspicion of a second malignancy metastasis	CSS, OS	9
Miller BL et al [15]	2018	USA	2003–2016	Retrospective	Single center data	135	PN, TA	AS	Histological diagnosis of oncocytoma or chRCC (cT1–2)	NA	CSS, OS	7
Tang DH et al [16]	2017	USA	2000–2013	Retrospective	Single center data	62	PN	AS	Age 80–89, cT1–2 renal mass	NA	CSS, OS	7
Larcher A et al [17]	2015	USA	2000–2009	Retrospective	SEER-Medicare-linked database	1860	TA	AS	T1aN0M0, unilateral RCC	RCC diagnosed only on death	CSS	9
Patel HD et al [18]	2015	USA	1995–2007	Retrospective	SEER-Medicare-linked database	2603	PN	AS	cT1aN0M0 renal cortical tumor	cT3–4, N1–2, M1, unknown classification, urothelial carcinoma, noncortical renal tumors, multiple procedures, bilateral tumors, previous diagnosis of another cancer, undergone TA	CSS, OS, CVSS	8
Patel N et al [19]	2012	UK	2005–2010	Retrospective	Cancer Research Uro-Oncology Database	161	PN	AS	cT1aN0M0 renal mass	NA	CSS, OS	7
Lane BR et al [20]	2010	USA	2000–2006	Retrospective	Single center data	391	open/ laparoscopic PN, TA (CA, RFA)	AS	Age > 75, cT1 renal tumor	Not suspicious renal tumor, PN for other reason	CSS, OS, CVSS	8

AS active surveillance, *CA* cryoablation, *CSS* cancer-specific survival, *CVSS* cadiovascular-specific survival, *NA* not available, *OS* overall survival, *PN* partial nephrectomy, *RCC* renal cell carcinoma, *RFA* radiofrequency ablation, *SEER* Surveillance, Epidemiology, and End Results, *TA* thermal ablation

$Chi^2 = 23.65$, $P = 0.0003$); thus, the random-effects model was utilized. The combined HR of these studies revealed that NSI was associated with better OS (HR = 0.46, 95%CI: 0.39–0.53, $P < 0.001$) (Fig. 2b). OS subgroup analysis revealed that PN was responsible for weighting the pooled estimate for a better OS (HR = 0.40, 95%CI: 0.34–0.47, $P < 0.0001$), while patients may not benefit from TA in OS (Table 3). When confined to studies with T1a renal tumor, the pooled results (HR = 0.43, 95%CI: 0.36–0.51, $P < 0.001$) indicated that NSI had a positive impact on the OS for these patients.

Cadiovascular-specific survival

No obvious heterogeneity was observed in the two studies focusing on CVSS ($I^2 = 0\%$, $Chi^2 = 0$, $P = 0.98$), thus the fixed-effects model was applied. The pooled HR for CVSS was 0.37 (95%CI: 0.24–0.57, $P < 0.001$), favoring NSI for patients with renal masses (Fig. 2c).

Publication bias

Funnel plots were conducted to detect the publication bias. As shown in Fig. 3, no obvious publication bias was found in our meta-analysis of included studies. And the

Table 2 Baseline characteristics of included studies in meta-analysis

Study detail	No. of patients, type	Sex, Male/ Female	Median age (years)	Median tumor size (centimeter)	Median follow-up duration (months)
Alam R et al 2018 [14]	PN 231	145/86	61.3	2.4	
	TA 27	13/14	71.8	2.1	36.0 (Total)
	AS 339	190/149	70.6	1.8	
	AS 1978	NA	NA	2.8	> 42.2
Miller BL et al 2018 [15]	PN 31	NA	Oncocytoma 69.5 chRCC 57.0	NA	
	TA 14	NA		NA	39.9 (Total)
	AS 90	NA		NA	
Tang DH et al 2017 [16]	PN 31	24/7	81.0	3.2	51.0 (Total)
	AS 31	18/13	83.0	2.7	
Larcher A et al 2015 [17]	TA 553	308/245	77.0	2.7	30.0 (Total)
	AS 1307	778/529	78.0	2.8	
Patel HD et al 2015 [18]	PN 1849	1070/779	65–69 589(31.5%) 70–74 569(27.5%) 75–79 463(25.2%) 80–84 191(19.5%) ≥85 37(8.9%)	< 2 cm 454(41.2%) 2- < 3 cm 776(31.8%) 3- ≤ 4 cm 614 (17.0%)	56.0 (Total)
	AS 754	399/355	65–69 589(31.5%) 70–74 569(27.5%) 75–79 463(25.2%) 80–84 191(19.5%) ≥85 37(8.9%)	< 2 cm 134(12.2%) 2- < 3 cm 258(10.6%) 3- ≤ 4 cm 361(10.0%)	
Patel N et al 2012 [19]	PN 90	NA	58.9	2.69	33.0
	AS 71	52/19	71.9	2.2	34.0
Lane BR et al 2010 [20]	NSI 286	200/86	78.0	3.0	46.8 (Total)
	AS 105	58/47	81.0	2.3	

AS active surveillance, *chRCC* chromophobe renal cell carcinoma, *NA* not available, *NSI* nephron-sparing intervention, *PN* partial nephrectomy, *TA* thermal ablation

Egger's test demonstrated that there was no publication bias for CSS (P_{egger} = 0.649, intercept − 0.55 with 95%CI − 3.50 to 2.40) and OS (P_{egger} = 0.129, intercept 2.49 with 95%CI − 1.13 to 6.10).

Discussion

The option for localized renal tumors has experienced extraordinary change with the advent of minimally invasive and nephron-sparing interventions. AS represents the least invasive management and has been exploited selectively among patients with limited life expectancy for renal tumors with low malignant potential. The effectiveness of PN, TA, and AS for patients with renal tumors has attracted extensive attention and been widely debated; however, the strength of evidence remains low to moderate, and the lack of data regarding AS rendered analysis largely insufficient to draw conclusions [21]. Thus, we reviewed the studies and the principal findings of our study are relevant to the management options for node-negative non-metastatic renal tumor.

To summarize, NSI was associated with better OS and CSS when compared with AS, and was even better when confined to T1a renal tumor. Both PN and TA showed an apparently better CSS when compared with AS. According to Lane BR *et al* [20], although no difference was observed in cancer-specific mortality between AS and NSI (PN and TA), there were apparent differences in characteristics of patients and tumors between the comparing groups, and the proportion of malignancy in AS might be diluted to an unknown extent. Nevertheless, a study by Larcher A *et al* [17] mentioned that after adjustment for other cause mortality and various characteristics of patients and tumors, TA seemed to be associated with a protective effect on cancer specific mortality

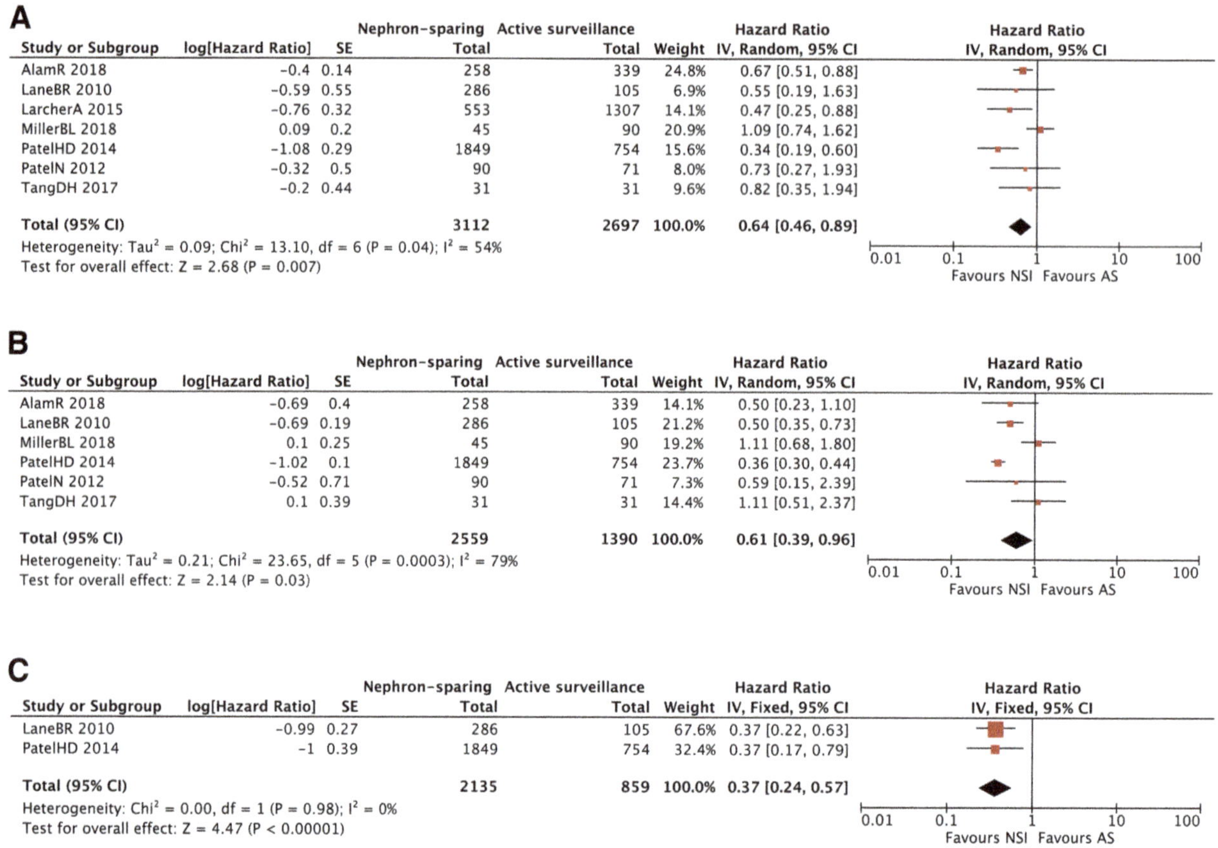

Fig. 2 Forest plot comparing cancer-specific survival in patients receiving nephron-sparing intervention versus active surveillance. **a** cancer-specific survival; **b** overall survival; **c** cardiovascular-specific survival

when compared with observation, and resulted in acceptable peri-operative morbidity [21]. We also noted that PN demonstrated better OS than AS, while TA did not. It was hypothesized that patients who underwent TA might be poor surgical candidates, as the current American Urological Association [22], European Association for Urology [23], and National Comprehensive Cancer Network guidelines [24] recommend. However, these recommendations are chiefly based on older TA data with higher local tumor recurrence rates and incomplete ablation rates [22–24]. Thus, with the development of improved ablative technologies, TA and PN could achieve comparable CSS. Additionally, relative long follow-up duration affirms the safety of AS compared to NSI among the selected population, who are usually older and have increased comorbidities. These factors probably explain the lower OS rate among AS patients and suggest that OS in AS group might be driven primarily by comorbidities [18, 25, 26]. Patel HD *et al* [18] stressed that patients who underwent nonsurgical management at the population-level in the SEER studies might not be representative of patients selected for AS in contemporary criteria. Besides, underestimating tumor stage might also contribute to the cancer-specific mortality in these nonsurgical management group. The elderly might also have a more aggressive tumor with the hypothesis that relative immunodeficiency associated with aging might facilitate rapid growth of RCC [27].

Interestingly, NSI was obviously associated with better CVSS, suggesting that cancer may be not the main cause of death for most patients undergoing AS. It is our hypothesis that the selection bias might contribute to this result. The AS group represents an extreme condition where patients did not experience intervention (especially surgery) for some reasons, but the most likely are age, comorbidities, tumor characteristics, and patient preference. A population-based competing risk analysis by Hollingsworth *et al* [28] demonstrated that the competing-cause mortality for elderly patients (aged >70 years) was 28%. In such cases, the surgeon and the patient would omit intervention and choose AS, which aims to reduce potential overtreatment without conceding oncologic outcomes [29] and may result in worse CVSS in the AS group. Therefore, patients at high cardiovascular risk are very reasonable candidates for AS [18].

Table 3 Subgroup analysis of CSS and OS by quality of the study, publication year, patient sample, number or type of intervention, and tumor size

Subgroup/co-variant	Coefficient	s.e.	*P* value	HR (95%CI); *P* value
CSS				
Quality	− 0.227	0.1580	*0.195*	
Publication year	0.598	0.2929	*0.096*	
≤ 2015				0.44 (0.31–0.64); < *0.001*
> 2015				0.76 (0.65–0.89); *0.03*
Patient sample	−0.688	0.2539	*0.030*	
Cancer registry or single center				0.78 (0.63–0.96); *0.02*
Population based				0.39 (0.26–0.60); < *0.001*
Type of intervention	−0.014	0.2628	*0.958*	
PN				0.67 (0.49–0.90); *0.008*
TA				0.68 (0.52–0.89); *0.005*
Tumor size	−0.567	0.2342	*0.046*	
T1a				0.68 (0.56–0.82); < *0.001*
Not only T1a				0.70 (0.36–1.38); *0.31*
OS				
Quality	−0.446	0.1986	*0.066*	
Publication year	0.560	0.3845	*0.196*	
≤ 2015				0.39 (0.33–0.46); < *0.001*
> 2015				0.93 (0.65–1.34); *0.70*
Patient sample	−0.658	0.4973	*0.234*	
Cancer registry or single center				0.68 (0.53–0.88); *0.004*
Population based				0.36 (0.30–0.44); < *0.001*
Intervention	0.625	0.2489	*0.049*	
PN				0.40 (0.34–0.47); < *0.001*
TA				1.05 (0.62–1.80); *0.85*
Tumor size	−0.681	0.3091	*0.070*	
T1a				0.43 (0.36–0.51); < *0.001*
Not only T1a				0.58 (0.42–0.82); *0.002*

CI confidence interval, *CSS* cancer-specific survival, *OS* overall survival, *PN* partial nephrectomy, *TA* thermal ablation

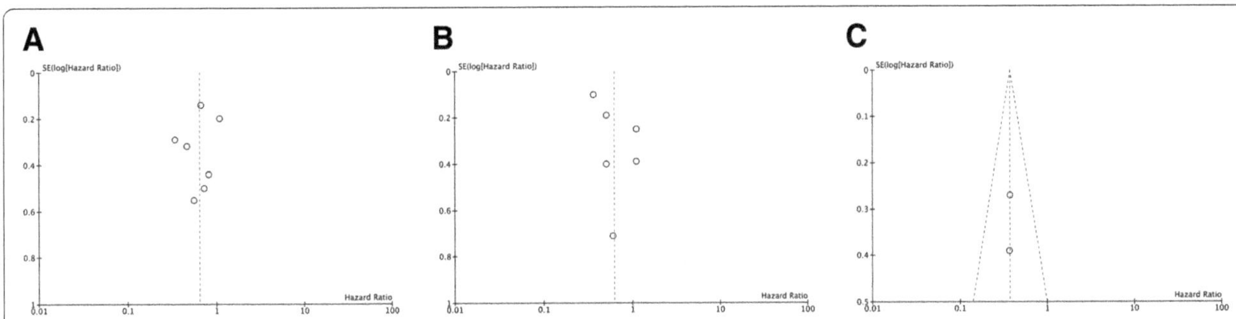

Fig. 3 Funnel plot for the evaluation of potential publication bias. **a** cancer-specific survival; **b** overall survival; **c** cardiovascular-specific survival

To the best of our knowledge, this is the first time that a comprehensive systematic review and meta-analysis has compared the effectiveness between NSI (PN and TA included) and AS for patients with renal masses; nevertheless, this meta-analysis has a few limitations to be noted. First, the sources of the publications were limited, and we failed to retrieve unpublished studies or studies written in other language, therefore potentially introducing inevitable publication biases. Second, only two studies in this research was prospective cohort studies. Despite the high quality (> 6 stars) of the seven studies, intrinsic bias might have rendered the results less trustworthy. Third, we failed to compare the survival according to age, Charlson comorbidity index and histology due to lack of information. Increased age and Charlson comorbidity index are associated with a higher hazard of all-cause mortality [17, 18, 30]. Fourth, there were only two studies compare CVSS between NSI and AS even after a systematic literature search, and the risk of random error might have inevitably increased; thus, larger prospective cohort studies are needed to further verify our findings. Furthermore, studies of TA and AS may include patients with benign tumors and may overestimate the efficacy of these management options. Improved diagnostics and judicious use of renal mass biopsy may improve the understanding of tumor biology. Finally, the outcomes were influenced by the quality of selected studies and the reporting bias that papers with significant outcomes were easier to be published than those with null or nonsignificant results might be unavoidable [31].

Conclusions

In conclusion, notwithstanding the limitations of this systematic review and meta-analysis, it seems that NSI is associated with better OS, CSS and CVSS when compared with AS for patients with renal masses. Further better prospective cohort studies with matched groups based on comorbidities and age are needed to make definitive statements about these different treatment methods.

Abbreviations

AS: Active surveillance; CI: Confidence interval; CSS: Cancer-specific survival; CVSS: Cardiovascular-specific survival; HR: Hazard ratio; NSI: Nephron-sparing intervention; OS: Overall survival; PN: Partial nephrectomy; RCC: Renal cell carcinoma; TA: Thermal ablation

Acknowledgements

Not applicable.

Authors' contributions

RQG participated project development, data collection, interpretation of the results, statistical analysis, and drafting of the manuscript. XGL participated in data collection, interpretation of the results, statistical analysis, critical revision and supervision. Both authors read and approved the final manuscript.

References

1. Kutikov A, Fossett LK, Ramchandani P, et al. Incidence of benign pathologic findings at partial nephrectomy for solitary renal mass presumed to be renal cell carcinoma on preoperative imaging. Urology. 2006;68:737–40.
2. Leibovich BC, Lohse CM, Crispen PL, et al. Histological subtype is an independent predictor of outcome for patients with renal cell carcinoma. J Urol. 2010;183:1309–15.
3. Ferlay J, Steliarova-Foucher E, Lortet-Tieulent J, et al. Cancer incidence and mortality patterns in Europe: estimates for 40 countries in 2012. Eur J Cancer. 2013;49:1374–403.
4. Siegel RL, Miller KD, Jemal A. Cancer statistics, 2018. CA Cancer J Clin. 2018;68:7–30.
5. Jewett MA, Mattar K, Basiuk J, et al. Active surveillance of small renal masses: progression patterns of early stage kidney cancer. Eur Urol. 2011;60:39–44.
6. Huang WC, Elkin EB, Levey AS, Jang TL, Russo P. Partial nephrectomy versus radical nephrectomy in patients with small renal tumors--is there a difference in mortality and cardiovascular outcomes? J Urol. 2009;181:55–61.
7. Kates M, Badalato GM, Pitman M, McKiernan JM. Increased risk of overall and cardiovascular mortality after radical nephrectomy for renal cell carcinoma 2 cm or less. J Urol. 2011;186:1247–53.
8. Miller DC, Schonlau M, Litwin MS, Lai J, Saigal CS. Urologic diseases in America P. renal and cardiovascular morbidity after partial or radical nephrectomy. Cancer. 2008;112:511–20.
9. Tierney JF, Stewart LA, Ghersi D, Burdett S, Sydes MR. Practical methods for incorporating summary time-to-event data into meta-analysis. Trials. 2007;8:16.
10. Wells G, Shea B, O'connell D, Peterson J, Welch V. The Newcastle-Ottawa Scale (NOS) for assessing the quality of nonrandomised studies in meta-analyses. 2012; http://www.ohri.ca/programs/clinical_epidemiology/nosgen.pdf. Accessed September 2018.
11. Higgins JP, Thompson SG, Deeks JJ, Altman DG. Measuring inconsistency in meta-analyses. BMJ. 2003;327:557–60.
12. DerSimonian R, Laird N. Meta-analysis in clinical trials. Control Clin Trials. 1986;7:177–88.
13. Higgins JP, Green S. Cochrane handbook for systematic reviews of interventions. Online Kensaku. 2014;35(3):154–5.
14. Alam R, Patel HD, Osumah T, et al. Comparative effectiveness of management options for patients with small renal masses: a prospective cohort study. BJU Int. 2018; [Epub ahead of print].
15. Miller BL, Mankowski Gettle L, Van Roo JR, et al. Comparative analysis of surgery, thermal ablation, and active surveillance for renal Oncocytic neoplasms. Urology. 2018;112:92–7.
16. Tang DH, Nawlo J, Chipollini J, et al. Management of Renal Masses in an octogenarian cohort: is there a right approach? Clin Genitourin Cancer. 2017;15:696–703.
17. Larcher A, Trudeau V, Sun M, et al. Population-based assessment of cancer-specific mortality after local tumour ablation or observation for kidney cancer: a competing risks analysis. BJU Int. 2016;118(4):541–6.
18. Patel HD, Kates M, Pierorazio PM, Allaf ME. Balancing cardiovascular (CV) and cancer death among patients with small renal masses: modification by CV risk. BJU Int. 2015;115:58–64.
19. Patel N, Cranston D, Akhtar MZ, et al. Active surveillance of small renal masses offers short-term oncological efficacy equivalent to radical and partial nephrectomy. BJU Int. 2012;110:1270–5.
20. Lane BR, Abouassaly R, Gao T, et al. Active treatment of localized renal tumors may not impact overall survival in patients aged 75 years or older. Cancer. 2010;116:3119–26.
21. Pierorazio PM, Johnson MH, Patel HD, et al. Management of Renal Masses and Localized Renal Cancer: systematic review and meta-analysis. J Urol. 2016;196:989–99.
22. Campbell SC, Novick AC, Belldegrun A, et al. Guideline for management of the clinical T1 renal mass. J Urol. 2009;182:1271–9.
23. Ljungberg B, Bensalah K, Canfield S, et al. EAU guidelines on renal cell carcinoma: 2014 update. Eur Urol. 2015;67:913–24.
24. National Comprehensive Cancer Network (NCCN). NCCN Clinical Practice Guidelines in Oncology (NCCN Guidelines) Kidney Cancer. Version 4. 2018. https://www.nccn.org/professionals/physician_gls/pdf/kidney.pdf. Accessed August 25, 2018.
25. Kutikov A, Egleston BL, Canter D, Smaldone MC, Wong YN, Uzzo RG. Competing risks of death in patients with localized renal cell carcinoma: a comorbidity based model. J Urol. 2012;188:2077–83.
26. Scoll BJ, Wong YN, Egleston BL, Kunkle DA, Saad IR, Uzzo RG. Age, tumor size and relative survival of patients with localized renal cell carcinoma: a surveillance, epidemiology and end results analysis. J Urol. 2009;181:506–11.

27. Zargar H, Atwell TD, Cadeddu JA, et al. Cryoablation for small renal masses: selection criteria, complications, and functional and oncologic results. Eur Urol. 2016;69:116–28.
28. Hollingsworth JM, Miller DC, Daignault S, Hollenbeck BK. Rising incidence of small renal masses: a need to reassess treatment effect. J Natl Cancer Inst. 2006;98:1331–4.
29. Patnaik JL, Byers T, Diguiseppi C, Denberg TD, Dabelea D. The influence of comorbidities on overall survival among older women diagnosed with breast cancer. J Natl Cancer Inst. 2011;103:1101–11.
30. Xing M, Kokabi N, Zhang D, Ludwig JM, Kim HS. Comparative effectiveness of thermal ablation, surgical resection, and active surveillance for T1a renal cell carcinoma: a surveillance, epidemiology, and end results (SEER)-Medicare-linked population study. Radiology. 2018;288:81–90.
31. Sutton AJ, Song F, Gilbody SM, Abrams KR. Modelling publication bias in meta-analysis: a review. Stat Methods Med Res. 2000;9:421–45.

Permissions

All chapters in this book were first published by BioMed Central; hereby published with permission under the Creative Commons Attribution License or equivalent. Every chapter published in this book has been scrutinized by our experts. Their significance has been extensively debated. The topics covered herein carry significant findings which will fuel the growth of the discipline. They may even be implemented as practical applications or may be referred to as a beginning point for another development.

The contributors of this book come from diverse backgrounds, making this book a truly international effort. This book will bring forth new frontiers with its revolutionizing research information and detailed analysis of the nascent developments around the world.

We would like to thank all the contributing authors for lending their expertise to make the book truly unique. They have played a crucial role in the development of this book. Without their invaluable contributions this book wouldn't have been possible. They have made vital efforts to compile up to date information on the varied aspects of this subject to make this book a valuable addition to the collection of many professionals and students.

This book was conceptualized with the vision of imparting up-to-date information and advanced data in this field. To ensure the same, a matchless editorial board was set up. Every individual on the board went through rigorous rounds of assessment to prove their worth. After which they invested a large part of their time researching and compiling the most relevant data for our readers.

The editorial board has been involved in producing this book since its inception. They have spent rigorous hours researching and exploring the diverse topics which have resulted in the successful publishing of this book. They have passed on their knowledge of decades through this book. To expedite this challenging task, the publisher supported the team at every step. A small team of assistant editors was also appointed to further simplify the editing procedure and attain best results for the readers.

Apart from the editorial board, the designing team has also invested a significant amount of their time in understanding the subject and creating the most relevant covers. They scrutinized every image to scout for the most suitable representation of the subject and create an appropriate cover for the book.

The publishing team has been an ardent support to the editorial, designing and production team. Their endless efforts to recruit the best for this project, has resulted in the accomplishment of this book. They are a veteran in the field of academics and their pool of knowledge is as vast as their experience in printing. Their expertise and guidance has proved useful at every step. Their uncompromising quality standards have made this book an exceptional effort. Their encouragement from time to time has been an inspiration for everyone.

The publisher and the editorial board hope that this book will prove to be a valuable piece of knowledge for researchers, students, practitioners and scholars across the globe.

List of Contributors

Alissar El Chediak, Deborah Mukherji, Sally Temraz and Ali Shamseddine
Department of Internal Medicine, Division of Hematology/Oncology, American University of Beirut - Medical Center, Riad El Solh, Beirut 110 72020, Lebanon

Samer Nassif, Sara Sinno and Rami Mahfouz
Department of Pathology and Laboratory Medicine, American University of Beirut - Medical Center, Beirut, Lebanon

Atsushi Okada, Shuzo Hamamoto, Kazumi Taguchi, Rei Unno, Teruaki Sugino, Ryosuke Ando, Kentaro Mizuno, Keiichi Tozawa, Kenjiro Kohri and Takahiro Yasui
Department of Nephro-urology, Nagoya City University Graduate School of Medical Sciences, 1 Kawasumi, Mizuho-cho, Mizuho-ku, Nagoya, Aichi 467-8601, Japan

Rui-hong Ma, Xiao-bing Luo and Hai-qiang Zhong
The Department of Clinical Laboratory, The Sixth People's Hospital of Nansha, Xingye Road No. 7, Dagang Town, Nansha, Guangzhou 511470, People's Republic of China

Qin Li
The Department of Pulmonary, Critical Care and Sleep, Yale School of Medicine, New Haven, USA

Forough Ebrahimtabar
Faculty of Medicine, Babol University of Medical Sciences, Babol, Iran

Hamid Shafi and Mohammad Mehdi Darzi
Department of Urology, Faculty of Medicine, Babol University of Medical Sciences, School of Medicine, Babol, Iran

Mohammad Ranaee
Department of Pathology, School of Medicine, Babol University of Medical Sciences, Babol, Iran

Andrea Schlegel and Philipp Kron
Division of Visceral and Transplantation Surgery, University Hospital, Zurich, Switzerland

Markus K. Muller
Division of Visceral and Transplantation Surgery, University Hospital, Zurich, Switzerland
Department of Surgery, Kantonsspital Frauenfeld, 8500 Frauenfeld, Switzerland

Jeannette D. Widmer
Department of Surgery, Kantonsspital Frauenfeld, 8500 Frauenfeld, Switzerland

Marc Schiesser
Department of Surgery, Kantonsspital St. Gallen, St. Gallen, Switzerland

Jens G. Brockmann
Department of Surgery, Kidney and Pancreas Transplantation, King Faisal Specialist Hospital, Riyadh, Kingdom of Saudi Arabia

Yongquan Tang
Department of Pediatric Surgery, West China Hospital, Sichuan University, No. 37 of Guoxue Xiang, Chengdu 610041, China

Zhihong Liu, Jiayu Liang, Kan Wu, Chuan Zhou, Fuxun Zhang and Yiping Lu
Department of Urology, Institute of Urology, West China Hospital, Sichuan University, Chengdu, China

Ruochen Zhang
Department of Urology, Fujian Provincial Hospital, Fuzhou, China

Zijun Zou
Department of Urology, the Third Affiliated Hospital, Sun Yat-sen University, Guangzhou, China

Yifei Lin
Department of Urology, Institute of Urology (Laboratory of Reconstructive Urology), West China Hospital, Sichuan University, Chengdu, Sichuan, People's Republic of China

Sike Lai
West China School of Medicine, Sichuan University, Guoxuexiang 37, Chengdu 610041, Sichuan, China

Jin Huang and Liang Du
West China Hospital, Sichuan University, Guoxuexiang 37, Chengdu 610041, Sichuan, China

Jie Yang, Jia-dong Xia, Jian-xin Xue, Ning-hong Song, Chao Liang, Di Xi, Ya-min Wang and Zeng-jun Wang
Department of Urology, First Affiliated Hospital of Nanjing Medical University, Nanjing 210029, Jiangsu, China

Yu-Li Jiang, Cheng-Xia Peng, Heng-Zi Wang and Lu-Jie Qian
Department of Urology, The Affiliated Hospital of Hang Zhou Normal University, Hangzhou 310015, China
School of Medicine, Hang Zhou Normal University, Hangzhou 310016, China

Mustufa Babar, Saad Hamdani and David S. Schnapp
DSS Urology, Queens Village, New York, USA

Corinne Liu
Department of Radiology, Memorial Sloan Kettering Cancer Center, New York, USA

Jogarao Vedula
Department of Pathology, NYU Winthrop Hospital, Mineola, New York, USA

Daisuke Motoyama, Yuto Matsushita, Hiromitsu Watanabe, Keita Tamura, Toshiki Ito, Takayuki Sugiyama, Atsushi Otsuka and Hideaki Miyake
Department of Urology, Hamamatsu University School of Medicine, 1-20-1 Handayama, Higashi-Ku, Hamamatsu 431-3192, Japan

Zhenxing Wang
Basic Medical College, Guizhou Medical University, Guiyang 550004, China
Department of Urology, Guizhou Provincial People's Hospital, No. 83 East Zhongshan Road, Guiyang 550002, Guizhou, China

Zhaolin Sun, Guangheng Luo, Ye Tian and Xiushu Yang
Department of Urology, Guizhou Provincial People's Hospital, No. 83 East Zhongshan Road, Guiyang 550002, Guizhou, China

Giuseppe Magistro, Philipp Weinhold, Frank Strittmatter, Christian G. Stief and Michael Staehler
Department of Urology, Ludwig-Maximilians-University of Munich, Marchioninistrasse 15, 81377 Munich, Germany

Patrick Bregenhorn
Department of Radiology, Ludwig-Maximilians-University of Munich, Munich, Germany

Bernhard Krauß, Dominik Nörenberg and Melvin D'Anastasi
Siemens Healthcare GmbH, Research and Development, Forchheim, Germany

Anno Graser
Gemeinschaftspraxis Radiologie München, Munich, Germany

Yu Liu, Liang Zhou and Donghui Ye
Department of Urology, Institute of Urology (Laboratory of Reconstructive Urology), West China Hospital, Sichuan University, No.37 Guo Xue Xiang, Chengdu, Sichuan 610041, People's Republic of China

Guan-Lin Huang, Hao-Lun Luo and Po-Hui Chiang
Department of Urology, Kaohsiung Chang Gung Memorial Hospital and Chang Gung University College of Medicine, 123, Ta-Pei Road, Niaosung, Kaohsiung, Taiwan

Kehua Jiang, Fa Sun, Jianguo Zhu, Peng Zhang, Yong Ban and Gang Shan
Department of Urology, Guizhou Provincial People's Hospital, Guiyang, China

Changxiang Liu
Department of Urology, The Affiliated Hospital of Guizhou medical University, Guiyang, China

Nariman Gadzhiev and Sergei Petrov
Department of Urology, Pavlov First Saint Petersburg State Medical University, Lva Tolstogo 17, Saint-Petersburg, Russian Federation 197342

Ullubiy Oibolatov, Leonid Kolotilov and Sergei Parvanyan
Department of Anesthesiology, The Nikiforov Center of Emergency Medicine, Optikov 54, Saint-Petersburg, Russian Federation 197448

Gagik Akopyan
Department of Urology, Sechenov First Moscow State Medical University, Optikov 54, Saint-Petersburg, Russian Federation 197448

Courtney M. Cottone, John Sung and Zhamshid Okhunov
Department of Urology, University of California, Irvine, 333 City Boulevard West, Orange, CA 92868, USA

O. Shoshany, S. Golan, J. Baniel and D. Lifshitz
Urology Department, Rabin Medical Center, Hasharon Hospital, 7 Keren Kayemet St, 49372 Petah Tikva, Israel
Sackler School of medicine, Tel Aviv University, Tel Aviv, Israel

T. Erlich, N. Kleinmann, B. Rosenzweig, A. Eisner, Y. Mor, J. Ramon and H. Winkler
Sackler School of medicine, Tel Aviv University, Tel Aviv, Israel
Urology Department, Chaim Sheba Medical Center, Ramat Gan, Israel

Dorit Esther Zilberman, Alon Lazarovich, Harry Winkler and Nir Kleinmann
Department of Urology , Chaim Sheba Medical Center, Affiliated to Sackler School of Medicine, Tel-Aviv University, Tel-Hashomer, Ramat-Gan, 52621 Tel-Aviv, Israel

C. Senger, A. Kluge, D. Pasemann, A. Grün, G. Kalinauskaite, V. Budach and C. Stromberger
Department of Radiation Oncology, Charité - Universitätsmedizin Berlin, Augustenburger Platz 1, 13353 Berlin, Germany
Charité CyberKnife Center, Charité - Universitätsmedizin Berlin, Augustenburger Platz 1, 13353 Berlin, Germany

A. Conti
Charité CyberKnife Center, Charité - Universitätsmedizin Berlin, Augustenburger Platz 1, 13353 Berlin, Germany
Department of Neurosurgery, University of Messina, Messina, Italy

M. Kufeld
Charité CyberKnife Center, Charité - Universitätsmedizin Berlin, Augustenburger Platz 1, 13353 Berlin, Germany

G. Acker
Charité CyberKnife Center, Charité - Universitätsmedizin Berlin, Augustenburger Platz 1, 13353 Berlin, Germany
Department of Neurosurgery and Center for Stroke research Berlin (CSB), Charité - Universitätsmedizin Berlin, Charitéplatz 1, 10117 Berlin, Germany
Berlin Institute of Health (BIH), Anna-Louisa-Karsch-Str. 2, 10178 Berlin, Germany

M. Lukas
Department of Nuclear Medicine, Charité – Universitätsmedizin Berlin, Charitéplatz 1, 10117 Berlin, Germany

J. Waiser
Department of Nephrology and Medical Intensive Care, Charité - Universitätsmedizin Berlin, Charitéplatz 1, 10117 Berlin, Germany

Christopher S. Hollenbeak
Department of Health Policy and Administration, The Pennsylvania State University, 604E Donald H. Ford Building, University Park, State College, PA 16802, USA

Eric W. Schaefer
Department of Public Health Sciences, College of Medicine, The Pennsylvania State University, Hershey, PA, USA

Justin Doan
Bristol-Myers Squibb, Princeton, NJ, USA

Jay D. Raman
Department of Surgery, College of Medicine, The Pennsylvania State University, Hershey, PA, USA

Mi Zhou, Xiang He, Yuelong Zhang and Weiwen Yu
Department of Urology, Zhejiang Provincial People's Hospital/People's Hospital of Hangzhou Medical College, Hangzhou, China

Peter Rehder, Marco Pedrini and Jannik Stühmeier
University Hospital for Urology, Department of Surgery, Medical University of Innsbruck, Innsbruck, Austria

Rafael Rehwald
Department of Radiology, University of Cambridge, Cambridge, UK
Queen Square Institute of Neurology, University College London, London, UK

Julia M. Böhm, Alexander Loizides and Bernhard Glodny
Department of Radiology, Medical University of Innsbruck, Anichstraße 35, 6020 Innsbruck, Austria

Astrid E. Grams
Department of Neuroradiology, Medical University of Innsbruck, Innsbruck, Austria

Abdelrahman Bashar
Urology Division, Tawam Hospital in affiliation with Johns Hopkins Medicine, Al Ain, UAE

Fayez T. Hammad
Department of Surgery, College of Medicine and Health Sciences, United Arab Emirates University, Al Ain, UAE

Qing He, Kaiwen Xiao, Yuntian Chen, Banghua Liao, Hong Li and Kunjie Wang
Department of Urology, Institute of Urology (Laboratory of Reconstructive Urology), West China Hospital, Sichuan University, No. 37 Guo Xue Xiang, Chengdu, Sichuan 610041, People's Republic of China

Emre Karabay, Serdar Duvar, Cagatay Tosun, Ahmet Ruknettin Aslan and Omer Ergin Yucebas
Department of Urology, Haydarpasa Numune Training and Research Hospital, University of Health Sciences, Tibbiye Street. No: 23 34668 Uskudar /, ISTANBUL, Turkey

Nejdet Karsiyakali
Department of Urology, Cukurca State Hospital, Cukurca Devlet Hastanesi, Uroloji Klinigi, Cukurca/, HAKKARI, Turkey

Yu-De Wang and Che-Rei Yang
Department of Urology, China Medical University Hospital, No. 2, Yu-De Rd., Taichung City 404, Taiwan, Republic of China

Chi-Ping Huang, Chao-Hsiang Chang and Po-Fan Hsieh
Department of Urology, China Medical University Hospital, No. 2, Yu-De Rd., Taichung City 404, Taiwan, Republic of China
School of Medicine, China Medical University, No. 91, Xueshi Rd., North Dist, Taichung City 404, Taiwan, Republic of China

Hsi-Chin Wu
School of Medicine, China Medical University, No. 91, Xueshi Rd., North Dist, Taichung City 404, Taiwan, Republic of China
Department of Urology, China Medical University Beigang Hospital, No. 123, Xinde Rd., Beigang Township, Yunlin County 651, Taiwan, Republic of China

Yu-Ping Wang
Department of Radiology, Taichung Veterans General Hospital, No. 1650, Sec. 4, Taiwan Blvd., Xitun Dist., Taichung City 407, Taiwan, Republic of China

Inkeun Park
Division of Medical Oncology, Department of Internal Medicine, Gachon University Gil Medical Center, 1198 Guwol-dong, Namdong-gu, Incheon 21565, Republic of Korea

Young Sup Shim
Department of Radiology, Gachon University Gil Medical Center, Incheon, Republic of Korea

Heounjeong Go
Department of Pathology, Ulsan University Asan Medical Center, Seoul, Republic of Korea

Bum Sik Hong
Department of Urology, Ulsan University Asan Medical Center, Seoul, Republic of Korea

Jae Lyun Lee
Department of Oncology, Ulsan University Asan Medical Center, Seoul, Republic of Korea

Run-Qi Guo and Xiao-Guang Li
Minimally Invasive Tumor Therapies Center, Beijing Hospital, National Center of Gerontology, No.1 Dongdan Dahua Street, Beijing 100370, People's Republic of China

Index

www.ingramcontent.com/pod-product-compliance
Lightning Source LLC
LaVergne TN
LVHW082208200926
848484LV00008B/2234
* 9 7 9 8 8 8 7 4 0 2 2 4 6 *